COGNITIVE-BEHAVIORAL THERAPY FOR BODY DYSMORPHIC DISORDER

Also from Sabine Wilhelm

For General Readers

Feeling Good about the Way You Look:
A Program for Overcoming Body Image Problems
Sabine Wilhelm

COGNITIVE-BEHAVIORAL THERAPY *for* BODY DYSMORPHIC DISORDER

A TREATMENT MANUAL

Sabine Wilhelm
Katharine A. Phillips
Gail Steketee

THE GUILFORD PRESS
New York London

A Division of Guilford Publications, Inc.
72 Spring Street, New York, NY 10012
www.guilford.com

Printed in the United States of America

This book is printed on acid-free paper.

Last digit is print number: 9 8 7 6 5 4 3 2 1

Library of Congress Cataloging-in-Publication Data

Wilhelm, Sabine.
Cognitive-behavioral therapy for body dysmorphic disorder : a treatment manual / Sabine Wilhelm, Katharine A. Phillips, and Gail Steketee.
pages cm
Includes bibliographical references and index.
ISBN 978-1-4625-0790-0 (paperback)
1. Body dysmorphic disorder—Treatment. 2. Cognitive therapy. I. Phillips, Katharine A. II. Steketee, Gail. III. Title.
RC569.5.B64W55 2013
616.89′1425—dc23

2012037824

About the Authors

Sabine Wilhelm, PhD, is Associate Professor of Psychology in the Department of Psychiatry at Harvard Medical School and Director of the Obsessive–Compulsive Disorder (OCD) and Related Disorders Program at Massachusetts General Hospital. She is Vice Chair of the Scientific Advisory Board for the International OCD Foundation, serves on the Scientific Council of the Anxiety Disorders Association of America, and is on the editorial boards of several journals. Dr. Wilhelm's clinical work and research focus on body dysmorphic disorder (BDD), OCD, and tic disorders. She is the author of more than 140 articles and book chapters and several books, including the self-help guide *Feeling Good about the Way You Look: A Program for Overcoming Body Image Problems*, which won the Self-Help Seal of Merit from the Association for Behavioral and Cognitive Therapies.

Katharine A. Phillips, MD, is Director of the BDD Program, Director of Research for Adult Psychiatry, and Senior Research Scientist at Rhode Island Hospital, and Professor of Psychiatry and Human Behavior at the Alpert Medical School of Brown University. A Fellow of the American College of Neuropsychopharmacology and a Distinguished Fellow of the American Psychiatric Association, she is the recipient of a Special Presidential Commendation from the American Psychiatric Association for her research on BDD. Dr. Phillips has repeatedly been included in Best Doctors in America and Castle Connolly's America's Top Doctors. She has more than 250 scientific publications and has written a number of books on BDD for professionals and the public, including *Understanding Body Dysmorphic Disorder: An Essential Guide*.

Gail Steketee, PhD, is Dean and Professor at the Boston University School of Social Work. She serves on the editorial boards of several journals and was Co-Chair of the World Congress of Behavioural and Cognitive Therapies in Boston in 2011. She has conducted many research studies on the psychopathology and treatment of anxiety and obsessive–compulsive spectrum disorders. These include projects on family factors that affect treatment outcome and the development and testing of cognitive and behavioral therapies for OCD, BDD, and hoarding. Dr. Steketee has published more than 200 articles and chapters and 12 books, including *Cognitive Therapy for Obsessive-Compulsive Disorder* (coauthored with Sabine Wilhelm). Her book *Buried in Treasures* (coauthored with David Tolin and Randy Frost) won the Self-Help Seal of Merit from the Association for Behavioral and Cognitive Therapies, and *Stuff: Compulsive Hoarding and the Meaning of Things* (coauthored with Randy Frost) was a finalist for the Books for a Better Life Award from the National Multiple Sclerosis Society.

Acknowledgments

We would like to thank several people who helped make this book possible. We are particularly grateful to our editors at The Guilford Press, Jim Nageotte, Kitty Moore, Barbara Watkins, Jane Keislar, and Marie Sprayberry, who provided us with helpful guidance at every step of the project. We would also like to acknowledge Drs. Jennifer Greenberg, Elizabeth Didie, and Ulrike Buhlmann for giving us excellent suggestions on earlier versions. We would like to thank Dr. Didie in particular for her contributions to the "Weight, Shape, and Muscularity" optional module (see Chapter 16). Thanks are due as well to the many therapists, evaluators, and research assistants who have helped us test the BDD treatment described in this manual. We are also grateful to Barbara Rosemberg and Michelle Silverman, who helped us with various steps along the way. We would like to thank Sarah Masnik for her assistance with the references. Our patients who shared their stories, successes, and feedback deserve a special thank-you; we have disguised their identities in this book to ensure confidentiality. Finally, we would like to thank our wonderful families for giving us the time and support to write this manual.

DISCLAIMER

The authors have checked with sources believed to be reliable in their efforts to provide information that is complete and generally in accord with the accepted standards of practice at the time of publication. However, in view of the possibility of human error or changes in behavioral, mental health, or medical sciences, neither the authors, nor the editor and publisher, nor any other party who has been involved in the preparation or publication of this work warrants that the information contained herein is in every respect accurate or complete, and they are not responsible for any errors or omissions or the results obtained from the use of such information. Readers are encouraged to confirm the information contained in this book with other sources.

SUICIDALITY IN BODY DYSMORPHIC DISORDER

Although research is limited, body dysmorphic disorder (BDD) appears to be characterized by high rates of suicidal thinking, suicide attempts, and completed suicide. Further information about suicidality in BDD can be found in other publications and in Chapters 1, 2, 3, 18, and elsewhere in this manual. Thus clinicians treating patients with BDD should carefully monitor the patients for suicidality throughout the treatment, and should keep in mind that additional treatment modalities (such as medication) or a higher level of care (e.g., hospitalization) may be indicated for more highly suicidal patients.

CONFIDENTIALITY

To ensure confidentiality, all patients' names and stories in this book have been modified, and much of the patient–therapist dialogue has been fictionalized.

Contents

List of Forms and Handouts

PART I

FUNDAMENTALS OF BODY DYSMORPHIC DISORDER AND ITS TREATMENT

This manual provides a guide for clinicians who are treating patients with body dysmorphic disorder (BDD). BDD is a common but often severe disorder that can be difficult to treat. Research to date indicates that cognitive-behavioral therapy (CBT) is often efficacious for BDD. We have written this manual to describe "CBT-BDD," the version of CBT we have developed for treating patients with BDD. We hope it will enable more patients to overcome this very distressing and impairing disorder.

This first part of the treatment manual provides information about BDD and its treatment, as well as guidance regarding the assessment of BDD. It also provides some tools to enhance motivation in patients who are ambivalent about starting treatment.

CHAPTER 1

INTRODUCTION TO BDD

Sometimes clinicians who want to work with patients who have BDD ask us: Why not just use CBT approaches that work for obsessive-compulsive disorder (OCD), social phobia, or eating disorders? Isn't BDD the same as—or pretty similar to—these other disorders? The answer is that BDD has important differences from all of these disorders (e.g., Allen & Hollander, 2004; Chosak et al., 2008). For example, compared to patients with OCD, patients with BDD have more delusional beliefs. Unlike patients with social phobia, patients with BDD tend to engage in extensive ritualistic behaviors. Compared to patients with eating disorders, patients with BDD are concerned with more body areas (typically not weight). Because BDD differs from other disorders, it requires treatment targeting its unique symptoms. For example, because many patients with BDD are convinced they are physically deformed and are thus reluctant to initiate or stay in psychiatric treatment, they need more intensive engagement and ongoing motivational interventions. In addition, exposure exercises and behavioral experiments are needed to address the prominent social avoidance in BDD, and these approaches differ from treatment for OCD and eating disorders. All these differences are reasons why we have written this manual. Although CBT-BDD overlaps in some ways with treatments for these other disorders, much of it is tailored specifically to BDD; we think that this tailoring will increase the likelihood of a successful outcome.

WHAT IS BDD?

BDD has been described for more than a century under such descriptors as "dysmorphophobia" (Morselli, 1891) and "dermatological hypochondriasis" (Ladee, 1966; Veale, 2009). However, BDD has been systematically researched for only the past 15 years or so. In the *Diagnostic and Statistical Manual of Mental Disorders*, fourth edition, text revision (DSM-IV-TR; American Psychiatric Association, 2000), BDD is defined as a preoccupation with an imagined defect in appearance; if the person does have a slight physical flaw, the concern is excessive. The appearance concern must be associated with considerable upset and/or impairment in functioning (including work and social functioning). In addition, the DSM reminds the reader that the body image concerns should not solely occur in the context of another psychiatric disorder (such as the weight and shape concerns in anorexia nervosa).

BDD occurs somewhat more often among women than among men. Although most of its clinical features appear generally similar in both genders, some gender differences have been found (Perugi et al., 1997; Phillips, Menard, & Fay, 2006). BDD usually begins during early adolescence, and appears to have a chronic and unremitting course unless it is appropriately treated (Phillips, 2002; Phillips, Pagano, Menard, & Stout, 2006).

Clinical Features of BDD

Prevalence of BDD

BDD has been found to occur in 1.7–2.4% of the general population in nationwide surveys (Koran, Abujaoude, Large, & Serpe, 2008; Rief, Buhlmann, Wilhelm, Borkenhagen, & Brähler, 2006), making it somewhat more common than schizophrenia or bipolar I disorder. BDD also occurs in 4–5% of college students (Bohne, Keuthen, Wilhelm, Deckersbach, & Jenike, 2002; Bohne, Wilhelm, et al., 2002) and is common in patients with other psychiatric disorders, such as major depressive disorder, substance use disorders, and anxiety disorders (Grant, Kim, & Crow, 2001; Wilhelm, Otto, Zucker, & Pollack, 1997). However, BDD often goes unrecognized. Because many patients are embarrassed and ashamed of their symptoms, they are reluctant to reveal them to family members, friends, or therapists (Conroy et al., 2008). They may worry that other people will consider them vain and dismiss their concerns. In addition, many patients seek and receive surgery or other cosmetic (e.g., dermatological) treatment, which does not address their underlying psychological problem and leaves the BDD inadequately treated.

Core BDD Symptoms

Appearance Preoccupations

Patients with BDD are preoccupied with the idea that one or more aspects of their appearance are unattractive, deformed, defective, flawed, or "not right" (Buhlmann & Wilhelm, 2004; Phillips, McElroy, Keck, & Pope, 1993). Some patients describe themselves as "unattractive," whereas others use stronger words (e.g., "ugly," "hideous," "repulsive," or "looking like a monster"). In reality, these body areas usually look normal. If an imperfection is present, it is slight and not anything that would typically be noticed at a conversational distance.

Preoccupations may focus on any area of the body. They commonly involve the face or head—most often the skin, hair, or nose (Marques, Weingarden, LeBlanc, & Wilhelm, 2011; Phillips, 1996, 2005; Phillips, Menard, Fay, & Weisberg, 2005). Patients may worry, for example, that their skin is terribly scarred, their hair is thinning, their teeth are not straight enough, or their nose is too big. They may be concerned that they are not muscular enough, their thighs are too fat, or their cheekbones are asymmetrical. On average, over the course of their illness, patients are excessively preoccupied with about five or six different body areas; however, some obsess about only one area, whereas others obsess about virtually every body area. The appearance preoccupations have an obsessive quality, in that they occur frequently (an average of 3–8 hours a day) and are usually difficult to resist or control (Phillips, Gunderson, Mallya, McElroy, & Carter, 1998). The thoughts are very distressing and are associated with low self-esteem, rejection sensitivity, anxiety, and depression, as well as feelings of defectiveness, unworthiness, embarrassment, and shame (Phillips, 2009; Rosen & Ramirez, 1998).

Rituals

Nearly all patients perform behaviors (rituals) that are intended to examine, improve, or hide the perceived defect (Phillips, Menard, Fay, & Weisberg, 2005; Rosen, 1995). Many of these behaviors (e.g., mirror checking and reassurance seeking) are considered compulsive, in that they are repetitive, time-consuming, and difficult to resist or control. Others (e.g., camouflaging the perceived flaw with a hat, clothing, or makeup) may be conceptualized as safety behaviors that are intended to prevent a feared consequence (e.g., being ridiculed by others). Table 1.1 lists the most common BDD behaviors and the percentages of people with BDD who have been found to engage in these behaviors over their lifetimes.

One behavior included in Table 1.1, skin picking, deserves special mention. More than one-third of individuals with BDD compulsively pick their skin to try to improve its appearance (Phillips & Taub, 1995). Because this behavior is difficult to resist and may occur for hours a day, it may cause noticeable skin lesions (Wilhelm et al., 1999), especially if implements such as needles or razor blades are used. Thus, unlike other patients with BDD, those who pick their skin may not look "normal" because the picking may cause skin lesions or scarring. In more extreme cases, this behavior can be life-threatening; for instance, one woman picked at her neck so forcibly that she exposed her carotid artery, requiring emergency surgery (O'Sullivan, Phillips, Keuthen, & Wilhelm, 1999).

TABLE 1.1. Common BDD Behaviors

Behavior	Percentage of people with the behavior
Camouflaging (e.g., with body position/posture, clothing, makeup, hand, hair, or hat)	91%
Comparing body part with that of others/scrutinizing the appearance of others	88%
Checking appearance in mirrors and other reflecting surfaces	87%
Seeking surgery, dermatological, or other cosmetic treatment	72%
Excessive grooming (e.g., combing or styling hair, applying makeup, shaving, removing hair)	59%
Questioning: seeking reassurance or attempting to convince others that the perceived defect is unattractive	54%
Touching the perceived defect	52%
Changing clothes	46%
Dieting	39%
Skin picking	38%
Mirror avoidance (avoidance of all mirrors for at least several days in a row)	24%
Tanning (BDD-related)	22%
Excessive exercise	21%
Excessive weight lifting	18%

Note. Adapted with permission of the publisher from Phillips, K. A. (1996; Revised and Expanded Edition, 2005). *The Broken Mirror: Understanding and Treating Body Dysmorphic Disorder.* New York: Oxford University Press.

During the assessment phase, you will need to ask patients carefully about BDD behaviors, because these will be targeted in treatment with response prevention (or habit reversal for skin picking or hair plucking). BDD behaviors are varied and limitless; Table 1.1 includes only the most common ones. One woman, for example, repeatedly tensed and relaxed her facial muscles to make them less "limp," and another frequently pushed on her eyeballs to change their shape. To make his face look fuller, a man with BDD slept without a pillow, ate large amounts of food, and drank more than three gallons of water a day (Phillips, 1996, 2005). Thus, in addition to asking patients about whether they engage in any of the behaviors in Table 1.1, you will need to ask whether they do any other things to check, fix, hide, or otherwise cope with their perceived flaws.

Avoidance Behaviors

Nearly everyone with BDD avoids at least some social situations, as they typically feel very self-conscious and embarrassed about how they look in the presence of other people; they believe that others consider them unattractive, ugly, or disfigured. A majority experience ideas or delusions of reference, believing that other people take special notice of them and single them out of the crowd in a negative way—for example, stare at them, talk about them, or laugh at them because of how they look.

As a result, many patients avoid social gatherings, dating, and/or sexual intimacy; places with lots of mirrors (e.g., stores); places where their bodies will be more exposed (e.g., the beach); or places with lots of people (e.g., shopping malls). Some people avoid only certain situations, whereas others avoid virtually any situation where other people might see them. Many patients avoid work or school, because they feel too ugly to be seen or feel too depressed and distracted by their appearance obsessions or rituals to focus on the task at hand. About one-third of patients have been completely housebound for at least 1 week because of their BDD symptoms (Phillips & Diaz, 1997; Phillips, Menard, Fay, & Pagano, 2005).

Impairment in BDD

It is easy to trivialize BDD by confusing patients' appearance concerns with vanity. However, BDD is very distressing and impairing (Hollander & Aronowitz, 1999; Marques et al., 2011; Phillips, Menard, Fay, & Pagano, 2005). Although levels of functioning vary, nearly all individuals with BDD experience impairment in social and occupational/academic functioning, often to a debilitating degree. They may avoid usual social and leisure activities, stop working, or drop out of school. As noted above, they often avoid dating and other social interactions, and some may even become housebound. A high proportion of patients require psychiatric hospitalization (Phillips & Diaz, 1997). On average, individuals with BDD appear to have poorer quality of life than either patients with clinical depression (major depression and/or dysthymia) or patients with a medical condition such as type II diabetes or a recent heart attack (Phillips, 2000; Phillips, Menard, Fay, & Pagano, 2005).

Poor Insight or Delusional Beliefs

Most patients with BDD have poor insight or have delusional BDD beliefs. That is, they do not recognize that the appearance flaws they perceive are actually minimal or nonexistent (Mancuso, Knoesen, & Castle, 2010; Phillips, 2004). Very few untreated patients have good insight.

They typically say things like "I'm pretty sure I'm right about my nose—it really looks strange," or "I'm certain I really do look deformed; otherwise, why would everyone be staring at me?" They also tend to think that most other people share their view of the supposed defects. It's usually hard to talk people with BDD out of their appearance beliefs. Whereas some patients realize that their appearance beliefs have a psychological or psychiatric cause, many do not; they simply think that their beliefs are true.

Patients with poor insight or delusional beliefs can be more difficult to engage and work with in treatment. Although delusional and nondelusional patients have many similarities, the former appear to have a greater likelihood of attempting suicide, a higher rate of substance use disorders, poorer social functioning, and more severe BDD symptoms (Phillips, Menard, Pagano, Fay, & Stout, 2006).

Co-Occurring Mental Health Problems

Most patients with BDD have other mental disorders. Major depressive disorder is most common, with the largest studies reporting a current prevalence of 38–58% and a lifetime prevalence of 74–76% (Gunstad & Phillips, 2003; Phillips, Didie, & Menard, 2007). In these studies, the BDD usually began before the depression, and the depressive symptoms often appeared to be secondary to the BDD. A longitudinal study found that improvement of BDD was often quickly followed by improvement of depression, and, conversely, that improvement of depression might also be quickly followed by improvement of BDD (Phillips & Stout, 2006).

Lifetime comorbidity of BDD with other disorders—including substance abuse or dependence (40%), social phobia (38%), and OCD (33%) (Gunstad & Phillips, 2003; Phillips, Menard, Fay, & Weisberg, 2005)—is also common. Other studies have reported lower comorbidity rates (Veale, Boocock, Gournay, & Dryden, 1996), which may reflect the treatment setting, referral sources, or other factors. Reported rates of a personality disorder in sizable samples of patients seen in psychiatric settings range from 40 to 72%, with avoidant personality disorder most common (Phillips & McElroy, 2000; Phillips, Menard, Fay, & Weisberg, 2005; Veale et al., 1996).

Suicidal Ideation and Suicide Attempts

An important consideration in treating patients with BDD is that suicidal ideation and suicide attempts are common (e.g., Buhlmann et al., 2010; Hollander & Allen, 2006). Lifetime rates of suicidal ideation are in the range of 78–81%, and 24–28% of patients have attempted suicide (Phillips, Coles, et al., 2005; Phillips & Diaz, 1997; Veale et al., 1996). The lifetime suicide attempt rate for BDD is an estimated 6–23 times higher than in the general U.S. population, and appears higher than for many other psychiatric disorders (Phillips, Coles, et al., 2005).

It is not known with certainty how many people with BDD commit suicide. However, completed suicides have been reported, and the suicide rate (though the data are limited) appears to be very high (Phillips & Menard, 2006). In a retrospective study of patients in two dermatology practices who were known to have committed suicide over 20 years, most had acne or BDD (Cotterill & Cunliffe, 1997). Furthermore, patients with BDD have many suicide risk factors, including (in addition to high rates of suicidal ideation and suicide attempts) psychiatric hospitalization; unemployment and/or disability; being single or divorced; poor social supports; and high rates of major depressive disorder, eating disorders, and substance use disorders (Phillips, 2009; Phillips, Menard, Fay, & Weisberg, 2005). Additional risk factors include high levels of anxiety and depression, feelings of shame and humiliation, and poor self-esteem. From a clinical perspective, patients' often delusional belief that they look deformed causes distress and self-loathing. This distress is further fueled by time-consuming intrusive obsessions about the "defect," as well as the belief that other people share their belief and even mock and ostracize them because of how they look.

Thus patients with BDD must be carefully monitored for suicidality. For patients with worrisome levels of suicidality, hospitalization may be required. Medication can also be considered in addition to CBT (see below), as suicidal thinking often diminishes in patients who receive appropriate medication for BDD (Phillips, 2009; Phillips & Kelly, 2009).

Research on Treatments for BDD

Cognitive-Behavioral Therapy

Data from available studies indicate that CBT is often efficacious for BDD. Most published studies of CBT have included both cognitive therapy and behavioral components consisting mainly of exposure and response prevention to reduce social avoidance and compulsive behaviors (e.g., mirror checking). CBT has led to consistently good outcomes in studies of individual treatment, studies of group treatment, and one study that used both individual and group treatment. These studies are described briefly below.

CBT was conducted in an individual intensive format by Neziroglu, McKay, Todaro, and Yaryura-Tobias (1996), who provided 20 daily 90-minute sessions to patients with BDD over 1 month. The treatment included exposure to perceived physical defects and social situations; prevention of compulsive behaviors; and cognitive therapy aimed at challenging faulty appearance-related beliefs, perfectionism, and concerns about social acceptance and attractiveness. This treatment produced a 50% reduction in BDD symptoms for 12 of 17 patients.

Veale et al. (1996) compared a less intensive individual treatment (12 sessions of 1-hour CBT) to a wait-list control condition; 90% of the patients were women. Their CBT focused on education about a cognitive-behavioral model for BDD to foster engagement in therapy, as well as Socratic questioning, cognitive restructuring, and exposure and response prevention. The investigators reported substantial improvement with CBT, compared to the wait-list condition.

In a third study, McKay, Todaro, Neziroglu, and Campisi (1997) used a 6-week intensive treatment of 30 sessions, but only included exposure and response prevention *in vivo* and in imagery, without cognitive therapy. Half of their 10 patients received a 6-month relapse prevention program after treatment, which included psychoeducation about lapses and relapses, exposure and response prevention assignments, and brief therapist contacts. Patients' BDD symptoms were significantly improved after treatment and remained stable at follow-up. The relapse prevention program did not confer more benefit at longer-term follow-up.

Although the McKay et al. (1997) study suggests that cognitive therapy may not be a necessary component of CBT for BDD, all other studies have included a cognitive component. In addition, in contrast to McKay et al.'s findings, some data suggest that exposure and response prevention alone may not be effective for BDD (Campisi, 1996). Poor treatment outcome with exposure and response prevention alone is perhaps due to the poor insight and depression characteristic of this disorder (Phillips, Didie, & Menard, 2007; Phillips, Menard, Pagano, Fay, & Stout, 2006; Phillips, Siniscalchi, & McElroy, 2004); these factors may also predict poor response to CBT in patients with OCD (Foa, 1979).

Further supporting the value of a cognitive approach, a preliminary report suggests that cognitive therapy alone may be efficacious for BDD (Geremia & Neziroglu, 2001). In this multiple-baseline study, four patients with BDD received cognitive therapy based on Beck's model (14 twice-weekly 75-minute sessions). Body satisfaction and mood improved for three of the four patients, and BDD symptoms improved for two patients. Consonant with our own clinical experience, the authors suggested that cognitive therapy may be advantageous in reducing inaccurate beliefs and increasing compliance with behavioral interventions. Future dismantling studies will be needed to identify specific effects of treatment components.

Rosen, Reiter, and Orosan (1995) compared group CBT to a wait-list control condition for 54 women with BDD. CBT was provided in 2-hour sessions for 4–5 patients per group; it consisted of education, perceptual comparisons, feedback from group members, exposure and response prevention, thought stopping, relaxation, cognitive correction, and relapse prevention. CBT was significantly more efficacious than no treatment on measures of BDD symptoms, body appearance, and self-esteem. BDD symptoms improved in 82% of the CBT group after treatment and 77% up to 5 months later. However, this study did not include men, and it focused mainly on concerns about body weight and shape.

In the second study of group CBT, Wilhelm et al. (1999) demonstrated significant improvement in 13 adults with BDD who received 12 group sessions of 90 minutes each. The dropout rate of 31% was high, probably because these patients were severely ill and impaired. Treatment led to moderate reductions in BDD symptoms and depressed mood, and longer treatment would probably have led to more gains. Finally, a retrospective study of 11 patients with BDD utilized a 6-week combination of daily CBT, medication, and psychosocial rehabilitation in a partial hospital setting (Saxena et al., 2001). Again, BDD symptoms improved after treatment.

We (Wilhelm et al., 2009; Wilhelm, Phillips, Fama, Greenberg, & Steketee, 2011) then conducted a study of individual CBT-BDD that was funded by the National Institute of Mental Health. This study used and tested the present manual. The study had three phases: (1) development of this manual, which was an expansion of the manual used in the Wilhelm et al. group study described above; (2) treatment of 12 patients, during which we further refined the manual on the basis of our experience with these patients; and (3) a study in which 18 patients treated with the revised manual were compared to a wait-list control group. We found that the majority of patients improved with respect to their BDD symptom severity, delusionality, and depression. Thus there is empirical support for the effectiveness of our manualized CBT-BDD.

In summary, the studies described above suggest that CBT specifically developed for BDD is very promising for patients with BDD. Patients improved not only with regard to BDD symptoms, but also with respect to associated features of BDD, such as depression. Nevertheless, these treatment studies leave many important questions unanswered. For example, it is not yet clear how many sessions at what frequency are most useful. Nor is it clear whether individual treatment is superior to group treatment. This treatment also needs to be compared to other types of therapy. Thus more research is needed.

Pharmacotherapy

Available data indicate that serotonin reuptake inhibitors (called SRIs or SSRIs) are often efficacious for BDD (Phillips, 2009; Phillips & Hollander, 2008). SRIs that are marketed in the United States at this writing include escitalopram (Lexapro), citalopram (Celexa), fluoxetine (Prozac), fluvoxamine (Luvox), sertraline (Zoloft), paroxetine (Paxil), and clomipramine (Anafranil). SRIs are currently recommended as the first-line medications for BDD. SRIs affect the neurotransmitter serotonin, which is one of the brain's natural chemicals used to communicate between brain cells. Specially, SRIs block the reabsorption (reuptake) of serotonin into the releasing nerve cells. This changes the serotonin balance in the brain, and more serotonin is made available to affect key brain areas.

Two randomized double-blind controlled studies of SRIs have been done. A randomized double-blind parallel-group study found that fluoxetine (Prozac) was more efficacious than placebo for BDD symptoms and psychosocial functioning (Phillips, Albertini, & Rasmussen, 2002; Phillips & Rasmussen, 2004). In a randomized double-blind crossover study, the SRI clomipramine (Anafranil) was more efficacious for BDD than the non-SRI tricyclic antidepressant desipramine (Hollander et al., 1999). This latter study is consistent with previous case series in indicating that SRI antidepressants may be more efficacious than non-SRI antidepressants for BDD.

Systematic, methodologically rigorous open-label studies with the SRIs fluvoxamine (Perugi et al., 1996; Phillips, Dwight, & McElroy, 1998), citalopram (Phillips & Najar, 2003), and escitalopram (Phillips, 2006a) found that these SRIs are also often efficacious for BDD. Although methodologically rigorous open-label studies of the SRIs sertraline (Zoloft) and paroxetine (Paxil) have not been conducted for BDD, our clinical experience indicates that they are often efficacious (Phillips, Albertini, Siniscalchi, Khan, & Robinson, 2001).

Among all six SRI studies, BDD response rates in intention-to-treat analyses (which included study dropouts, who may not have had adequate time to improve) ranged from 53 to 77%, and BDD symptoms significantly improved. Response rates were higher than this among those patients who completed the studies. In addition to improving BDD symptoms, these medications also often significantly improved suicidal ideation, depressive symptoms, anxiety, anger/hostility, somatization, psychosocial functioning, and mental-health-related quality of life in patients with BDD. Of note, SRIs alone also appeared to be efficacious for patients who were completely convinced that they looked ugly or deformed (i.e., who had delusional BDD beliefs).

SRI doses that are needed for successful treatment of BDD are often higher than those typically needed for many other disorders, such as depression. Also, BDD may require a longer time to respond (sometimes as long as 12–14 weeks) than many other disorders require. If one SRI is not adequately helpful for BDD, another SRI may be. Alternatively, some patients improve when a different type of medication is added to an ineffective or partially effective SRI.

Although less is known about the efficacy of serotonin–norepinephrine reuptake inhibitors for BDD, a small open-label trial (Allen et al., 2008) and our clinical experience suggest that venlafaxine (Effexor) may be helpful for some patients (Phillips, 2009), although it is not currently considered a first-line treatment for BDD. And a recent open-label pilot study suggested that the antiepileptic medication levetiracetam (Keppra) may also be efficacious for BDD, although this medication is also not considered a first-line treatment (Phillips & Menard, 2009). No medications currently have U.S. Food and Drug Administration approval for the treatment of BDD, because not enough placebo-controlled studies have been conducted.

Medication can be used in combination with CBT; the two are compatible treatments. For more severely ill patients who are having difficulty engaging in CBT because they are so ill, medication may enable patients to improve to the point where they are more willing or able to participate meaningfully in CBT. A combination of CBT with medication should especially be considered for patients who appear at high risk of committing suicide. Detailed guidelines about treating BDD with medications may be found elsewhere (National Collaborating Centre for Mental Health, 2006; Phillips, 2009; Phillips & Hollander, 2008).

Surgical, Dermatological, and Other Cosmetic Treatments

A majority of patients with BDD seek and receive cosmetic treatment (e.g., surgical, dermatological, dental) for their BDD concerns (Cotterill, 1996; Crerand, Phillips, Menard, & Fay, 2005; Fukuda, 1977; Marques et al., 2011; Phillips, Grant, Siniscalchi, & Albertini, 2001). In fact, studies have found that 9–12% of patients in dermatology clinics and 3–53% in cosmetic surgery clinics have BDD (Ishigooka et al., 1998; Phillips, 2006b; Sarwer, Wadden, Pertschuk, & Whitaker, 1998). Not surprisingly, they may request extensive procedures (Fukuda, 1977). Some patients even attempt their own surgery, as in the case of a patient who attempted to replace his nose cartilage with chicken cartilage in the desired shape (Phillips, 1996); another patient used a staple gun to do a facelift (Veale, 2000).

The outcomes of cosmetic treatments usually appear to be poor. In fact, they can lead to increased or new appearance preoccupations and multiple medical procedures without improvement (Cotterill, 1996; Crerand et al., 2005; Fukuda, 1977; Koblenzer, 1994; Phillips, Grant, Siniscalchi, & Albertini, 2001). Occasionally, dissatisfied patients have committed suicide or become violent toward treating physicians (Cotterill, 1996; Phillips, 1991). Thus we do not recommend these treatments for BDD. Our CBT-BDD includes a treatment module for patients who are receiving or considering cosmetic treatment.

THEORIES FOR UNDERSTANDING BDD

What Causes BDD?

The cause of BDD is currently largely unknown, although some possible risk factors have been identified. Like other mental disorders, BDD is likely to be multifactorial—that is, to result from a complex interplay of genetic and environmental risk factors (Buhlmann & Wilhelm, 2004; Phillips, 2009; Wilhelm, 2006). Preliminary data indicate that the $GABA_A$-γ2 gene may be implicated in BDD (Phillips & Kaye, 2007). Environmental risk factors may include perceived childhood neglect and/or abuse, teasing, an overemphasis on appearance, and low parental warmth. Sociocultural factors (such as the emphasis on looking attractive) and evolutionary factors may also play a role.

Individuals with BDD score very high on measures of neuroticism and very low on measures of extroversion (Phillips & McElroy, 2000), and it is possible that these traits are risk factors for the development of BDD. Dysfunction in various brain circuits—such as the amygdala, striatum, and other brain regions involved in processing of body image, faces, and facial emotions—may also be involved in BDD. Of more direct relevance to our CBT-BDD, neuropsychological studies have found that people with BDD tend to focus overly on details of visual and verbal stimuli (such as abstract drawings, and word lists), rather than on more global, configural attributes of these stimuli (Deckersbach et al., 2000). Visual processing of faces is also characterized by a focus on detail, at the expense of a more holistic processing style (e.g., Feusner, Townsend, Bystritsky, & Bookheimer, 2007). These findings are consistent with clinical observations that patients selectively attend to and overly focus on specific aspects of their appearance or minor flaws (Wilhelm, 2006). This manual's perceptual retraining exercises help patients learn to "see the big picture" and focus less on disliked details of their appearance.

Studies of cognitive and emotional processing suggest that people with BDD tend to misinterpret ambiguous social situations, and other situations, as threatening (Buhlmann et al.,

2002). They also tend to misinterpret self-referent facial expressions as contemptuous and angry (Buhlmann, Etcoff, & Wilhelm, 2006). Interpretive biases such as these may possibly combine with traits of perfectionism, overestimation of the attractiveness of others (Buhlmann, Etcoff, & Wilhelm, 2007), rejection sensitivity, and an overestimation of the importance of beauty to contribute to the development of BDD. The approaches described in this manual target misinterpretations, biases, and traits such as these.

A Cognitive-Behavioral Model for Understanding BDD

Several writers have contributed to a cognitive-behavioral model for understanding BDD (Rosen et al., 1995; Veale et al., 1996; Wilhelm & Neziroglu, 2002). This model is similar to models proposed for OCD and other disorders. People's behaviors and emotions are thought to be determined by their interpretation of events. Thus it is not a situation itself that determines what a person feels, but how the person perceives it. Most people uncritically accept their perceptions of situations or events as true, and may not even be aware that they are making interpretations because this happens so automatically and quickly. Instead, most people notice only the shift in emotion that follows the interpretation. But why does one person interpret the same situation differently from another? Different interpretations spring from different beliefs.

Beliefs about Appearance and the Self

Beginning in childhood, people develop beliefs or understandings about themselves, other people, and their personal worlds. Healthy individuals attribute little importance to minor appearance flaws or negative intrusive thoughts about their appearance. Therefore, they experience little discomfort when they have such thoughts, easily ignoring or dismissing them. Those who develop BDD, however, pay excessive attention to perceived flaws, perhaps especially at times of stress or low mood. They interpret minor imperfections in appearance as signaling major personal flaws, because they hold predisposing beliefs or assumptions learned previously. As Geremia and Neziroglu (2001) have noted, patients with BDD endorse negative beliefs such as the following:

> "If my appearance is defective, I am inadequate/worthless."
> "If I am unattractive, I will be alone and isolated all my life."
> "Others will notice [my defect] and be appalled by it."

They also confuse physical attractiveness with happiness and self-worth:

> "If I looked better, my whole life would be better."
> "How I feel about myself is based on how I feel about the way I look."
> "If only I can change my appearance, I will be able to achieve what others can do."

"Core beliefs" (or "schemas") are central ideas about the self and others. Most people have relatively adaptive core beliefs, such as "I am a functional person." Negative core beliefs have an absolute, global, or overgeneralized quality. Patients with BDD usually have very negative core beliefs pertaining to their personal worth, which underlie their negative view of their appearance. Here are some examples of patients' core beliefs about themselves:

"I am defective."
"I am worthless."
"I am different."

Patients with BDD may also have negative core beliefs about others, such as "People only like attractive people," which feed their core beliefs that they themselves are worthless and unlovable. When a negative core belief is activated, most people easily process information consistent with this core belief, but ignore or distort information inconsistent with the belief. Like patients with schizophrenia who have delusional beliefs, patients with BDD tend to jump to conclusions without considering alternative explanations for their negative interpretations of situations. For example, if others are glancing in the direction of a person with BDD, the person may assume that the other people are thinking, "You are ugly and therefore defective." These negative interpretations provoke anxiety, depressed mood, and increased attention to the perceived flaws, in an increasing spiral of negative beliefs, emotions, and perceptions. Although the causes of this distorted cognitive processing are unknown, possible causes include fear of negative evaluation and sensitivity to rejection; childhood experiences of feeling unloved; and family and cultural values about attractiveness and self-worth. Stress and current mood may also contribute to emotional reactions to perceived flaws.

Perfectionistic beliefs may also play a role in BDD thinking (Buhlmann et al., 2007; Neziroglu, Anderson, & Yaryura-Tobias, 1999). Veale et al. (1996) observed that about 70% of individuals with BDD endorsed the belief "I have to have perfection in my appearance." In our clinical experience, this typically refers to the "defective" body areas, but for most patients it doesn't imply a desire to be unusually attractive; most simply want to look normal. From an evolutionary perspective, flaws and asymmetries in appearance may interfere with mating success in animals and humans (Feusner, Hembacher, & Phillips, 2009). Because good looks increase the odds of finding a biologically fit partner, it makes sense that humans, as well as animals, are concerned about it. Nevertheless, beliefs about symmetry or good looks are held rigidly in BDD, and they contribute to extreme negative evaluation and heightened attention to minor flaws in appearance (Neziroglu & Yaryura-Tobias, 1997; Veale et al., 1996). Extreme and perfectionistic views about appearance might include the following:

"If there is one flaw in my overall appearance, then I feel unattractive."
"If my [body part] is not beautiful, then it must be ugly."

Progression of Dysfunctional Beliefs to Rituals, Avoidance Behaviors, and More Negative Thinking

As shown in the CBT model of BDD presented in Chapter 7, the negative emotions (e.g., fear, anxiety, depression, and shame) that are triggered by negative appearance-related thoughts and beliefs provoke efforts to neutralize these feelings with avoidance behaviors and ritualistic actions. As discussed above, avoidance behaviors include (but are not limited to) avoiding social contacts and other situations where the person can be seen. Rituals (also discussed above) include mirror checking, skin picking, reassurance seeking, repeated plastic surgery, comparing one's body with that of other people, and excessive grooming. Unfortunately, these efforts have a rebound effect in which the negative thoughts about appearance actually increase after attempts to block them. In addition, they keep a patient focused on the BDD. Because these rituals and avoidance behaviors may temporarily diminish painful emotions, they are negatively reinforced and actually maintain the dysfunctional BDD beliefs and behaviors.

CBT-BDD as described in this manual is based on this model. This treatment's cognitive and behavioral components target different components of the BDD model. For example, cognitive restructuring focuses on developing more accurate and helpful beliefs about appearance. Other cognitive approaches focus on developing more positive core beliefs. Ritual prevention helps patients cut back on or stop repetitive rituals, and exposure and behavioral experiments decrease the avoidance of anxiety-provoking situations and help patients feel more comfortable around other people.

CHAPTER 2

TREATMENT OVERVIEW AND ROADMAP

This chapter provides a treatment overview and roadmap to orient you, the therapist, to CBI-BDD. We recommend reading the whole manual, or at least Chapters 1–6, before your first meeting with a patient you are considering for this treatment.

WHO IS QUALIFIED TO CONDUCT THIS TREATMENT?

Mental health professionals who wish to conduct CBT-BDD should have at least 1 year of training and experience in conducting general psychotherapy, as well as some formal training in CBT. In addition to attending workshops and courses on the basics of CBT, training could include reading books such as *Cognitive Therapy of Anxiety Disorders: A Practice Manual and Conceptual Guide* by Adrian Wells (1997) or *Cognitive Behavior Therapy: Basics and Beyond* by Judith Beck (2011).

Additional psychotherapy and CBT experience will be needed to treat more severely ill patients. A sound knowledge of BDD symptoms is essential—not only to treat the presenting problems successfully, but to enable patients to feel well understood. For therapists who are not too familiar with BDD, we recommend additional reading on this disorder. Because patients with BDD often have comorbid mood disorders or symptoms, including suicidal thinking and low self-esteem, therapists using this manual must be able to establish a strong therapeutic alliance and be fully familiar with procedures for managing complex cases, including those of suicidal patients. Readers who feel uncertain about the adequacy of their background in these issues should seek supervision if they decide to conduct CBT-BDD, especially with more severely ill or suicidal patients.

WHO IS APPROPRIATE FOR THIS TREATMENT?

We have developed CBT-BDD for a broad range of adults with BDD who are suitable for treatment in an outpatient setting. Our goal has been to develop a treatment that is widely applicable to a broad range of patients with this disorder, rather than only a small or selected subset of patients. In our clinical work and research with the present manual, we have treated both women and men, people from a variety of racial and ethnic groups, and a broad range of ages; however, for patients younger than 18 the treatment needs to be modified somewhat (Greenberg et al., 2010). We have treated patients with different levels of BDD (from mild to severe), and with a broad range of typical BDD symptoms as well as less common presentations, such as muscle dysmorphia. We have treated patients who have some insight, as well as patients with delusional BDD, who can be especially challenging to treat. Finally, patients treated with this manual have had a broad range of comorbid disorders, reflecting the range that therapists encounter in the "real world" (although patients with certain disorders were excluded, as discussed below).

Nonetheless, you will need to consider whether CBT-BDD is appropriate for a particular patient. Here we provide some general considerations regarding which patients are, and which may not be, appropriate for this treatment. It is impossible, however, to provide a comprehensive guide on this issue. You will need to draw on your clinical experience, judgment, and understanding of each particular patient to determine whether CBT-BDD seems appropriate for the patient.

Diagnosis of BDD

First, it is important to ascertain that the patient actually has BDD. Chapter 1 of this book provides some information on BDD's clinical features and diagnosis. In our view, CBT-BDD is appropriate for patients with mild, moderate, or severe BDD. It can be used alone as well as in combination with medication. Research on combination treatments in BDD has not yet been done, but our clinical experience suggests that combination treatments can be very beneficial, especially for treatment-refractory, highly delusional, or suicidal patients.

Suicidality Considerations

It is beyond the scope of this manual to provide comprehensive guidelines on the treatment and management of suicidal patients; such guidelines are available elsewhere (American Psychiatric Association, 2003). We do, however, say more about this important issue later in this chapter and in Chapters 3 and 18. For patients with mild suicidal ideation, but no intent or plan, you can cautiously proceed, but you must carefully assess suicide risk and other safety risks throughout the treatment. More concerning degrees of suicidality may warrant treatment strategies in addition to CBT-BDD (American Psychiatric Association, 2003), especially if the patient's suicidality does not appear entirely or largely due to the BDD symptoms. Experience, judgment, and knowledge of each particular patient are needed when you are deciding how to best manage suicidal patients. Consultation or supervision may be helpful in such cases.

Level of Care Required

A further consideration is what level of care is most appropriate for each patient. Some patients with BDD can be successfully treated in an outpatient setting. Others, however, may have BDD symptoms that are too severe, or may be too suicidal, to be safely or effectively treated as outpatients. In such cases, a higher level of care (e.g., day hospital, inpatient, residential) and more intensive treatment may be needed. We have developed this treatment for an outpatient setting and have not tested it in other settings. However, in our view it would be appropriate for inpatient or other settings if more frequent and/or longer sessions are used as needed.

Comorbid Problems

If a patient has another mental health disorder or other problem (e.g., a relationship crisis) that is currently more problematic than BDD, it is often more appropriate to treat that problem before embarking on, or continuing with, CBT-BDD. For example, if the patient has a severe eating disorder that is causing significant medical problems, it may be more appropriate to treat the eating disorder first. If the patient is actively psychotic or manic, it probably would not be appropriate or feasible to do CBT-BDD.

A more complicated situation arises with patients who are actively misusing substances. We recommend that these patients receive additional concurrent treatment focused specifically on their substance use. It is often appropriate to conduct CBT-BDD while patients are still using a substance—especially if the patients attribute their substance use to their BDD, as an attempt to self-medicate the emotional distress resulting from BDD. However, it may be very difficult, if not impossible, to make progress in CBT-BDD if patients are intoxicated during their sessions or don't do homework because of their substance use. In such cases, CBT-BDD may need to be deferred until the substance use is under better control.

In cases where severe or disruptive psychosocial stressors or relationship problems exist, to what extent do they appear due to the BDD? If they seem entirely or largely attributable to the BDD (e.g., marital discord because a patient is too ashamed because of a perceived defect to leave the house), it makes sense to try to continue CBT-BDD. Additional therapeutic strategies may be needed, however, to manage the problem or crisis. If the crisis or problem is extremely disruptive, it may not be appropriate or possible to do CBT-BDD at the present time, as this is a highly structured treatment that requires completion of homework. In such cases, CBT-BDD may need to be deferred, and other therapeutic strategies used, until the crisis is resolved.

You will need to use your judgment about other patient characteristics or factors that may make CBT less appropriate, if not impossible, to conduct. For example, untreated attention-deficit/hyperactivity disorder (ADHD) may make it hard for a patient to focus on treatment sessions or do homework. Cognitive impairment or certain personality disorders may also interfere with implementation of the treatment. If the interfering problem is adequately addressed, successful CBT-BDD may become feasible.

Treatment Characteristics

Session Length

To best meet the needs of clinical settings, CBT-BDD uses 50- to 60-minute individual sessions. However, if possible, we recommend 90 minutes for the first session, to allow more time to get to know the patient.

Session Frequency

The optimal session frequency is unclear. Research studies have used a broad range of frequencies, with no clear indication of which is best. We recommend at least weekly sessions. Some patients, however, especially those who are more severely ill, may benefit from more than once-a-week sessions. To get the treatment going more quickly, consider scheduling two sessions per week for Sessions 1–4. The final two relapse prevention sessions are spaced 2 weeks apart, so that patients can learn to maintain treatment gains independent of meetings with the therapist.

Treatment Duration and Brief Overview

The treatment in this manual lasts for 22 sessions on average. It starts with *three introductory sessions (Part II)*, which focus on psychoeducation, case formulation, motivational enhancement, and setting treatment goals. These three introductory sessions lay important groundwork for the rest of the treatment and should not be skipped.

The manual then focuses on *core treatment components (Part III)* that are used with all patients: cognitive restructuring, exposure/behavioral experiments, ritual prevention, and perceptual retraining, all of which are tailored specifically to BDD's unique features. New core treatment components are typically introduced until Session 11 or later (depending on when advanced cognitive strategies begin). The patient and you will then keep using and practicing these core components in all sessions until Session 20. The patient will also continue to practice all of these core components as part of homework exercises until the treatment ends. Over time, the patient will engage in increasingly challenging exercises (e.g., increasingly challenging exposures).

In addition to these core treatment components, the manual includes *optional treatment modules (Part IV)* that can be used with selected patients to supplement the core interventions. These modules are used for patients who have specific symptoms (e.g., cosmetic treatment seeking, skin picking, depression) that require specific treatment strategies. For example, the module on weight, shape, and muscularity teaches treatment strategies designed for these specific concerns and related symptoms. The module on skin picking or hair pulling/plucking helps patients with these compulsive BDD-related symptoms by teaching them modified habit reversal. Use of the optional modules thus ensures that the treatment can be personalized for individual patients (i.e., tailored to problem areas that are characteristic of some but not all patients with BDD). After the supplemental modules have been introduced, they are used in subsequent sessions and homework assignments for as long as necessary.

The last two treatment sessions (typically Sessions 21 and 22) focus on *relapse prevention*, which is used with all patients before their treatment ends.

Although our research indicates that 22 treatment sessions are adequate for most patients, you should keep the number of sessions for the patients in your clinical practice somewhat flexible, as some patients may need more sessions or possibly fewer sessions.

Patients who have made gains in treatment are good candidates for booster sessions after formal CBT-BDD ends, to prevent relapse. The frequency of booster sessions can be gradually reduced over time. For example, the first booster session might occur 1 month after the end of treatment, and the second session might occur 3 months after the end of treatment. If the booster sessions seem useful, you can offer additional ones—for example, once per season, then once a year. *The frequency of booster sessions should be tailored to the needs of each patient.*

Components of the CBT-BDD Program

Before Starting Therapy (Chapters 3 and 4)

As with any patients, you will need to develop diagnostic impressions, obtain a psychosocial and medication treatment history, as well as to complete the standard intake assessment. This manual does not cover these aspects of initial assessment, but assumes that you have completed an intake evaluation to determine that this treatment is appropriate for your patient. Chapter 3 discusses special issues that should be considered before you begin treatment, and Chapter 4 provides guidance in the initial diagnosis and assessment of BDD in particular. You can then ask the patient to return for an additional session that focuses in more detail on assessment and diagnosis (see Chapter 6, which covers the first session).

Enhancing Motivation (Chapter 5)

For many if not most patients with BDD, assessing motivation and using motivational strategies are essential for enabling the patients to cooperate with and benefit from treatment. Many patients with BDD are ambivalent about receiving mental health treatment, believing that their problem is physically based and that they need corrective cosmetic treatment, not therapy. Others believe that their situation is hopeless and that nothing can help them. Some misunderstand CBT, thinking it is too hard or scary. Providing psychoeducation and offering hope that most patients with BDD get better with the right treatment are helpful but not always adequate.

Derived from Miller and Rollnick's (2002, 2013) *Motivational Interviewing*, motivation enhancement strategies are designed to resolve ambivalence about seeking and receiving treatment or reducing symptoms. Motivational strategies may be particularly useful during the introductory treatment sessions (see below). Other patients may exhibit ambivalence later in treatment—for example, by expressing uncertainty or reluctance about being or staying in treatment, by not doing homework, or by missing sessions. Chapter 5's discussion of motivational methods does not include a session-specific agenda, because these strategies are intended for use during any session whenever signs of ambivalence appear. These strategies can cover an entire session, or parts of sessions, at any point during the treatment.

Introductory Sessions

Before you start treating a patient, it's essential to set the stage by (1) doing further assessment and providing psychoeducation about BDD and the treatment process; and (2) developing a case formulation, a CBT model of the patient's symptoms, and clear goals for treatment. These tasks will take approximately three sessions. We strongly recommend that you not skip over or shorten this part of the treatment. These early sessions are an essential foundation for treatment; without them, the treatment may not succeed. You may not adequately understand the patient's symptoms, and the treatment may not focus on key symptoms or have realistic goals that are shared by the patient.

The strong therapeutic alliance and collaborative working relationship that are forged during these initial sessions will be critical to learning subsequent strategies and techniques. It often takes more time to cover this material than it does in CBT for other disorders, since patients with BDD may not accept treatment as easily because of their poor insight. You may need to be gentler, move less quickly through the sessions, and use motivational techniques (see above) during these early sessions. If the patient complains that things are moving too slowly at the outset, emphasize the importance of first understanding the BDD and deciding on goals to increase the likelihood that treatment will be successful.

Further Assessment and Education (Chapters 6 and 7)

Session 1 of CBT-BDD (Chapter 6) is devoted to assessing the patient's BDD in further detail, providing feedback about BDD symptoms, orienting the patient to treatment, assessing and enhancing motivation as described above, and answering the patient's initial questions. Session 2 (Chapter 7) offers an opportunity to provide psychoeducation about BDD in general and the patient's own symptoms in particular, as well as to give further feedback.

Case Formulation and Goal Setting (Chapters 7 and 8)

You will then move on to case formulation and goal setting. Case formulation focuses on developing a model to understand the elements that constitute and contribute to each individual patient's body image problem. It also determines the specific treatment strategies that will be needed to address each contributing element for that particular patient. This work is usually completed during Sessions 2 and 3, right after psychoeducation is completed. You and the patient will also review your patient's values and set goals for the treatment. It's important for the goals to represent progress for the patient, but also to be realistic.

Core Treatment Components for All Patients

The core interventions follow education, case formulation, and goal setting, with motivational strategies (Chapter 5) inserted as needed during these and subsequent interventions. Core interventions cover the basic components for treating all patients with BDD, although the specific strategies used will vary somewhat, depending on each patient's particular presentation. The core interventions should be used in the order presented in this manual, as each session builds on and reinforces the skills taught in previous sessions. In rare cases, patients will not display any rituals that need to be addressed, obviating the need for the ritual prevention component (Chapter 11).

Evaluating Thoughts (Chapter 9)

In this chapter, patients learn to identify problematic thoughts about their appearance and examine them. Methods such as identifying cognitive errors, using Socratic questioning to examine the evidence for and against beliefs, and taking a more accurate and helpful perspective are used. We recommend doing this cognitive work before beginning exposure, as cognitive therapy skills are integrated into exposure exercises. In our experience, this makes exposure less anxiety-provoking and increases its effectiveness.

Exposure (Chapter 10)

Exposure to feared and avoided situations is highly effective for reducing discomfort in a wide variety of disorders. We apply it to BDD by generating patient-specific hierarchies of situations for gradual exposure. Some exposure is completed during the session if possible, and exposure is also assigned as homework, so that a patient can observe the natural decrease of anxiety over time.

Preventing Rituals (Chapter 11)

Compulsive, ritualistic behaviors (e.g., mirror checking) that patients perform to try to reduce their anxiety are the targets of this chapter. Although it would be optimal to reduce those behaviors all at once, this is often not possible, and therefore a gradual approach will probably be needed. Exposure and response prevention are often combined, and exposures can be planned as behavioral experiments in which patients gather evidence for and against their beliefs.

Perceptual Retraining (Chapter 12)

To help them manage intrusive thoughts about their appearance, patients learn mindfulness exercises. These skills train patients to observe and describe negative thoughts related to their BDD (e.g., "My skin is so red, I better put on some makeup.") without immediately jumping to react to them. In essence, they learn to tolerate unpleasant experiences that led them to engage in BDD behaviors in the past. These mindfulness exercises are combined with perceptual retraining done in front of the mirror. To counteract selective attention to disliked body areas, as well as rituals like mirror checking and excessive grooming, patients learn to observe and describe their entire bodies while looking in the mirror (not just the perceived flaws) in a more holistic, objective, and nonjudgmental way.

Advanced Cognitive Strategies (Chapter 13)

This chapter covers cognitive strategies to address deeper-level core beliefs. Ordinarily, these skills will be covered after patients have learned skills for evaluating thoughts, exposure, response prevention, and mindfulness/perceptual retraining skills, and can combine them flexibly. Advanced cognitive strategies include the downward arrow, metaphors, the self-esteem pie, turning the tables, and the survey method. These methods usually work well after some basic exposures have been completed, and they may be used to prepare patients for more difficult exposures.

Relapse Prevention (Chapter 14)

The last two treatment sessions focus on preventing relapse. They begin with a review of the treatment techniques that patients have found most helpful and a discussion of how to practice these after the end of treatment. You will also review remaining problems and help patients address their fears about ending therapy; enhance self-efficacy by attributing progress to new knowledge and skills the patients have acquired; and encourage patients to anticipate possible stressors and setbacks and think ahead about how to manage these with techniques learned in therapy. In addition, you will decrease the frequency of treatment sessions, to ensure a more gradual transition to the end of treatment. Booster sessions are provided, at a minimum, 1 month and 3 months after the end of treatment. The content of these sessions follows that of the relapse prevention sessions.

Optional Modules

The core interventions described above are likely to be relevant for all patients. However, they may not adequately target or reduce certain symptoms (e.g., skin picking, seeking surgery/dermatological treatment) that some, but not all, patients with BDD have. So, in addition to the core skills, you can select any of the specialized treatment modules described in Chapters 15–18 to suit particular patients' needs and to increase the flexibility of the treatment. Some patients may not need any of the specialized modules, whereas others will potentially benefit from more than one.

Usually you will select specialized modules some time after patients have learned the core CBT-BDD skills and you are fully familiar with their symptoms. However, some patients may require administration of a specialized module earlier in treatment, because this module addresses their chief complaint or a major concern. For example, if a patient is self-inflicting serious skin damage from BDD-related skin picking, consider using this module earlier in the treatment—for example, concurrent with Preventing Rituals (Chapter 11) and possibly even before Evaluating Thoughts (Chapter 9). When weight or muscularity concerns are key symptoms or the patient's only area of concern, plan to incorporate this module (Chapter 16) early in the treatment (before covering all of the core treatment elements). We have also occasionally worked on core beliefs by using advanced cognitive strategies (Sessions 11–20, Chapter 13) early in treatment with some patients who requested this and were at risk of dropping out of treatment because of the intensity of these core beliefs.

Determining whether your patients need one or more of these specialized modules should be based on the patients' input about symptoms they consider problematic, your own clinical judgment, and elevated scores on aspects of BDD measures. Below are brief descriptions of each specialized module.

Skin Picking and Hair Pulling (Chapter 15)

More than one-third of patients with BDD compulsively pick their skin to try to remove tiny imperfections (e.g., pimples, bumps). They may use their fingers or other implements, such as pins, needles, razor blades, staple removers, or knives. This behavior can consume hours a day and can cause visible disfigurement and tissue damage, even though the patients' intent is *not* to damage their skin or harm themselves. Hair pulling or plucking (e.g., to make eyebrows even or to remove "excessive" hair) may also occur. This module builds upon the ritual prevention techniques presented in Chapter 11, and also teaches some new skills (e.g., habit reversal).

Weight, Shape, and Muscularity (Chapter 16)

About one-quarter of patients with BDD have excessive concerns about their weight, shape, and/or muscle development. Women are more likely to worry that they're too fat, whereas men are more likely to have muscle dysmorphia (i.e., to think that their bodies are too thin, too small, or inadequately muscular). They may excessively exercise, excessively lift weights, diet, and use anabolic steroids or other substances to build bulk and muscle. This module provides additional psychoeducation on these problems and tailors core interventions (e.g., cognitive restructuring, response prevention, exposure) to this particular presentation of BDD.

If a patient is actually overweight, use your judgment as to whether this module is appropriate. It may be helpful if the patient is just slightly overweight and has a distorted view of the extent of the overweight. On the other hand, if the patient is actually very overweight or obese, we recommend that you not use this module. It may not be helpful or appropriate, for example, to have such patients do exposure, as they may actually be stared at or ridiculed because of how they look.

Cosmetic Treatment (Chapter 17)

About two-thirds of patients with BDD obtain cosmetic treatment, most commonly dermatological treatment or plastic surgery. They may also pursue dental treatment, other nonpsychiatric medical treatment (e.g., seeing an endocrinologist for "excessive" body hair), or paraprofessional treatment (e.g., electrolysis) for their perceived flaws. These treatments are rarely helpful and can even make BDD symptoms worse. This module provides additional psychoeducation, tailors core interventions (e.g., cognitive restructuring, response prevention, exposure) to this issue, and provides additional CBT approaches to prevent pursuit of such treatment.

Managing Depression (Chapter 18)

Many patients with BDD have comorbid major depressive disorder. About three-quarters have had a current or past major depressive episode, and about one-third to two-thirds meet DSM-IV-TR (American Psychiatric Association, 2000) criteria for current major depressive disorder. These patients often score in the moderate or high range on measures of current depressive symptom severity. Severe depression can interfere with treatment of BDD. For example, patients may have trouble attending sessions or doing CBT homework because of low energy or low motivation due to depression. Patients may also have suicidal ideation that requires a treatment focus on hopelessness. This module offers approaches that are tailored to patients with this problem, such as behavioral activation and scheduling pleasant and achievement-oriented activities.

Examples of Treatment Schedules

Most patients will receive the treatment components in the order presented in this manual—first the core interventions, and then any specialized treatment modules that are relevant. Motivational techniques are used as needed throughout the treatment. We provide session numbers as general guidelines, but it is important to recognize that some patients learn treatment skills faster than others do. You will need to use your own judgment in deciding how quickly you can cover the material presented here with a particular patient. Adam's treatment, described below, followed the usual sequence. However, in some cases, you'll need to use relevant modules earlier in treatment if they target prominent symptoms. Jane's treatment, also described below, illustrates the flexibility that may be needed in pacing the treatment and sequencing its components.

Adam's and Jane's Treatment Schedules

Adam has typical BDD symptoms. He obsesses about his supposedly thinning hair and long face. He compulsively checks his appearance in mirrors, compares his appearance with that of other people, and excessively combs and styles his hair, trying to get it to "look right." As a result of these concerns and behaviors, he's often late for work. Because he is self-conscious about how he looks, he feels anxious around other people and is reluctant to see friends or go out with his girlfriend. Adam is moderately depressed because of his appearance concerns and has occasional passive suicidal ideation. He's considering getting a hair transplant at some point in the future, but not within the next 6 months. His appearance-related insight is fair to poor; he is fairly motivated for treatment.

Jane obsesses about tiny pimples on her skin and compulsively picks at her skin for 4–5 hours a day. She considers her skin picking a major problem. She also obsesses about the size of her nose and is considering seeing a surgeon for a consultation within the next 6 months. Because of her appearance concerns, Jane is currently unemployed and is not dating. She is moderately depressed and has chronic passive suicidal ideation. She has poor insight regarding her appearance concerns, and her motivation for CBT-BDD is fairly low; as she states, "Why should I see you? You can't make my nose any smaller!"

Adam's and Jane's treatment schedules are presented in Figure 2.1. (These schedules assume that a standard clinic assessment has already been conducted and that a clinic record has been opened.)

Later in the treatment, after all of the core intervention skills have been covered, there is more flexibility in deciding what to work on. (Notice in Figure 2.1 how Jane's treatment schedule deviates from Adam's at various points, particularly from midtreatment onward. While Adam's treatment continues to focus on core interventions, Jane's focuses on skin picking and motivational interventions.) Generally, it's helpful to focus on techniques that need more practice, problems that a patient is still having, or especially helpful techniques that it may be beneficial to reinforce.

Once each component of the treatment is learned, it is integrated into most subsequent sessions and most homework assignments. For example, once Adam and Jane learn cognitive restructuring, both patients continue to complete thought records and to do cognitive restructuring as part of all of their future homework assignments.

If a patient doesn't seem engaged in the treatment, isn't improving despite adequate motivation, or appears to be clinically deteriorating despite good adherence to treatment, consider a change in treatment. This requires a discussion with the patient. Changes may include refining the cognitive-behavioral model that guides the treatment (Chapters 7 and 8), implementing motivational strategies (Chapter 5), or using relevant specialized treatment modules (Chapters 15–18) earlier in treatment. You can also consider a reassessment of the patient's treatment goals.

Standard Session Format

Each treatment session follows the same general format. We offer suggested times for each session component, to help you stay on track and complete all session components. Too much time with the initial brief check on symptoms, for example, may limit discussion of agenda items or leave too little time for assigning homework. The times provided below are general guidelines that you may need to modify for certain sessions. We also offer suggested language that you can use to introduce new concepts in therapy. Don't recite these suggestions sentence by sentence, but rather try to cover the recommended content in your own words.

Session No.	Adam	Jane
1	Diagnosis and assessment	Diagnosis and assessment (plus some motivational interviewing)
2	Education (plus brief motivational interviewing)	Completion of diagnosis and assessment (plus some motivational interviewing)
3	Case formulation, discussion about values, and goal setting	Education
4	Evaluating self-defeating thoughts (cognitive restructuring)	Case formulation and goal setting
5	Evaluating self-defeating thoughts (cognitive restructuring)	Evaluating self-defeating thoughts (cognitive restructuring) (plus additional motivational interviewing integrated into thought records)
6	Exposure	Evaluating self-defeating thoughts (cognitive restructuring)
7	Exposure, response prevention	Exposure
8	Exposure, response prevention	Exposure, response prevention
9	Exposure, response prevention	Response prevention (with a focus on skin picking)
10	Perceptual retraining	Skin-picking/hair-plucking module
11	Practice of all learned skills	Response prevention and skin-picking/hair-plucking module
12	Practice of all learned skills	Perceptual retraining
13	Core beliefs	Cosmetic treatment
14	Core beliefs	Practice of all learned skills (plus more motivational interviewing)
15	Continued work on all learned skills plus motivational interviewing focusing on homework completion	Core beliefs
16	Continued work on all learned skills	Core beliefs
17	Continued work on all learned skills	Continued work on all learned skills
18	Continued work on all learned skills	Continued work on all learned skills
19	Continued work on all learned skills	Continued work on all learned skills
20	Continued work on all learned skills	Continued work on all learned skills
21	Relapse prevention	Relapse prevention
22	Relapse prevention	Relapse prevention

FIGURE 2.1. Adam's and Jane's treatment schedules.

Encourage Patients to Take Notes during Sessions

In the first session, provide patients with a notebook, binder, or folder in which to keep all forms and handouts from the therapy, so they can bring these to each session. You may need to help patients keep this binder or folder organized by content, to avoid confusion and time wasted during sessions in searching for information needed during the sessions. For example, patients might put key handouts in one section and completed homework, blank homework forms, and personal session forms in other separate sections.

In addition, give patients a *Personal Session Form* (Form 2.1) at the beginning of each session for taking notes about important points. Patients can use this form to record their homework for the upcoming week and any questions or problems that arise during the week. Encourage them to place these forms in their treatment folder or binder, so that by the end of therapy they have a complete record of the CBT-BDD activities. This becomes important in reminding patients what to do during therapy and in working on relapse prevention at the end of treatment.

Check Mood and BDD Symptoms (1–5 Minutes)

Begin sessions by asking patients how they're doing with regard to current and recent mood (e.g., depression, anxiety, anger, frustration) and the severity of BDD symptoms since the previous session. Patients will also complete an inventory such as the *Beck Depression Inventory–II* (BDI-II), a short self-report measure of depression that is discussed further in Chapter 4, in the waiting room before each session. This will provide a general indication of depressed mood and help you determine whether there is a significant risk of suicidal behavior (see item 9). If so, discuss the need to develop a safety plan during the coming days, and establish a formal plan to monitor suicidality. If a patient refuses to agree to contact you if he or she feels unsafe, or if you believe that the patient is at significant risk, take immediate measures to ensure safety. Always take as much time as needed to ensure the patient's safety. We say more about suicidal thinking in later chapters.

In addition, briefly ask about events during the intervening week and the patient's reactions. This brief check-in (1–5 minutes) may yield items for the session's agenda. If needed, take a little time to talk about any material that seems important or needs clarification. But don't spend too much time on this initial step, as it will take time away from working on the agenda.

Briefly Review the Previous Session (2 Minutes)

The purpose of briefly reviewing the previous session is to check patients' perception and understanding of that session. For example, you might ask, "What did you get out of the last session, and what seemed important about it?" Or "Did anything bother you about the session?" Such questions provide an opportunity to obtain feedback. Once your patients know that you'll ask them about the previous session, they will be more motivated to prepare by thinking about what happened and what they learned from it. This becomes a good springboard for the current session. Patients are more likely to remember the content of the last session if you encourage them to write down important points during the sessions.

Set the Agenda Jointly with the Patient (2–3 Minutes)

Together, you and each patient will set the agenda for each session. Early in the treatment, you will need to put concepts or treatment strategies on the agenda yourself (e.g., learning about cognitive errors, preventing rituals). However, patients can contribute by noting particular situations or experiences they'd like to work on. For example, suppose Mary mentions that she rarely leaves the house, but this week she went outside and thought that someone laughed at her because of her messy hair, so she ran back home to check the mirror and frantically combed her hair. If you're doing cognitive restructuring that day, you could work on the thoughts and beliefs she had during that episode. If Mary is scheduled to work on exposure and response prevention during the session, you could weave in a relevant exposure. For example, she could walk around your office building or waiting room with slightly messed-up hair, while also doing response prevention by not checking the mirror or combing her hair before or during the exposure.

Later during the treatment, especially after the core components have all been covered, patients should have more input into the agenda—with regard not only to specific situations to cover, but to the overall focus of the session.

In one of the first sessions, you might say something like this:

> "Usually we set an agenda for what we want to cover in the session. Especially for the early sessions, I have a pretty good idea of what we'll want to cover. I also want to invite you to put on the agenda any problems you've had over the past week that you'd like to work on. How does that sound?"

At a later stage in treatment, you might say something like this:

> "OK, let's set our agenda for today. I'd like to discuss. . . . What's on your list to talk about? . . . Sure, that sounds good. Oh, also, I want to ask about your homework from last week, and I have that information we talked about for you. Anything else?"

If the agenda seems too full, you and the patient can prioritize what to cover that day and what might wait till next time. If a pressing issue arises that isn't on the agenda, you can deviate from the agenda (with the patient's permission).

Review Homework (10 Minutes or Longer)

After setting the agenda, review homework the patient has worked on since the previous session. Homework assignments should appear on every agenda for discussion early in the session, to emphasize the importance of homework and to reinforce efforts to work on BDD problems soon after they have occurred. Studies of other disorders have found that patients who regularly do homework improve more than those who do not do homework. Thus it's important to let patients know this, to encourage compliance with homework, and review it during the session.

First, ask patients how their homework went, and inquire about their thoughts about this. Then review the previous homework assignment and reinforce or correct the patients' efforts. If they did a good job, be sure to comment positively. If you spot mistakes, use Socratic questioning to help your patients consider possible solutions. If they had any problems completing the homework, focus on these to resolve the problem before continuing with other parts of therapy.

Although homework review will usually take only about 10 minutes, it may sometimes take longer than this, especially when agenda items for the current session are contained in the previous homework assignment or when patients are having difficulty with homework. Also, more experienced therapists may wish to integrate the homework review with the next step (working on the agenda). In doing this, however, it's important not to get sidetracked and forget the homework review.

Work on the Agenda (25–35 Minutes)

Focus on the agenda items for the bulk of the session. Here you will work on a few problems the patient wishes to work on, while interweaving training in new CBT-BDD skills, and reinforcing previously learned ones. You might develop homework assignments during your session, rather than waiting to assign them at the end of the session. It's also helpful to relate the agenda items to the patient's therapy goals, to reinforce the CBT model of BDD, and to reinforce previously learned skills.

Early in the treatment, the agenda will focus on education and on new skills to be learned, although it's good to incorporate items the patient would like to cover (e.g., a distressing social interaction from the previous week) to the extent possible. Later in the treatment, after all of the skills have been covered, there is more flexibility in deciding what to work on (as shown in the Figure 2.1 treatment schedules).

Assign Homework (5 Minutes)

Recommendations for homework assignments appear at the end of each therapy chapter. Homework assignments will vary widely, depending on the phase of treatment and the specific material being covered. However, once certain core skills are introduced (such as exposure, response prevention, and mirror retraining), we recommend that practice of all previously learned skills be included in all future homework assignments.

When choosing homework for the upcoming week, a useful strategy is to ask the patient, "Do you think there's at least a 70% chance that you can successfully complete the task?" If the percentage is lower than this, it may be too challenging and unlikely to be completed, and it's probably wise for you and the patient to come up with an alternative assignment. If all of the homework is too easy, however, it may not help the patient make gains.

Rather than assigning new homework in the last few minutes of a session, it's preferable to agree on or plan homework over the course of the session, as new skills are being learned or as areas that require practice become evident. However, it's good to include a brief reminder at the end of the session about what the homework is. This is also an opportunity to assign additional homework that may not have come up during the session.

It's important to have patients write the homework down on their *Personal Session Form* (Form 2.1) so they remember it. Some patients may find it helpful to schedule the homework (which may include the specific assignments for each day) in their calendars as a reminder to get it done.

Summarize the Session (2 Minutes)

Either you or your patient will briefly summarize the major points covered in the session, in order to have a clear understanding of what has been accomplished that day. This enhances your patient's learning of the material covered in the session, and also gives you a recap of how your patient interprets the session content. It's best to refrain from activating negative thoughts at this late point in the session and to be more positive and upbeat. Early in treatment, you can do the summary to model for the patient. Then shift this role to the patient as the treatment progresses. If the patient has taken notes during the session, this will facilitate the summarizing.

Ask for Feedback (1–2 Minutes)

End the session by asking the patient to provide feedback on the session. If the patient has difficulty doing this, you could ask what was helpful about the session and what wasn't helpful, whether you said anything that bothered the patient, whether the session was too challenging or not challenging enough, or similar questions.

FORM 2.1

Personal Session Form

Name: ______________________________ Date: ____________ Session no.: ______

Agenda:

Main points:

Homework:

To discuss next time:

Adapted with permission of the publisher from Wilhelm, S., & Steketee, G. (2006). *Cognitive Therapy for Obsessive-Compulsive Disorder.* Oakland, CA: New Harbinger Publications.

CHAPTER 3

Special Considerations in Treating Patients with BDD

This manual is written for therapists who have training and experience in CBT. Nonetheless, we highlight here a few key points that are especially important for CBT-BDD.

Guidelines for CBT-BDD

Orienting Patients to CBT-BDD

Session 1 (Chapter 6) provides details to help you orient your patients to the treatment methods. You'll also explain the treatment at various points, especially when you build a model of a patient's symptoms. This orientation should help patients become comfortable with what happens in treatment and be more effective collaborators.

Educating Patients about BDD

It is essential to take some time to provide education about BDD, primarily in Session 2 (Chapter 7). Many people are unaware that BDD is a relatively common and treatable problem. It's important to convey this and to let patients know that they are not alone. Many are enormously relieved to learn this and to hear that there is hope for them.

Taking a Scientist's or Detective's Perspective

Much of CBT emphasizes taking the perspective of a scientist or a detective. Patients learn that just because they think something, this does not necessarily mean it's true. Thoughts and beliefs are hypotheses that can be tested. You'll repeatedly find yourself asking your patients, "What is the evidence for this particular belief? And what is the evidence against it?" Patients learn to open up their mind to other possibilities and set out to discover for themselves what is true. It's especially helpful to emphasize this when doing exposure/behavioral experiments, during which patients go out and actually collect evidence to see whether their beliefs and predictions are true. This approach is especially important for patients with BDD, since they may assume that you—like so many other people—will simply try to talk them out of their beliefs.

Emphasizing a scientist/detective perspective conveys that you will not fight with your patients to change their appearance beliefs or try to convince them that you're right and they're wrong. Rather, you will teach them skills to enable them to learn things and figure things out for themselves. Many patients with BDD have had the upsetting experience of others trying to tell them how wrong they are—which doesn't work.

Using a Socratic Style

Using a Socratic style involves asking a series of questions about a particular issue (e.g., an incident or a specific behavior pattern) to explore a patient's thoughts/beliefs and gently expose contradictions in these thoughts/beliefs. Patients with BDD typically have poor insight; they are convinced that their appearance-related thoughts and beliefs are accurate. Thus it is especially important to ask questions and explore, rather than try to talk patients into accepting your view.

Keeping Treatment Focused on Learning and Practicing CBT-BDD Skills

Patients who have had previous "talk" therapy may need more socialization to CBT-BDD. As a result of their past therapy experiences, they may try to fill sessions with discussions of what's going on in their lives, the meaning of their BDD symptoms, or other issues not central to the agenda. If such discussion is lengthy, it will derail session agendas and impede the learning of CBT-BDD skills. If this becomes a problem, gently redirect clients after the first couple of sentences to the agenda at hand:

> "I'm sorry to interrupt. It sounds like that might be important for us to discuss later on, but right now I'd like to stick with our agenda for today. We have a lot to do, so let's get back to . . . "

Avoiding Overinterpretation of Symptoms

It is helpful to develop some understanding of possible reasons for a patient's BDD symptoms—for example, early experiences with family and peers—when building a model of the patient's BDD (Chapters 7 and 8). However, the purpose of this understanding is to facilitate learning core CBT-BDD skills. Avoid extensive exploration of the origins of the problem, as this takes time away from training in core skills and strategies. Instead, focus treatment on resolving the problem by using CBT techniques the patient can learn to apply.

Forging a Strong Therapeutic Alliance

Effective treatment requires a strong therapeutic alliance and a collaborative effort between you and each patient. Starting with the first few sessions, you'll be demonstrating your attitude toward the patient and the BDD symptoms, as well as your approach to treatment and expectations of the patient.

Effective CBT therapists are respectful, empathic, interested, encouraging, and appropriately challenging. They are also clear communicators with a nondisparaging sense of humor. The need to be gently challenging and explicit about expectations is more typical of CBT than of other forms of psychotherapy. Some patients have commented that it's very helpful to have a therapist directing the treatment who encourages them to make their best effort. A sense of humor can be useful in planning difficult homework assignments and helping patients step back to gain perspective on their problems.

Of course, you must use humor judiciously, to avoid implying a casual attitude toward or disrespect for patients and their struggles. A particular caveat about BDD is in order: It's important to avoid humor about aspects of patients' appearance (including their clothing) or their appearance concerns. Remember that many patients with BDD are extremely sensitive to slights, even if intended positively.

The therapeutic alliance is greatly enhanced when you attempt to understand patients' BDD symptoms so well that you can anticipate their responses. You figuratively step into the patients' shoes. For example, if you feel that you need to get a better understanding of a patient's daily life, you can ask the patient to describe his or her activities and BDD symptoms from morning to night on a given day. With such efforts, patients feel well understood and encouraged about the therapy process.

Helping Patients See the "Big Picture"

A major theme of this treatment is helping patients learn to see the "big picture," which patients with BDD have a hard time doing. We've found that patients like this phrase and find it helpful, so we encourage you to refer to it throughout the treatment. CBT-BDD helps patients learn to see the big picture in many ways:

- *Cognitive restructuring* helps patients to broaden their views of themselves and the world, and to consider other possibilities, rather than automatically assuming that their negative thoughts are correct.
- *ERP* enables patients to collect actual evidence during exposure as to whether their negative thoughts and predictions are true. Collecting evidence involves observing the world in a broader and more open-minded way than the patients are used to doing.
- *Work on comparisons and other rituals* encourages patients to "turn on their senses" by noticing aspects about others besides their appearance, and by noticing what's going on around them in their environment.
- *Perceptual retraining*, by helping patients observe and describe their entire bodies in a holistic and nonjudgmental way, enables them to avoid zeroing in on perceived flaws.
- *Advanced cognitive strategies* involve work on core beliefs that affect self-esteem, to enable patients to acknowledge themselves as whole people—including positive traits rather than only negative ones about their appearance.

Harnessing the Power of Writing

Writing helps patients clarify and process thoughts. We strongly encourage patients to write things down on the *Personal Session Form* (Form 2.1) and to complete a variety of worksheets that are presented in later chapters (e.g., forms for describing the patient's BDD model and goals). Sometimes patients say they "did" their homework (e.g., a thought record) but didn't write it down. In this case, consider asking them to complete the relevant form during the session. Convey how important actually filling out the forms is to getting the most out of this treatment.

Later in treatment, patients will do more and more of the treatment "in their heads" without writing it down, as they incorporate the CBT-BDD strategies into their everyday thoughts and actions. For example, they will eventually want to do cognitive restructuring and prepare for exposures in their minds. With more and more practice, these skills become overlearned, "automatic," and integrated into their lives. But throughout this treatment program, especially early in the treatment, writing is key.

Ensuring That Patients Complete Homework

It is critically important for patients to do homework, including written homework, between sessions. In general, we recommend at least 30–60 minutes of homework ("skills practice") a day for 6–7 days a week. This may sound like a lot, but keep in mind that homework for treatment is different from homework for school, as patients do not necessarily have to sit at a desk to complete it. In fact, as treatment progresses, it is increasingly important that they incorporate the skills they learn into their daily lives. Especially later in treatment, homework often means that they do things they have to do anyway, but that they now incorporate their new treatment strategies. Thus even a trip to the supermarket can "count" as a homework exercise if a patient uses it as an opportunity to practice new skills. Patients need to commit to doing homework at the very beginning of treatment; if they don't, CBT-BDD is probably not the right treatment for them.

Explain to patients that the more homework they do, the more it will increase their chances of getting better. If they don't do the homework, they're unlikely to improve. It can be helpful to use an analogy of a skill requiring practice to learn that you think a patient will resonate with (e.g., learning a sport or learning to play an instrument).

Although most therapists want their patients to like them, being overly permissive or overly tolerant can foster dependency and impede progress. Therapists who let patients avoid homework or make less than a good effort reduce the patients' motivation to work hard and their chances of improving. If patients have difficulty following through on homework between sessions, investigate carefully to determine why the problem occurred and how it can be corrected. If this is a more significant or continuing problem, it may be helpful to use the motivational techniques described in Chapter 5.

Matching Treatment to Patients' Emotional States

You must encourage and even gently push patients toward working on their symptoms, while also recognizing times when patients are overwhelmed and cannot move forward. The best compromise is probably to push mildly, but, when this meets with resistance, to back off and empathically encourage patients to describe their feelings. Problem-solving methods may prove useful in helping overwhelmed patients break tasks down into smaller steps. You can be warm and caring while also expecting your patients to try their hardest and make progress.

Giving Praise for Even Small Gains

Be authentic in making positive statements. Remember that changing an apparently simple thought or behavior can be an enormous accomplishment for some patients. Use both verbal and nonverbal expressions of praise: A smile, a nod of encouragement, and expressions of pleasure or pride ("Nice job," "Good for you," "I'm impressed") can provide powerful reinforcement for patients to keep working on their problems.

Looking at the Big Picture When Assessing Progress

Especially with more severely ill patients, it's easy to become discouraged by what seems like lack of progress. In such cases, ask yourself whether your patients are *generally* moving in the right direction. Are they gradually engaging in rituals less, and going out and doing other things more? Try not to judge progress on a day-to-day basis; instead, look at the big picture.

Progress is not a straight line that moves steadily in the right direction. It is a wiggly line with ups and downs while a patient is moving toward improvement. (See Handout 8.2 in Chapter 8, which is used to illustrate improvement to patients during the initial sessions.) BDD symptoms typically wax and wane, and a period of improvement can be followed by some bad days. It can help to remind your patients (and yourself!) that occasional setbacks do not mean they have lost all their gains. However, if a setback persists or is severe, it's wise to consider whether a change in the treatment may be needed.

Helping Patients Become Their Own Therapists

Although you initially need to adopt the role of expert, gradually transfer decision making to patients as they gain understanding and experience with CBT-BDD techniques. In other words, ask patients to take an increasingly greater role in selecting techniques to challenge thinking and modify actions during homework assignments. The goal is to gradually prepare patients to be their own therapists after the treatment with you ends.

Maintaining Hope

Let your patients know that you cannot predict with certainty how much better they will get with treatment. This will depend in large part on the effort they make. However, most patients with BDD do get better with CBT-BDD.

Special Challenges in Treating BDD

Working with patients who have BDD can be challenging. Patients with milder symptoms and some insight into the fact that they have a psychiatric illness are easier to engage and keep in treatment. With many others, however, this is difficult. Some patients are so depressed that it's hard for them to get motivated to come to sessions or do assigned homework. Many have such poor insight into the inaccuracy of their appearance beliefs that they cannot understand how you or CBT-BDD could possibly help them. To use two examples from Chapter 2, how can CBT make Jane's nose smaller or give Adam more hair? After all, it isn't surgery or hair replacement. Some patients are dragged to treatment by family members who are desperate for help. Because you can't fix their perceived appearance flaws, such patients may be reluctant to see you. In addition, patients with BDD tend to be sensitive to rejection, so you must be careful to convey a sense of acceptance and concern without reinforcing their inaccurate beliefs about their appearance and its importance.

Taking BDD Symptoms Seriously

Approach BDD as you would any other serious mental illness. Don't confuse BDD with vanity. Resist any temptation to dismiss patients' concerns or to reassure them that they look fine. Avoid telling them that something else (such as low self-esteem or relationship fears) is their "real" problem. Responses like these usually make patients feel very misunderstood—even humiliated. Some patients may drop out of treatment because they think you don't understand and won't help them deal with their appearance concerns.

Dealing with Delusionality/Poor Insight

A major challenge in treating BDD is that before treatment, most patients have poor insight. About one-third currently have delusional beliefs about their appearance. It can be especially challenging to engage and to retain delusional patients in treatment. They may think that the solution to their problem is a physical change in how they look (e.g., with surgery) rather than therapy. They may feel that you misunderstand them, because you are not recommending cosmetic treatment or agreeing that they look bad.

Certain elements of the treatment may be harder for delusional patients. For example, it will probably be more difficult for them to identify cognitive errors and come up with more accurate alternative beliefs during cognitive restructuring. They may find exposures more anxiety-provoking than patients with some insight do, because they truly believe that they look horrendous and that other people mock or reject them for this reason. Similarly, the mirror exercises may provoke more anxiety, because they hate their appearance so much or even find it frightening to look at themselves.

We recommend being gentle and less challenging with these patients. If you push too hard, delusional patients may feel misunderstood or even drop out of CBT-BDD. You may have to move through certain parts of the treatment a little more slowly, because it may be harder for them to grasp and master the skills; also, you may risk frightening them by moving too fast or pushing too hard. On the other hand, you will probably need to encourage, cheerlead, and even push (gently!) as necessary to help your patients progress through the treatment. You'll need to find the best balance for each patient. It's important to check in with your patients from time to time about how the treatment is going for them. You will also want to listen carefully to their feedback at the end of each session, so you can modify your approach if necessary.

Not Trying to Talk Patients Out of Their BDD Beliefs

Especially early in treatment, some patients want your opinion on how they look. They may try to convince you that they are right (i.e., that they are really ugly) and that you are wrong. This is a potential trap that can wound patients and even end the treatment before it starts. The main thing is to avoid struggling with patients over what they actually look like. Try to avoid convincing them that you are right and they are wrong. Also try to avoid reassuring them that they look fine. They usually won't believe you anyway. Even if you say something positive about how they look, telling them that they look "fine" or even "attractive" can upset perfectionistic patients who want to look unusually good. Or, if you say that that certain body areas look good, they may interpret this to mean that other areas are really ugly.

A common mistake is to say something like this: "Well, your nose is a little big, but it isn't that bad," or "Your legs aren't really thin, but they aren't fat either." Comments such as these, while meant to reassure patients, usually backfire. Patients can be devastated by them and may become more convinced than ever that they look abnormal. We also recommend that you not make even casual comments to patients about their appearance or clothes—for example, "Oh, you got a new haircut!"—as many patients will interpret even neutral or positive comments in a negative way.

We suggest offering a simple response that to some extent sidesteps a potential disagreement or argument. First, tell patients that they have BDD, and explain what this means. Don't be dismissive of their distress and anxiety. You can validate their feelings, but don't reinforce their distorted beliefs. You can agree with patients who already recognize that their appearance views are distorted (i.e., patients who have good insight). You can also tell them that CBT-BDD aims to help them maintain healthy beliefs like this and to develop even more helpful ones.

However, relatively few patients have good insight about their appearance beliefs prior to treatment. For patients with poor insight or for those who are actively delusional, you could respond emphatically with something like this:

> "I wouldn't have diagnosed you with BDD if I thought there was something wrong with how you look. Your symptoms are very typical for someone with BDD. [Elaborate if necessary.] People with BDD view themselves differently than other people do: They think there's something wrong with how they look, when other people don't perceive this. If you try to convince other people that you look [deformed, flawed, . . . use a patient's own words], you probably can't convince them. Has this been your experience? . . . When other people try to convince you that there's nothing wrong with how you look, they probably can't convince you either. Has that been true for you? . . . For the time being, we probably just need to agree to disagree about what you look like. But in your treatment, this is one of the things we'll work on—finding ways for you to develop a healthier body image, suffer less, and enjoy your life more."

Focusing on Patients' Suffering, Poor Functioning, and Poor Quality of Life

Focus on the potential for CBT-BDD to diminish patients' suffering and improve their quality of life. Many patients can acknowledge that they spend too much time thinking about their appearance and that their concerns are making them suffer. Early in treatment, it's important to convey that the general goals of CBT-BDD are to help them do these things:

- Obsess less about their appearance.
- Reduce their discomfort when obsessive thoughts occur.
- Gain better control over their compulsive rituals and avoidance behavior.
- Feel less depressed and anxious because of their appearance concerns.
- Function better in their lives.
- Suffer less and enjoy their lives more.

Focusing on these components of the illness, rather than on how they actually look, may help motivate patients to engage in CBT-BDD and keep them engaged in the treatment.

Dealing with Depressive Symptoms

As discussed in Chapter 1, many patients with BDD experience depression, which can range from mild to severe. Severe depression can interfere with therapy by decreasing energy or motivation to come to sessions or do homework. Depressive cognitions involving hopeless or pessimism (e.g., "This treatment will *never* work!") can also interfere.

It's important to assess each patient's depressive symptoms carefully and determine the extent to which these seem due largely or entirely to BDD. If they are BDD-related, CBT-BDD is likely to be helpful for depressive symptoms as well as BDD symptoms. It is also possible that some of the skills patients learn will generalize to depressive symptoms that are less strongly associated with BDD. If depressive symptoms interfere with your ability to conduct CBT-BDD, we recommend that you use the module for managing depression (Chapter 18) when you realize this. You can also focus on depressive cognitions when you are doing cognitive restructuring or working on core beliefs.

Monitoring Suicidal Ideation and Behavior

One of the biggest challenges in treating patients with BDD is that many are suicidal. You must carefully monitor suicidal thinking and plans, especially if your clinical interview or pretreatment measures (see Chapter 4) indicate that a patient is very depressed or has suicidal thinking. If suicidal thinking is passive and the patient has no plan and no intent, simply reassessing his or her status from time to time may be all that is necessary. If a patient talks about the possibility of attempting suicide, ask about a plan, how serious the intent is, whether these thoughts are likely to interfere with treatment progress, or whether suicidal thinking is likely to improve as BDD improves. For patients whose suicidal thinking is primarily due to BDD, this thinking may very well decrease with CBT-BDD.

Patients with more worrisome suicidal thinking require more intensive monitoring. Such a patient must agree formally not to act on these thoughts during therapy. Make it clear that you will ask about the patient's level of depression and suicidal thoughts at every session. You and the patient will need to agree that if the patient becomes actively suicidal or develops a plan, he or she will inform you immediately. For such a patient, review instructions of your workplace for managing suicidal thoughts and discuss resources in case of difficulty, including contact information for you and for providers of acute psychiatric care.

Most therapists are unwilling to work under conditions in which they feel uncertain about a patient's safety. If the patient remains at high risk, a change in treatment may be indicated. Consider referring the patient for medication, outpatient therapy that directly targets the suicidal thinking (especially in cases where the suicidality is not BDD-related), or inpatient hospitalization.

Common Problems and How to Avoid Them

You will inevitably encounter problems that interfere with patients' ability to apply treatment methods. In this section, we discuss some of these behaviors and provide recommendations for addressing them.

Missing or Canceling Sessions or Arriving Late

Missed/canceled sessions or late arrivals may be indicators of various problems. Patients may be unconvinced that treatment will help, fearful of therapy, or overwhelmed by other life responsibilities that they aren't managing effectively. The first of these may indicate ambivalence that requires exploration through motivational strategies (see Chapter 5). You can also probe to determine whether patients feel they have something to lose by getting better, or whether the time is right for them to work on their therapy goals. If other circumstances are too pressing and it is not feasible for them to put in the effort that CBT-BDD requires, this problem should be discussed. In some such cases, it may be better to postpone the therapy. Irregular sessions will be frustrating for both you and patients, because they may not produce steady progress. In addition, a problem-solving strategy may be useful. Encourage patients who are uncomfortable with the therapy or with you or your approach to discuss their concerns directly, to see whether they can be addressed.

Not Doing Homework

It is important for patients to understand that completing homework is central to making progress on the problem. Emphasize the importance of working between sessions, and address this therapy-interfering behavior before moving on. You can begin by showing empathy with a patient's emotional reluctance:

> "I understand that you feel . . . "
> "I know homework may be unpleasant."

Then proceed with a statement like this:

> "I'm afraid we have to resolve this before we can make any progress. What interfered with your getting this done?"

The following line of questioning focuses attention on the problem and aims to resolve it:

> "Do you think this will be a regular problem?"
> "What do you think you could do about this?"
> "Let's brainstorm a bit. Can you think of any way you might have found time to do the homework?"
> "Did we set too hard a goal?"
> "How will we know next time that you'll be able to accomplish the assignment?"

It may help patients to put the homework in a calendar or appointment book if writing down the homework on the *Personal Session Form* (Form 2.1) isn't a sufficient reminder. You can have them fill in a calendar during the session, or create a schedule together during the session if they don't have one. If lack of homework completion becomes a more persistent problem, consider using the motivational approaches in Chapter 5 to enhance motivation to do the homework. You can use cognitive restructuring if patients have thoughts such as "Why do the homework? I'll never get better."

As we've recommended for other patient problems (Wilhelm & Steketee, 2006), a metaphor may help acknowledge the emotional strain of letting go of usual coping methods. Here is an example:

> "Therapy can be like using a life preserver when you're afraid of drowning. You have to let go of the sinking boat to try a better option, but the only way to know whether the life preserver works is by trying it."

For patients who are doing very little homework and aren't responding to the suggestions above, you could try more creative approaches. For example, you could try an experiment of not doing the homework for a week and then doing it for a week, and seeing which works better. Or you could have a patient leave a message for you each day, briefly telling you how the homework went (if you feel this is clinically appropriate for that patient). You could also try a role play in which you portray the patient and the patient plays you, to see how the patient would handle your not wanting to do the homework. If you think part of the problem is with the word "homework" (which some patients may react negatively to), you could use other terms instead, such as "skills practice," "skills training," or "home exercises."

Being Ambivalent about Treatment

As we have often noted, patients with BDD may be ambivalent about treatment. Poor insight, the belief that they need cosmetic treatment rather than therapy, and depressive symptoms can all contribute to this problem. If motivational problems are interfering with treatment, it is crucial to address them. When these problems occur, we recommend using the motivational techniques in Chapter 5, which can be used at any point during the treatment as needed.

Some patients are reluctant—or even refuse—to do certain parts of the treatment, often because the tasks seem scary. As noted earlier, exposure exercises can be anxiety-provoking, especially for delusional patients who are convinced that they look deformed and that other people mock them because of how they look. If a patient is reluctant or refuses to do an element of the treatment, we recommend using a combination of techniques to address this. First, listen and try to understand the patient's reluctance and fears. Some psychoeducation can help. We suggest explaining that you will carefully prepare the patient for the exposure; and that you and the patient will plan the exposures carefully together, to be reasonably certain that he or she can tolerate the anxiety and do the exposure successfully. If it does not go well, you'll both use what you have learned from the experience to plan the next one better. Motivational techniques may also be helpful for avoidance of specific therapy tasks. We provide more specific advice about helping patients prepare for exposure exercises in Chapter 10.

Not Staying Focused on BDD

Patients can have problems staying focused on BDD for any number of reasons. For example, they may have attention deficit problems or outright ADHD. Attention problems may require you to obtain permission from patients to interrupt and redirect them when the problem occurs. Patients who have had unstructured therapy in the past (e.g., supportive therapy) may find it difficult to make the transition to CBT-BDD, which is a much more structured and faster-paced treatment. In such cases, you can remind the patients that CBT-BDD is different and that if it is too unstructured, the patients are less likely to learn and benefit from the skills.

Making Requests for Reassurance

One therapist who treated a patient with severe BDD told us that for several years his three-times-a-week sessions consisted largely of the patient's asking him repeatedly whether her nose looked OK and his telling her that it looked fine. Clearly, the treatment wasn't very helpful! The therapist was frustrated and tried every way he could think of to get out of this trap, to no avail.

Do *not* respond to requests for reassurance with reassurance. If a patient repeatedly asks you whether he or she looks OK, consider the following refusal:

> "I know you feel a very strong urge to ask, but I don't think it will be helpful answer this question. When people tell you that there's nothing wrong with how you look, how do you feel? . . . And how long does that last? . . . So it sounds as though it doesn't really help, at least not for very long. [See whether the patient agrees.] The other problem is that by answering you, I'll just be feeding your BDD by keeping you focused on how you look. [If you've already developed a model of the patient's BDD, refer to it here, noting that reassurance seeking is a ritual that feeds BDD symptoms.] So it seems we both agree that it's best for me not to reassure you. Let's try to develop some ways to get better control over this behavior, since it really doesn't make you feel much better and takes up lots of your time."

The response above is most appropriate early in treatment. For patients who have already learned cognitive restructuring, ask why they are seeking reassurance, and help them identify cognitive errors associated with this urge. For those who have learned response prevention, you can target this behavior as homework or during your sessions.

Arguing

Occasionally patients will directly challenge your statements or homework assignments. Arguing is definitely not helpful, as it only solidifies this adversarial stance. Instead, try to understand and discuss patients' concerns, and then engage in collaborative problem solving. As discussed above, it's especially important to avoid arguing with patients about how they "really" look.

Getting Discouraged Despite Progress

Patients who discount or minimize evident progress may be doing so because they're depressed or are holding themselves hostage to perfectionistic standards or core beliefs about being "a failure." Advanced cognitive strategies (Chapter 13) are most likely to be useful for these problems. You can also show such patients changes in their scores on measures of BDD symptoms and discuss these (if the scores have indeed improved).

Some of the strategies discussed earlier in this chapter, such as looking at the big picture, may also be helpful: Overall, if not day to day, are the patients gradually improving? If patients' expectations of treatment are too high, you can discuss the value of partial change. It can also be helpful to remind patients that progress in CBT-BDD can take some time and lots of practice, as there are many skills to learn. Most patients who stick with the treatment, complete it, and practice their skills do improve.

CHAPTER 4

DIAGNOSING AND ASSESSING BDD AND ASSOCIATED SYMPTOMS

This chapter provides tools for diagnosing and assessing BDD and associated symptoms (e.g., depressive symptoms). A standard intake evaluation (e.g., family history, medical history, previous treatments) is not included here. Once you have determined that CBT-BDD is appropriate for your patient, we recommend the measures described in this chapter for the following uses:

- To evaluate BDD symptoms (diagnosis, clinical features, severity) in detail before you start treatment.
- To evaluate the patient's progress in treatment (severity of BDD clinical features).
- To enhance your understanding of important aspects of your patient's symptoms before you begin core interventions.
- To help you select specialized modules for selected problems.

Before discussing these measures, however, we first discuss a few basic guidelines for diagnosing and assessing BDD.

BASIC DIAGNOSTIC/ASSESSMENT GUIDELINES

Diagnostic Criteria for BDD

The DSM-IV-TR (American Psychiatric Association, 2000) criteria for BDD specify that the person must be preoccupied with a perceived defect in his or her physical appearance; if a small anomaly is present, the person's concern must be notably excessive. The preoccupation must cause considerable distress or interfere in social, occupational, or other important areas of functioning. In addition, it must not be accounted for by another mental disorder, such as anorexia nervosa. Although DSM-5 is currently in preparation, the DSM-5 criteria for BDD are likely to be similar to the current ones. Once you suspect that BDD is present, the diagnosis is relatively straightforward (see Form 4.1 *BDD Questions*). When you find that a patient has BDD, it is important to ask about the symptoms as you would any other disorder, resisting any urge to reassure the patient that he or she looks fine or imply that BDD isn't the "real" problem. Instead, verify that the diagnostic criteria are fulfilled, and ask about the patient's symptoms and experience with the illness.

Detection of "Secret" BDD

A big challenge is to recognize that a patient has BDD. Many people with BDD are remarkably secretive about their symptoms. Most are too embarrassed and ashamed of their concerns to reveal them to a clinician or even a family member or friend. In fact, a number of studies have found that BDD often goes undetected in clinical settings (Grant, Kim, & Eckert, 2002; Phillips, Nierenberg, Brendel, & Fava, 1996). Thus clinicians usually need to screen patients for this disorder and to be alert to clues for it in the clinical presentation. Despite patients' reluctance to describe their symptoms of their own volition, studies have found that people with BDD want their clinicians to ask about the symptoms so they can discuss them (Grant et al., 2002).

Astute clinicians may suspect that BDD is present from patients' appearance or behaviors. For example, they may notice skin lesions or scarring caused by skin picking, or may observe that a patient always wears a baseball cap. Indeed, appearance-related compulsive behaviors and camouflaging are clues to possible BDD. Whereas most patients with BDD look normal, some wear noticeable camouflage, such as hats, bulky clothing or multiple layers of clothing even in hot weather, heavy makeup, heavy-rimmed glasses, or wigs. Some patients have unusual hairstyles or hair that covers their faces; others are always very tanned (in an attempt to minimize perceived blemishes or to darken "pale" skin).

Additional clues include the following:

- Ideas or delusions of reference, which some patients describe as "paranoia" (because they think that people are looking at them, talking about them, or laughing at them because they are ugly).
- Panic attacks due to BDD (e.g., when looking in the mirror or thinking people are laughing at them because of how they look).
- Depression, social anxiety or other forms of anxiety, substance abuse, and suicidal ideation.
- Being housebound.

Differential Diagnosis

BDD or an Eating Disorder?

According to DSM-IV-TR, BDD should not be diagnosed if the symptoms are better accounted for by another disorder, such as an eating disorder. For example, if a woman's only body image concern is that she is too fat, and she meets full diagnostic criteria for anorexia nervosa, BDD would not be diagnosed. However, many patients meet criteria for both BDD *and* an eating disorder, in which case both disorders should be diagnosed. In such cases, patients have both weight/fat-related appearance concerns and non-weight/fat-related concerns. To determine whether a patient with an eating disorder also has BDD, you can use *BDD Questions* (Form 4.1) while "excluding" weight concerns from your questions.

BDD or OCD?

In our experience, BDD is often misdiagnosed as OCD, because BDD consists of obsessional preoccupations and compulsive behaviors. However, if the obsessions focus on appearance, BDD is the more accurate diagnosis. It's important not to misdiagnose BDD as OCD, because these disorders differ in some important ways that have implications for treatment. First, BDD involves body image disturbance, and thus many symptoms differ from those of OCD (e.g., patients with BDD may use anabolic steroids to increase muscularity and are likely to seek cosmetic treatment). Patients with BDD also have poorer insight; in other words, they are more likely to believe that their beliefs (e.g., that they're ugly) are really true. These patients also appear more likely than those with OCD to have suicidal thinking, depression, and substance abuse or dependence. In addition, in our clinical experience, patients with BDD are more likely to have underlying core beliefs involving feeling unlovable, worthless, inadequate, and ashamed. Some patients have both BDD and OCD, and in treatment we tend to focus first on whichever is the more severe and distressing problem.

BDD or Depression?

In our clinical experience, people with BDD are often diagnosed as having depression rather than BDD. BDD symptoms may be missed or mistakenly attributed to depression. Although depressive symptoms and comorbid major depressive disorder are common in patients with BDD, BDD should be diagnosed when the diagnostic criteria for it are met.

BDD or Social Phobia?

Patients with BDD tend to be introverted and to have high levels of social anxiety, distress, fear, avoidance, and physiological arousal in social situations. In addition, both disorders involve feelings of inadequacy, shame, preoccupation with how other people see them, and fear of being negatively evaluated, embarrassed, humiliated, and rejected. However, unlike social phobia, BDD preoccupations focus specifically on perceived physical flaws, and nearly all patients with BDD have compulsive behaviors. BDD and social phobia are frequently comorbid.

BDD or Schizophrenia?

Because some people with BDD (about one-third currently and one-half at some point in their lives) have delusional beliefs and referential thinking, they can be misdiagnosed as having schizophrenia. But BDD and schizophrenia have many important differences. Most notably, people with BDD typically do not have other positive or negative symptoms of schizophrenia.

Assessment of Comorbid Conditions

BDD commonly coexists with major depressive disorder, substance use disorders, social phobia, OCD, and eating disorders. It is therefore important to screen for comorbid conditions by using a clinical interview or structured interview measure such as the *Structured Clinical Interview for DSM-IV* (SCID; First, Gibbon, Spitzer, Williams, & Benjamin, 1997; First, Spitzer, Gibbon, & Williams, 1996). It can be helpful to ask patients to what extent they believe these associated problems are accounted for by their appearance concerns. If they appear secondary to

BDD, treatment focused on BDD may alleviate them. However, if a comorbid disorder appears very problematic, or more problematic than the BDD, it may be more appropriate to treat that disorder before the BDD or concurrently with the BDD. For example, if substance abuse is problematic, it is probably wise to encourage patients to obtain additional treatment focused on the substance use itself.

MEASURES OF BDD AND DEPRESSIVE SYMPTOMS

The following measures of BDD and depressive symptoms (summarized in Table 4.1) should be used before treatment starts. Some of these measures will also be helpful later during treatment.

TABLE 4.1. Measures for BDD and Associated Symptoms

Measure	Measure description	Clinician versus self-report	When to use
Diagnostic Questions	Diagnoses BDD	Clinician	• During the initial intake evaluation, if BDD is suspected Or • During Session 1 of CBT-BDD
Body Checklist	Assesses body parts of concern	Self-report	• During Session 1 of CBT-BDD
BDD-SS	Assesses severity of symptoms; organizes symptoms into conceptually similar clusters that map onto CBT-BDD modules and other treatment targets	Self-report	• During Session 1 of CBT-BDD • Monthly, when doing all core interventions • Monthly, when working on core beliefs • At least monthly, when selecting these specialized modules: skin picking/hair pulling, weight/shape/muscularity, cosmetic treatment
BDD Information-Gathering Form	Obtains information on key clinical features of BDD	Clinician	• During Session 1 of CBT-BDD
BDD-YBOCS	Assesses BDD severity during the past week	Clinician	• During Session 1 of CBT-BDD • Monthly, and before starting Relapse prevention
BDI-II, IDS, or QIDS	Assesses depression and suicidality, and may assist you in the selection of the depression management module	Self-report	• Weekly

BDD Questions

The questions provided in *BDD Questions* (Form 4.1) follow the DSM-IV-TR criteria for BDD as described above. These questions are similar to those included in other measures, such as the SCID (First et al., 1996, 1997). It's important to ask for examples of interference in social, academic, occupational, or role functioning, to determine whether any such interference is clinically significant.

Helpful Hints

When you are attempting to diagnose BDD, it is important *not* to ask patients whether they have an imagined defect in their appearance; many of those with the disorder have poor insight or no insight and do not realize that their view of their appearance is distorted. We also recommend not starting out by using words that some patients might perceive as "too strong" to describe their concern—for example, "deformed" or "hideous." Whereas some patients will endorse these terms, or even stronger terms (such as "monstrous"), others will use milder words such as "unattractive" or "not right." It's best to ask patients what words they themselves would use to describe how they look. It's also important to ask specifically about physical appearance, not just bodily functioning more generally.

BDD Clinical Features and History

The following measures should be used before treatment begins. In addition, portions of them will be useful later during treatment.

Body Checklist

The *Body Checklist* (Form 4.2) is a self-report form that identifies the body parts with which the patient is preoccupied.

BDD Symptom Scale

The *BDD Symptom Scale* (BDD-SS) (Form 4.3; Wilhelm, 2006) is a self-report measure that identifies and rates the severity of specific BDD symptoms. The scale organizes symptoms into conceptually similar clusters of problem behaviors that map on to the treatment modules and other treatment targets.

BDD Information-Gathering Form

The *BDD Information-Gathering Form* (Form 4.4) enables therapists to gather details about BDD to guide the treatment, including the following:

- *Body areas of concern.* Follows up on information the patient provided in the *Body Checklist* (Form 4.2) and determines whether body areas identified on the *Body Checklist* reflect excessive and problematic (as opposed to normal) appearance concerns.
- *Course of BDD symptoms.* Obtains information on the patient's history of appearance concerns.

- *Interference in functioning due to BDD.* Obtains information on recent and past functioning.
- *Treatment history.* Asks whether the patient has obtained, or is planning to obtain, treatment from a surgeon, dermatologist, dentist, other health professional, or paraprofessional (e.g., electrolysis) for the perceived defect.

BDD Severity

The *Yale–Brown Obsessive Compulsive Scale Modified for BDD* (BDD-YBOCS; Phillips, Hollander, Rasmussen, & Aronowitz, 1997) is a semistructured, clinician-administered scale that assesses average BDD severity in the past week. Items 1–5 rate thoughts, and items 6–10 rate compulsive behaviors (Phillips et al., 1997). Item 11 rates insight (delusionality), and item 12 rates avoidance of activities and situations. The interviewer should ask the questions provided, but can ask further questions to obtain additional information or clarify responses. Two methods of scoring can be used to identify clinically significant BDD symptoms:

1. Score on all 12 items ≥ 20 → current BDD.

or:

2. Score on first 3 items ≥ 5 → current BDD (the first 3 items mirror the DSM-IV-TR diagnostic criteria for BDD).

Depressive Symptoms

The *Beck Depression Inventory–II* (BDI-II; Beck, Steer, & Brown, 1996), *Inventory of Depressive Symptomatology* (IDS; Rush et al., 1986; Rush, Gullion, Basco, Jarrett, & Trivedi, 1996), and *Quick Inventory of Depressive Symptomatology* (QIDS; Rush et al., 2003) are all widely used measures of depression severity. We usually use the BDI-II, which must be purchased from Pearson Assessments. The IDS and QIDS are available online, and you can download, copy, and use them, with proper citation. No matter which depression measure you choose, it should be given weekly to assess the effects of CBT-BDD on depressed mood and to monitor suicidal ideation. Furthermore, you can use it to inform selection of the treatment module for managing depression (Chapter 18). In later text we refer to the BDI-II, but feel free to substitute the IDS or the QIDS for this.

The SCID (First et al., 1996, 1997) determines whether the patient meets DSM-IV criteria for past or current major depressive disorder. It can also be used to diagnose other disorders.

Measures for Treatment Planning

The measures discussed above provide information that will guide treatment from the outset. Some measures will also help later to assist with core interventions or to help select specialized treatment modules for your patient (see Table 4.1). We recommend that you use all of these measures. Some of them may be needed more frequently than shown in Table 4.1 for a particular patient. Or a patient may have additional problems that require assessment and monitoring. For example, a patient with comorbid depression (and even suicidal ideation) will require initial assessment and ongoing monitoring as clinically indicated. Therefore, we typically ask our patients to come 10 minutes before each session begins, to allow time to fill out a depression questionnaire.

FORM 4.1
BDD Questions

Name: ______________________ Date: ______________

1. Ask the patient, "Are you very worried about your appearance in any way?" Or "Are you unhappy with how you look?"

2. Invite the patient to describe his or her concern by asking, "What don't you like about how you look?" Or "Can you tell me about your concern?"

3. Ask whether there are other disliked body areas—for example, "Are you unhappy with any other aspects of your appearance, such as your face, skin, hair, nose, or the shape or size of any other body area?"

(cont.)

Adapted with permission of the publisher from Phillips, K. A. (1996; Revised and Expanded Edition, 2005). *The Broken Mirror: Understanding and Treating Body Dysmorphic Disorder.* New York: Oxford University Press.

4. Ascertain that the patient is preoccupied with these perceived flaws by asking, "How much time would you estimate that you spend each day thinking about your appearance, if you add up all the time you spend?" Or "Do these concerns preoccupy you?"

5. Ask, "How much distress do these concerns cause you?" Ask specifically about resulting anxiety, social anxiety, depression, feelings of panic, and suicidal thinking.

6. Ask about effects of the appearance preoccupations on the patient's life—for example, "Do these concerns interfere with your life or cause problems for you in any way?" Ask specifically about effects on work, school, other aspects of role functioning (e.g., caring for children), relationships, intimacy, family and social activities, household tasks, and other types of interference.

FORM 4.2

Body Checklist

Name: ______________________________ Date: ______________

Put a check next to each body part you are especially concerned about currently, or have been concerned about in the past.

Body part	Current	Past	Comment
Face			
Skin			
Ears			
Eyes			
Eyebrows			
Hair			
Forehead			
Nose			
Cheeks			
Lips			
Mouth			
Teeth			
Jaw			
Chin			
Head size or shape			
Neck			
Shoulders			
Arm/wrist			

Adapted with permission of the publisher from Wilhelm, S. (2006). *Feeling Good about the Way You Look: A Program for Overcoming Body Image Problems*. New York: Guilford Press.

(cont.)

Body Checklist *(page 2 of 2)*

Body part	**Current**	**Past**	**Comment**
Hands			
Fingers			
Back			
Breasts/pectorals			
Waist			
Stomach			
Buttocks			
Hips			
Penis			
Testicles			
Female genitals			
Legs			
Thighs			
Knees			
Calves			
Ankles			
Feet			
Toes			
Body build			
Weight			
Height			
Other (*specify*):			

FORM 4.3

BDD Symptom Scale (BDD-SS)

Name: ____________________________ Date: ______________

Each box below contains several behaviors or thoughts you may have experienced recently. For each symptom in each box, please check whether you have had it in the *past week*. Then rate the combined severity of all symptoms in one box on the scale on the right of each box. Severity refers to the average amounts of frequency and distress that have occurred during the *past week*.

EXAMPLE:

Yes	No	Symptom	If you checked "Yes" for any symptoms in the box on the left, please mark the overall severity of these symptoms during the past week on the following scale:
☐	☑	Visiting plastic surgeons, dermatologists, or dentists to improve appearance.	0 1 2 3 4 5 6 (7) 8 9 10
☐	☑	Obtaining cosmetic surgery.	0 = No problem; 5 = Moderately severe (frequency and distress); 10 = Very severe (frequency and distress)
☑	☐	Using medications or topical treatments to correct defects (e.g., skin, baldness).	
☑	☐	Applying self-surgery.	

Please look at the example above. This person indicated using medications or topical treatments to correct defects and applying self-surgery by checking "Yes" for those symptoms. Then the combined severity of the two symptoms was rated as "Very severe" (referring to frequency and distress) by marking 10 on the rating scale.

Yes	No	Symptom	If you checked "Yes" for any symptoms in the box on the left, please mark the overall severity of these symptoms during the past week on the following scale:
☐	☐	Checking or inspecting certain parts of my body.	0 1 2 3 4 5 6 7 8 9 10
☐	☐	Measuring or counting body part.	0 = No problem; 5 = Moderately severe (frequency and distress); 10 = Very severe (frequency and distress)
☐	☐	Touching or feeling body part.	
☐	☐	Asking questions about my appearance over and over again, even though I understood the answer the first time.	
☐	☐	Mentally reviewing past events, conversations, and actions to find out how people reacted to my appearance.	

Adapted with permission of the publisher from Wilhelm, S. (2006). *Feeling Good about the Way You Look: A Program for Overcoming Body Image Problems*. New York: Guilford Press.

(cont.)

Yes	No		
☐	☐	Checking mirrors repeatedly.	
☐	☐	Comparing my appearance to others' appearance (in person, in pictures, or in the media).	
☐	☐	Scrutinizing others.	

Yes	No		If you checked "Yes" for any symptoms in the box on the left, please mark the overall severity of these symptoms during the past week on the following scale:
☐	☐	Grooming myself longer than necessary.	0 1 2 3 4 5 6 7 8 9 10
☐	☐	Spending a lot of money to improve my appearance.	0 = No problem; 5 = Moderately severe (frequency and distress); 10 = Very severe (frequency and distress)
☐	☐	Tanning.	
☐	☐	Combing hair.	
☐	☐	Applying makeup.	
☐	☐	Shaving.	
☐	☐	Dieting.	
☐	☐	Changing clothes.	

Yes	No		If you checked "Yes" for any symptoms in the box on the left, please mark the overall severity of these symptoms during the past week on the following scale:
☐	☐	Lifting weights.	0 1 2 3 4 5 6 7 8 9 10
☐	☐	Using steroids.	0 = No problem; 5 = Moderately severe (frequency and distress); 10 = Very severe (frequency and distress)
☐	☐	Exercising excessively.	
☐	☐	Eating in special ways.	

Yes	No		If you checked "Yes" for any symptoms in the box on the left, please mark the overall severity of these symptoms during the past week on the following scale:
☐	☐	Picking skin.	0 1 2 3 4 5 6 7 8 9 10
☐	☐	Pulling or plucking hair.	0 = No problem; 5 = Moderately severe (frequency and distress); 10 = Very severe (frequency and distress)

(cont.)

BDD Symptom Scale (BDD-SS) *(page 3 of 4)*

<table>
<tr><td>

Yes No
☐ ☐ Avoiding mirrors or reflective surfaces.
☐ ☐ Avoiding social situations where family, friends, acquaintances, coworkers are present (work, parties, family gatherings, meetings, talking in small groups, having a conversation, dating, speaking to boss or supervisor).
☐ ☐ Avoiding public areas (shopping, stores, busy streets, restaurants, movies, buses, trains, parks, waiting in lines, public restrooms).
☐ ☐ Avoiding intimate or close physical contact with others (sexual activity, hugging, kissing, dancing, talking closely).
☐ ☐ Avoiding physical activities like exercise or recreation because of concern about appearance.
☐ ☐ Avoiding being seen nude or with few clothes on.
☐ ☐ Hiding appearance (with makeup, clothing, hairstyle, jewelry, hats, hands, or body position).
☐ ☐ Changing appearance (e.g., getting a haircut).
☐ ☐ Discounting compliments.
☐ ☐ Becoming upset by compliments.

</td><td>

If you checked "Yes" for any symptoms in the box on the left, please mark the overall severity of these symptoms during the past week on the following scale:
0 1 2 3 4 5 6 7 8 9 10
No problem — Moderately severe (frequency and distress) — Very severe (frequency and distress)

</td></tr>
</table>

<table>
<tr><td>

Yes No
☐ ☐ Visiting plastic surgeons, dermatologists, or dentists to improve appearance.
☐ ☐ Obtaining cosmetic surgery.
☐ ☐ Using medications or topical treatments to correct defects (e.g., skin, baldness).
☐ ☐ Applying self-surgery.

</td><td>

If you checked "Yes" for any symptoms in the box on the left, please mark the overall severity of these symptoms during the past week on the following scale:
0 1 2 3 4 5 6 7 8 9 10
No problem — Moderately severe (frequency and distress) — Very severe (frequency and distress)

</td></tr>
</table>

(cont.)

BDD Symptom Scale (BDD-SS) *(page 4 of 4)*

Yes	No	
☐	☐	I believe others are thinking of my appearance.
☐	☐	The first thing people notice about me is what's wrong with my appearance.
☐	☐	I think that others are staring at or talking about me.
☐	☐	I believe others treat me differently because of my physical defects.
☐	☐	If my appearance is defective, I am worthless.
☐	☐	If my appearance is defective, I will end up alone and isolated.
☐	☐	If my appearance is defective, I am helpless.
☐	☐	No one can like me as long as I look the way I do.
☐	☐	If my appearance is defective, I am unlovable.
☐	☐	I must look perfect.
☐	☐	I look defective or abnormal.
☐	☐	I am an unattractive person.
☐	☐	What I look like is an important part of who I am.
☐	☐	Outward appearance is a sign of the inner person.
☐	☐	No one else my age looks as bad as I do.
☐	☐	If I could look just the way I wish, I would be much happier.
☐	☐	People would like me less if they knew what I really looked like.
☐	☐	My appearance is more important than my personality, intelligence, values, skills, how I relate to others, and my performance at work or in other settings.
☐	☐	If I learn to accept myself, I'll lose my motivation to look better.

If you checked "Yes" for any symptoms in the box on the left, please mark the overall severity of these symptoms during the past week on the following scale:

0	1	2	3	4	5	6	7	8	9	10
No problem					Moderately severe (frequency and distress)					Very severe (frequency and distress)

FORM 4.4

BDD Information-Gathering Form

Name: ______________________________________ Date: ____________________

Current BDD Symptoms

Body areas of concern:

Avoidance of places, people, or activities (review BDD-SS and discuss):

Problematic BDD behaviors/rituals (review BDD-SS and discuss):

BDD-relevant beliefs about self and others, including feared consequences of BDD concerns (e.g., rejection by others, job failure):

Adapted with permission of the publisher from Wilhelm, S. (2006). *Feeling Good about the Way You Look: A Program for Overcoming Body Image Problems*. New York: Guilford Press.

(cont.)

Estimated probability of feared BDD consequences (0–100%; if >5%, verify and check perception of others' agreement):

Course of BDD

Age and circumstances of BDD onset (e.g., trauma, accidents, problems with appearance [such as acne], teasing, parental preferences, parental and cultural values); course of BDD symptoms:

Patient's causal explanation for BDD symptoms and onset:

Impairment

Interference in functioning (home, family, social, employment, leisure) due to BDD symptoms:

(cont.)

BDD-Related Treatments

Cosmetic treatment from surgeon, dermatologist, dentist, other health professional:

Medications (type, dosage, effects, side effects—past and current):

Psychotherapy (type, effects—past and current):

Self-treatment (including self-surgery):

Any planned interventions (cosmetic, psychiatric, etc.):

(cont.)

Comorbid Conditions

Other Relevant Aspects of the History

Medical history:

Family history:

Social history:

Current Context

Daily activities and how they are affected by BDD concerns (e.g., family, friends, social life):

CHAPTER 5

ENHANCING MOTIVATION

As discussed throughout Part I to this point, BDD can be a very challenging disorder to treat because of patients' limited insight and consequent low motivation to engage in psychotherapy. This chapter offers practical strategies for engaging these reluctant and ambivalent patients by using the motivational interviewing (MI) methods developed and described by Miller and Rollnick (2002, 2013). We recommend applying these techniques during the first two sessions to increase motivation for trying the treatment, and using them later in treatment whenever patients express ambivalence about resolving their problem or fail to participate fully in treatment.

The amount of time spent in using these methods will depend on the degree of patients' ambivalence. Some patients enter treatment under pressure from a family member; they are convinced that their concerns are real and that what they need is surgery, dermatological treatment, or other cosmetic treatment, not psychotherapy. In such a case, you can begin with MI and continue until the patient expresses clear statements indicating interest in change ("change talk"). Examples of change talk include "I'd probably be happier if I didn't worry so much about my nose," or "I'd like to be more like my friend Susan—she puts on makeup and stuff, but it's real quick, and mirrors just don't bother her." Such statements may express a desire to feel less upset or have fewer symptoms more clearly than a desire to resolve the BDD symptoms with CBT. Nevertheless, at this point you can move forward cautiously with CBT-BDD, returning to MI methods whenever ambivalence recurs.

Especially when the going gets harder—that is, when patients begin to confront their fears (see Chapter 10) and stop their rituals (see Chapter 11)—they may express more uncertainty about the need to change their behavior. This often appears as a statement of conviction about the existence of a physical defect and/or the need for physical treatment of the problem, as in this assertion: "What I really need is treatment for my thinning hair. I'm thinking about going to a dermatologist." In such a case, you can begin by simply affirming what has prompted the patient's statement. ("You've been thinking more about your hair. It's bothering you a lot.") and then revert immediately to MI until your patient confirms his or her interest in moving forward with therapy.

Thus, even in the middle of a session and during any part of treatment, you may need to switch to MI techniques when a patient's reluctance threatens to interfere with progress. You may also need to use these methods if the patient starts missing sessions, doesn't do assigned homework, or is thinking about dropping out of treatment. We strongly recommend taking the necessary time to do MI, especially if a patient seems likely to drop out of treatment. Although it's understandable to want to start the treatment right away—or to move on to the next skill if treatment has already begun—it's better to take the time to do MI so that you have a patient to treat!

This chapter first discusses how to recognize ambivalence and resistance, continues by describing the basic assumptions and principles of MI, and then provides specific MI strategies. We recommend that you read Miller and Rollnick's (2002, 2013) books to learn MI most effectively. Using MI requires a different approach to interactions with a patient and can be hard to apply if it is new to you. In using standard CBT-BDD as described in this manual, you will become accustomed to directing a patient about what to do (in collaboration with the patient). In contrast, MI methods require you to avoid directing your patient, but instead to be empathic, reflective, questioning, and affirming at critical points. We recommend paying close attention to the style as well as the methods described below until you become comfortable shifting gears into MI whenever your patient displays ambivalence about treatment.

Recognizing Ambivalence and Resistance

Some patients with BDD are so unmotivated for treatment that they simply refuse to engage in therapy, despite considerable pressure from family or friends. Others soon drop out. Beyond these obvious manifestations, motivation problems among those who do attend therapy may be reflected in many ways. During sessions, patients may directly express ambivalence by stating their uncertainty about their need or wish for treatment. As noted above, many believe that their actual appearance is the problem, not their thinking or behavior. Some are angry and frustrated with family members who have insisted they get CBT-BDD.

Here are examples of different forms of ambivalence and resistance:

- Arguing: "You know, I'm not just making this up. My nose is just awful! Nobody should have to live with this nose."
- Challenging the accuracy of therapist statements: "That doesn't make sense to me. Why would I want to leave the house without makeup?"
- Questioning or discounting the therapist's expertise: "How many patients like me have you treated?"
- Interrupting, talking over, or cutting off the therapist.
- Sidetracking the conversation to other topics.
- Not responding to questions or comments.
- Appearing bored.
- Denying the negative effects of the symptoms: "Yeah, but it doesn't take long to check the mirror."
- Blaming others (e.g., people who may have teased a patient in the past): "This really all comes down to my sister. If she hadn't made fun of me in front of her friends . . . "
- Making excuses or minimizing the problem: "It's not so bad to pluck my eyebrows, really. It doesn't take long to do it."
- Expressing reluctance to change: "It's not really worth all that effort. I just need to see my skin doctor."
- Conveying a sense of helplessness: "It's just so awful. I'll never get over this."

In addition to these behaviors in sessions, patients may avoid fully engaging in treatment (while giving lip service to working on the problem) in various ways:

- Arriving late.
- Missing sessions.
- Not completing agreed-upon homework assignments.
- Misremembering the homework plan.

Statements and behaviors such as these should be considered signals to institute MI strategies aimed at identifying the ambivalence or resistance and strengthening patients' commitment to change and confidence about making changes.

ASSUMPTIONS OF MI

Rollnick and Miller (1991) described MI as "a directive, patient-centered counseling style for eliciting behavior change by helping patients explore and resolve ambivalence" (p. 325). The spirit of MI is considered as important as the techniques for accomplishing motivation to change. MI is based on a client-centered model, in which the therapist collaborates with the patient to take advantage of the patient's own resources, capacity for self-direction, and informed choices to meet his or her personal goals. The basic assumptions of MI include the following:

- *Motivation to change cannot be imposed, but must be elicited.* Patients who enter treatment because they are pressured by others are unlikely to change their behavior unless they first decide they would be better off if they did so.
- *The patient's job is to articulate and resolve resistance or ambivalence; the therapist's job is to facilitate this process by making sure all sides of the patient's reactions are expressed.* Many people with BDD experience some desire to change, but when they are faced with the task of confronting feared situations, their motivation may wane. Encouraging patients to discuss their ambivalence or resistance sets the stage for treatment and helps clarify beliefs likely to interfere with recovery.
- *Ambivalence or resistance cannot be resolved by direct persuasion.* Changes in attitudes are elicited by using Socratic techniques and other methods described below.
- *The style for MI is quiet and eliciting.* Directive or authoritative methods will not work well for MI. Examples of Socratic interviewing methods are given in Judith Beck's (2011) *Cognitive Behavior Therapy: Basics and Beyond* or Miller and Rollnick's (2002, 2013) *Motivational Interviewing.*
- *The therapist aims to elicit, explore, and resolve resistance of ambivalence.* Ambivalence about or resistance to change must be identified and discussed. Otherwise, a lack of common goals will undermine the aims of the activities, exercises, and discussions of treatment.
- *Readiness to change emerges from the interpersonal interaction of the therapist and patient.* A trusting relationship is essential for this therapy. The therapist must not impose his or her own views on patients.
- *Therapy is a partnership, not a relationship between an expert and a recipient.* The therapist cannot make decisions for the patient or take responsibility for these decisions.

The therapist and patient must form an alliance to help the patient develop the ability to make these decisions.

PRINCIPLES OF MI

There are four basic principles of MI.

Expressing Empathy

Patient–therapist interactions should convey respect and a combination of understanding and shared purpose. This is best expressed through reflective listening. The expression of empathy is based on the assumption that ambivalence or resistance is normal. Therapists express empathy by attending to feelings, indicating acceptance, trying to understand, reflecting feelings, reinforcing courage, expressing caring or concern, and valuing patients' views.

Developing Discrepancy

Motivation for change is based on a patient's perception of a discrepancy between current circumstances and important personal goals and values. Heightened awareness of this discrepancy is therefore a central goal of MI, so that the patient, *not* the therapist, presents the arguments for change. For patients with BDD, the wish to engage in activities that are currently inhibited (e.g., socializing comfortably, dating, looking directly at others, getting to work on time, improving work or school performance) may help them become aware of the limitations imposed by their symptoms. As the therapist, you can also help patients clarify their values by asking what they consider most important. For example, you might ask, "What's the hardest part of this? What don't you do that you'd like to be doing?"

Rolling with Resistance

In MI, the therapist avoids arguing for change or directly confronting resistance. Rather, resistance is seen as an attempt to cope with anxiety and as a set of beliefs that can be examined. The therapist invites new perspectives, employing the patient as the primary resource for finding solutions. Patient resistance becomes a cue to respond differently. For instance, you might comment, "You are really upset about your nose and you aren't sure you want to try anything different."

Supporting Self-Efficacy

Don't get caught in arguing with the patient about whether they have an actual physical flaw or not. Instead try to agree with the patient that they are really suffering because of the way they feel about their appearance. That's the problem you can help them with in therapy. Patients must not only agree that they have a problem; they must also believe that they can do something to solve it. As the therapist, you cautiously express your belief that your patients are capable of making positive changes; the patients are responsible for choosing and carrying out change. For example, you might say, "You've done a lot of hard work on some other problems in your life. Your preoccupation with your appearance seems like a big one, but you seem to have some good problem-solving skills."

Strategies for Enhancing Motivation

The key goal of MI is to elicit self-motivational statements from patients that indicate the following:

- Recognition of the problem (i.e., that the patient suffers as a result of his or her appearance concerns).
- Concern about their behavior (e.g., avoidance behavior and appearance rituals).
- Intention to do something about their problem and related behaviors.
- Optimism about the possibilities for change.

These goals are pursued by using a variety of strategies described below. Throughout, you should emphasize patients' personal choice to engage in treatment and personal control over aspects of the therapy. At no time should you confront, pressure, blame, use sarcasm, or imply that you have all the answers, as these methods are entirely inconsistent with the respectful and collaborative spirit of MI.

Open-Ended Questions

Ask patients "what," "why," and "how" questions to get them to provide information about themselves. Here are examples:

"What led you to decide to come for treatment?"
"How can I be of help to you?"
"Why do you think your concerns about your appearance have become so important to you?"

Reflective Listening

Reflective listening is expressed in statements indicating that you have heard patients or noticed their reactions. They help patients feel understood and constitute a good fallback strategy if you don't know where to go next or you need more information about a patient. Reflective listening can also be very useful for crossing cultural boundaries when you and a patient come from very disparate backgrounds.

Simple reflections include repeating, rephrasing, paraphrasing, and reflecting feelings. They may be direct comments about feelings or reflections of personal statements:

"You didn't like that."
"These things are important to you."
"You don't want your mother to interfere."

Complex reflections provide new information by amplifying what patients have said and providing hypotheses about what they are thinking or feeling. Often what is amplified is ambivalence or resistance:

"You've considered that, but aren't sure it will help."

Double-sided reflections point directly to conflict and ambivalence:

"On the one hand, you feel . . . ; on the other hand, you. . . . "

In listening and commenting reflectively, you omit unnecessary words or cautious statements (e.g., "It seems like . . . ," "So . . . , " or "Maybe . . . "). Instead, you make simple, direct statements that reflect patients' thoughts, feelings, and behaviors. This enables the patients to hear the observations clearly, consider whether they are true, and respond accordingly.

Summarizing

Summarizing what patients have said helps to remind them of what they have said and to gain perspective on their own experience. In such a summary, you can reinforce some parts of the discussion more than others to emphasize important points. Summaries can also be used to change direction and/or to tie up loose ends and move on. Summaries should be brief and without qualifications or extra words, and may begin with "Let me see if I have this right," or "Let me see if I have a complete picture." Here is an example of a summary:

"You're angry with your parents for interfering with your plan to get surgery. Although you know this will be very expensive, you don't understand why they can't see your point of view. You'd like them to let you make your own decisions."

Summaries can be followed with open-ended questions, such as "What do you think of all this?"

Affirming Self-Efficacy

You can affirm patients' self-efficacy through supportive and appreciative statements that convey respect for the patients' actions, feelings, struggles, and accomplishments, and are based on your own genuine feelings. Such statements must not be contrived. For patients who feel that change requires more willpower or self-discipline than they possess, you can reframe weakness as a strength and express appreciation simply for their effort to come to the appointment, as in these examples:

"This must be very difficult for you."
"I respect what you have accomplished so far."
"You've made a huge effort."
"You've been dealing with a lot."
"I can tell you really make a strong effort to understand what's happening to you."

Evocative Questions

Evocative questions aim to elicit statements from patients that reflect recognition of the problem, feelings of concern or distress, intentions to change, and/or optimism about their capacity to do so. These questions direct patients to discuss the effects of their symptoms on themselves and on others. When patients have made tentative motivational statements, you can help strengthen them by asking:

"Why would you want to work on this?"
"In what ways has this been a problem for you?"
"What are your concerns?"
"How has your problem affected others?"
"How does this fit with your values?"
"What are the victories or good things that you can use to help you?"

Exploring Pros and Cons

You can help patients explore the pros and cons of a problem by asking questions that help elucidate both positive and negative elements (or advantages and disadvantages) of the problem and efforts to change it. Here are examples:

"What do you like about working out so much? What are the not-so-good parts of working out as much as you do?"
"What are the advantages of worrying so much about your hair? What about the disadvantages?"

In describing the advantages of these BDD symptoms, patients often say something like "Working out keeps me in shape," or "Worrying about my hair prevents me from looking like a complete slob!" This is helpful information for you, as it shows what might be maintaining the BDD-related beliefs, and what kinds of obstacles and fears these patients might face when giving up some of the BDD-related behaviors. You can simply accept your patients' answers at this time, but feel free to address any of the issues raised by these answers later in treatment. Your patients might mention some of the following when considering the disadvantages of their BDD:

"Low self-esteem."
"Feeling bad about my body."
"Feeling anxious when someone looks at me."
"Not able to get to work on time."
"Not able to go to the beach and parties and enjoy it."
"Not able to focus on anything other than my appearance when I'm at work."
"Surgery costs a lot of money."

Following this step, patients can make a list to consider the pros or advantages of getting treatment to resolve the BDD fears and symptoms. Do not strong-arm patients into listing certain pros and cons. A list of the advantages of change might look like this:

"Improved self-esteem."
"More respect for myself."
"Feeling better about my body."
"Less anxiety when someone looks at me."
"Able to get to my classes on time."
"Able to go to the beach and parties and enjoy it."
"Able to think about other things that are more important than my appearance."
"Able to go camping with friends."

"More energy to build relationships, paint, write."
"Save money to travel to Europe."
"Able to have other people see me close up."
"Able to enjoy having my boyfriend touch my face and stomach."
"Able to concentrate on my work and do much better in school."
"Be more outgoing and make new friends."

Asking for Elaboration

Another type of questioning is usually aimed at elaborating the negative consequences of the symptoms, once these have been mentioned. Such questions can also be requests to enhance commitment to change (see below under "Enhancing Change Talk"). Here are examples:

"Can you give me an example of how the surgery might complicate things for you?"
"When was the last time this happened?"
"What exactly did you do?"

Using Extreme Contrasts

You can also ask questions to pull for hypothetical situations that will amplify potential concerns about BDD symptoms and the benefits of working on the problem. Using such hypothetical situations can encourage patients to talk:

"What's the worst thing that can happen if you go along as you have been?"
"What are the best things that could come out of changing this?"
"If you were to decide to work on your preoccupation with your appearance seriously, what is most likely to happen?"
"If you were going to change, what would you do?"

Looking Forward and Looking Back

"Looking forward" questions are intended to amplify concerns by asking patients to project themselves into the future. This strategy elicits what patients care about, their basic values. Consider these examples:

"Think 5 years ahead. What would you like your life to be like? How does having another surgery fit with this? How does starting CBT-BDD fit with this?"
"What are you hoping for in the future?"
"What would it take for you to decide this was a problem you wanted to work on?"
"Suppose you were planning to commit time to therapy for this problem. What would that mean for your relationships?"
"How does what you are doing now fit in?"
"What do you want people to say about you at your funeral?"
"Do you want them to talk about how symmetrical your sideburns were?"

"Looking back" questions are similar, but they ask patients to reflect on the past, before the current problems began or became so severe:

"Contrast now with how you felt before these problems began. What was your life like then?"
"When was the last time things were going well?"

Reframing

Reframing typically involves making a statement that emphasizes positive aspects of working on the problem, in a way that changes the meaning or a patient's interpretation of an event. That is, you take something the patient is unhappy about and change this into a strength. For example:

"You think that her nagging about you rarely leaving the house is annoying, but it may indicate that she has real concern for you."

Enhancing Change Talk

As noted at the start of this chapter, "change talk" refers to statements about the desire, capacity, reasons, and need for change, as well as commitment to change. Readiness to change is often evident when patients stop arguing about whether they need a psychiatrist and appear calmer. Some may express sadness and/or ask questions about the future and about treatment options. You should avoid providing too much detail at this point about specific treatment methods, as this may provoke feelings of being overwhelmed and low self-efficacy.

Siding with the Negative

You can strengthen patients' commitment and confidence in their ability to change their BDD symptoms by making comments or asking questions that take the negative side of commitment to change. Doing this is akin to taking a "devil's advocate" position. Taking the negative side may get the patients out of defending their resistance and open a window for change. This strategy may not work for patients who are very delusional. Also, do not use this method until you have a very good rapport with a patient, and never express a negative view of the problem or your patient's capacity to resolve it. Here is an example of siding with the negative:

"Why would you want to try to change this with therapy? Regardless of what your family thinks, you really believe that something is wrong with your looks."

Emphasizing Personal Choice

You can clearly indicate that a patient is the one who makes the decisions, as in these examples:

"It's your choice whether you want to try this treatment or not."
"That is something you need to decide."

Cautious Interest

Cautious interest in change talk can be expressed via questions about how important it is to them to make changes and how confident they are that they can make the changes. Simply acknowledge the situation; do not prescribe more.

Rating Importance of and Confidence in Change

Expressions of cautious interest can be carried further by asking patients how important it is to change their problem (e.g., their preoccupation with their appearance, their appearance rituals, or their avoidance behavior) on a scale from 0 (not at all) to 10 (extremely). Next, you ask why they chose that number, and encourage change talk with questions that look both forward and backward. For a moderate score, ask, "What would it take for you to move from a 4 to an 8 on the scale?" For a low score, ask, "Why did you pick a 4 rather than a 1?" Then summarize the replies. A similar strategy can be used to determine how confident patients are about being able to change.

You then inquire about the next step:

"Where does that leave you now?"
"What are you thinking about your problem at this point?"
"What's the next step?"
"Where do your concerns about your appearance fit into your future?"

You can reinforce change talk by indicating your appreciation of patients' willingness to talk about how much pain their appearance concerns have caused them and expressing confidence that they will be able to make changes once they put their mind to it.

Predicting Outcome

When patients do decide to commit themselves to a psychiatric treatment such as CBT-BDD, versus a dermatological or surgical intervention, use their own knowledge of themselves to help them decide what to do (e.g., "Tell me what you think will happen, based on your own experience. How many times have you seen dermatologists? How well has this worked for you? How many times have you had CBT-BDD? What do you have to lose by trying CBT-BDD? What could you gain?"). You can reinforce or gently challenge the accuracy of their thinking about treatment as necessary. For patients who fear that after much effort they will not improve with the treatment program and "will feel like a failure," you can ask what they already know about CBT-BDD and its effects, and/or about themselves when they put their minds to a task.

Negotiating a Plan and Consolidating Change

The main goal of the final phase of MI is shifting to an action plan. Patients are probably ready to change when they begin to envision what the future may be like without the problem. They exhibit fewer behaviors indicating resistance or ambivalence, and they are likely to become quiet and contemplative, even resigned. They may start asking questions about change or state that they are tired of their behavior.

At this point, it's wise to summarize what a patient has said and to ask an open question:

"Now what do you think you need to do next?"
"What are you most concerned about?"

The patient's answer to this question, plus further inquiry as necessary about what needs changing, can lead to the start of a change plan. If the patient is unable to offer a plan, you can describe various options from which the patient can choose. In this case, it is wise to ask the patient's permission to give an opinion:

> "If it is OK with you, I can tell you of a plan that one person I know developed. [After the patient confirms that it is OK to proceed:] She agreed to come in every week and to try out a variety of homework assignments that we first worked on in the sessions. For example, in one session, she worked on looking in mirrors and focusing on her whole face and whole body rather than just the parts of her body she disliked. We practiced this together in the office first, and then she decided how often she could do it at home. She also began to observe her thoughts whenever she felt upset, and she kept some records of her thoughts at home to discuss in sessions."

You can write down the patient's plan of action, including behaviors and timetables, with a summary at the end. It will be helpful to emphasize that this plan is a work in progress rather than a single event, and that questions or changes in the plan may arise later on. You should ask for a commitment to work in treatment on the problem, but if the patient is not yet ready to give one, this can wait for the next session. MI sessions should end on a positive note:

> "I can see how hard this is for you, but I believe you're moving in the right direction with this plan. I think you're strong, and I'm sure you can do it."

As patients approach taking action to alter their symptoms, many begin to fear that if they decrease their efforts to improve their appearance, their fears will be confirmed. That is, they will no longer take care of their appearance, they will look awful as a result, and they will be rejected by others. The idea here is that their appearance will somehow get out of control. This can be addressed by asking whether they have evidence of this in their past behavior, and, if not, what evidence they have that this would suddenly occur. You can also reassure patients that other patients in CBT-BDD have not shown such tendencies, but that it is common for patients to fear making changes, because change is inherently uncomfortable for most people. This discomfort usually disappears once patients begin to make changes and become comfortable with the shifts in behavior and thinking. You can also note that the goal of treatment isn't for them to disregard their appearance completely or "let themselves go," but rather to get better control over their appearance obsessions and time-consuming behaviors.

DON'TS DURING MI

The following are *not* recommended during MI work:

- *Confrontation.* Avoid arguing the case for why change should happen. Arguments that champion change only make patients more defensive.
- *Insistence on labeling the problem.* Patients do not need to admit or declare that they have BDD. Although you will have already educated them about BDD and the fact that they have this illness, if they are reluctant to accept the diagnosis, it isn't necessary to push it or to argue about it. Typically, even patients who do not agree with the BDD diagnoses will agree that they are suffering because of their appearance concerns. You can use an alternative label that they find more acceptable, such as "body image

concerns." Using the term "BDD" isn't required for patients to become motivated or succeed, although many do eventually find it helpful to have a formal diagnosis, as this enables them to realize that others suffer similarly. Use labels only when patients indicate that these are helpful.

- *Blaming.* No one is at fault for the development of BDD. Undoubtedly, many factors have contributed to it. Don't side with a patient against someone else (e.g., a parent, sibling, or schoolmate) for causing the problem, as this can lead the patient to have to defend the other person, especially if it's a close family member. Also, the causes of BDD are not that simple. It's better to defuse the situation and suggest that no one is to blame.
- *Rapid-fire questions.* Avoid asking many questions at the outset; instead, listen closely to what a patient says. The general rule of thumb is never to ask three questions in a row.
- *Expert role.* You shouldn't set yourself apart from patients by adopting the role of expert, although you can use your experience to enhance patients' own expertise and self-understanding. This means that you should avoid lecturing. The patient–therapist relationship should feel like a partnership, in which the patient is the expert about him- or herself and the therapist is the expert about empirical information on BDD and others who have it.

MI and Delusional Beliefs

Almost by definition, most patients with BDD will have mixed feelings about trying to address their appearance concerns by engaging in a psychiatric treatment. Some mistaken beliefs about body imperfections are, by definition, part of the disorder. However, some patients hold delusional beliefs about their appearance that are closely linked to their identity. They are convinced that they are ugly, worthless, unlovable, and worse. Motivational methods alone will not alter these beliefs; they will simply provide the opening for patients to consider, if only briefly, that thinking and behaving a little differently might be valuable. Remember not to try to convince delusional patients with very low self-esteem that they are mistaken. MI methods work best and come most easily when you think of yourself as sitting next to a patient, or even inside his or her skin. Try hard to understand a patient's viewpoint from the patient's particular perspective before engaging in MI methods. This will help you avoid counterproductive efforts to "talk patients out of their beliefs and fears," in which you pit your views against theirs. Such efforts will merely produce disagreement and an adversarial relationship, rather than a trusting alliance.

PART II

INTRODUCTORY SESSIONS

Laying the Foundation for Successful Treatment

In this section of the manual (Part II), we describe the first three treatment sessions, which focus on assessment, orientation to CBT-BDD, psychoeducation, case formulation, motivational enhancement, and setting treatment goals. We also show you how you can teach your patients to assess their maladaptive thoughts. These three *introductory sessions* lay important groundwork for successful treatment.

From here on in this manual (i.e., throughout Parts II–IV), we alternate between "she" and "he" for an individual patient.

CHAPTER 6

SESSION 1

ASSESSING BDD, ORIENTING THE PATIENT TO CBT-BDD, AND ASSESSING MOTIVATION

SESSION SUMMARY

- ☐ Work on the agenda.
    - ☐ Welcome the patient.
    - ☐ Check mood.
    - ☐ Further assess BDD.
    - ☐ Provide feedback about BDD symptoms.
    - ☐ Orient the patient to CBT-BDD.
    - ☐ Provide the patient with a binder and the *Personal Session Form* (Form 2.1).
    - ☐ Assess and enhance motivation.
    - ☐ Answer your patient's questions.
- ☐ Assign homework.
- ☐ Ask for summary of/feedback on the session.

SESSION FORMS AND HANDOUTS

Self-Report Measures (already completed)

Body Checklist (Form 4.2)

BDD Symptom Scale (BDD-SS) (Form 4.3)

BDI-II (or other depression inventory)

Clinician-Administered BDD Measures

BDD Information-Gathering Form (Form 4.4)

Personal Session Form (Form 2.1)

Therapist Session Form (Form 6.1)

What Is Body Dysmorphic Disorder? (Handout 6.1)

A Message to Current Patients from Past Patients (Handout 6.2)

Introduction to This Session

This chapter covers Session 1, during which you will meet with the patient to introduce her to this treatment. You will need to prepare for this session by reviewing all assessment measures completed by the patient, and it might be helpful for you to have the BDD-SS (Form 4.3) and the *Body Checklist* (Form 4.2) in front of you during this session. During the session, you can ask your own questions to probe further.

However, you'll need to use clinical judgment to decide the order in which to complete the activities and the time that will be needed for each. Some patients may be so ambivalent about engaging in therapy that the motivational strategies described in Chapter 5 will be needed before you can proceed much further.

Your General Approach

To ease a patient's anxiety at the first therapy meeting, assume an active role by structuring the session and answering questions directly. Your goal is to encourage the patient to view you as helpful, caring, empathic, knowledgeable, and confident. The first few sessions should activate a sense of hope and optimism about treatment, diminish anxiety, and create openness to change.

Most patients are anxious and uncomfortable in the first few therapy meetings, for fear that you will judge their appearance negatively, consider them vain, dismiss their concerns as trivial, or force them to do something in therapy that goes against their wishes. Because many patients with BDD lack insight and are ambivalent about getting treatment, your primary goals are to get them to return for subsequent sessions and to accept the idea that therapy can help them.

Achieving these goals can be quite challenging. Some patients will think you cannot really help them, because you can't change how they actually look. Some do not yet accept the idea that they have a mental disorder that therapy can help. Some patients will have had negative experiences with past therapy, and these may interfere with their ability to process information you give them about BDD or its treatment. Others may feel that they have been pushed too quickly or too hard into treatment. Anticipate these potential problems by asking open-ended questions as needed early in the treatment. Avoid asking rapid-fire questions about patients' symptoms, so that they will not feel "grilled" about their problem. Also, see Chapter 5 for additional guidelines on how to engage patients and develop a therapeutic alliance.

Work on the Agenda

Welcome the Patient, Check Mood, and Further Assess BDD

As discussed in Chapter 4, we typically ask our patients to arrive 10 minutes before the start of the session, to allow time to fill out a depression questionnaire. We typically use the BDI-II, but as described in Chapter 4, you can also use the IDS or the QIDS. After welcoming the patient, check the BDI-II (or other depression inventory) that was completed in the waiting area. Pay particular attention to the suicidality item of the questionnaire.

Next, explain that the main focus of today's session is to achieve a clear understanding of the patient's symptoms and experience, in order to set the foundation for her treatment. Explain that today you will also give her feedback, tell her about the treatment, and answer her questions. The bulk of today's session will focus on further assessing BDD. Tell the patient that you have reviewed the questionnaires she has completed already, and that you will now ask some additional questions about her symptoms and experiences. The *BDD Information-Gathering Form* (Form 4.4) will guide you through this process. Use responses on the patient's self-report measures as a springboard for your use of the *BDD Information-Gathering Form.*

Take the time to understand the patient's experiences and her "story." This is essential not only for building a therapeutic alliance and getting a full picture of her experiences, but for treatment planning.

Provide Feedback about BDD Symptoms

Briefly give the patient feedback about her symptoms. For example, explain that the information she has provided on the forms and in session indicates that she has BDD, a relatively common and treatable disorder. Briefly explain that BDD is a preoccupation with a perceived defect in appearance (e.g., a large nose, large ears, thinning hair, facial scarring) that others believe is unimportant, nonexistent, or slight. Tell her why you think she has BDD (e.g., because she worries a lot about her appearance, checks mirrors a lot, etc.). You can explain that people with BDD see themselves differently than other people do, for reasons that are not well understood.

Tell your patient that she will learn a lot more about BDD in the next session. As described earlier, some patients may have difficulty accepting a BDD diagnosis, because they are convinced that they have an actual appearance flaw. If this is the case for this patient, don't try to talk her out of her beliefs, but rather use some of the language we have described earlier. If you and your patient disagree on the BDD diagnosis, focus on your patient's suffering, functioning, and quality of life. Most patients will agree that they are spending too much time thinking about their appearance and that their concerns are making them suffer.

Orient the Patient to CBT-BDD

Briefly orient the patient to CBT-BDD. Explain that CBT (as well as certain medications) is often effective for BDD is the most frequently recommended type of therapy for BDD. Briefly explain that the goal of CBT-BDD is to help her evaluate her thinking and develop more helpful ways of thinking. It should also give her more control over her compulsive behaviors and help her feel more comfortable around other people. Convey that anxiety, depression, and overall functioning usually improve as well. Describe the number of sessions and the frequency and length of each session.

Here are some additional points you can make:

- The patient will learn lots of skills to overcome BDD; she will not just talk about her problems.
- CBT-BDD is different from many other types of therapy. It's focused on a specific problem, so not all of the patient's problems will be solved.
- The sessions and treatment are very structured. Explain that all sessions will have a similar structure, and describe this structure.
- CBT-BDD is time-limited. (We usually estimate that patients might need about 22 sessions; however, certain patients may require more or even less time.)

- Homework between sessions is essential, so that the patient can build skills and practice them until they are mastered. As time goes on, she will take more of a role in deciding on homework assignments.
- Over time, the patient will learn to be her own therapist. At the end of the treatment, the patient will not need your help anymore and will continue to implement the skills on her own, although you and she may decide to engage in a few booster sessions.
- The patient needs to put effort into the treatment and to be an active collaborator with you. Your role as the therapist is more like that of a coach or a teacher who helps the patient learn new skills.

As you are explaining all this, it can help to use an analogy from sports, music, or another skills-based activity that is relevant to the patient. For example, if the patient enjoys figure skating, you could say something like this:

THERAPIST: Do you remember what was it like the first time you went out on the ice and tried to skate?

PATIENT: Oh, I was so wobbly; it was hard even TO skate in a straight line, and I couldn't do any turns or anything.

THERAPIST: So how did you learn to skate so well?

PATIENT: Well, it took lots of practice. I went out and practiced every day, and gradually I got pretty good at it.

THERAPIST: So it took lots of regular practice. That makes sense. It doesn't seem like you could learn a skill like that in a day! CBT-BDD will be a lot like that. In your sessions with me, you'll learn lots of useful skills and strategies, but it's only by practicing between treatment sessions that you'll really learn the skills and get good at them.

PATIENT: That makes sense.

For someone who's had therapy other than CBT in the past, point out how different CBT-BDD is, including the fact that it is much more structured than other types of therapy. Explain that the earlier sessions will have an educational focus, and you will be more like a teacher imparting knowledge; these sessions will provide a very important foundation for the rest of the treatment. Later, the treatment will be more collaborative and will focus more on skills building; in this phase, you will be more of a coach. The last two sessions will be devoted to anticipating and planning for difficult times that may occur in the future, so that the patient can successfully cope with these (i.e., relapse prevention).

Finally, tell your patient that in the coming sessions she will learn a lot more about what CBT-BDD is and how it works.

Provide the Patient with a Binder and the *Personal Session Form* (Form 2.1)

Provide your patient with a binder or folder in which to keep the handouts she'll get during the treatment, her homework forms, and the notes she takes during sessions. Ask her to bring it to all of her sessions. It can help to organize this folder according to content, to minimize confusion and wasted time during sessions when previously completed forms are needed (e.g., treatment goals).

In addition, give the patient a *Personal Session Form* (Form 2.1), and tell her that you will give her a copy of this form at the beginning of each session. Explain that she will use this form to take notes about important points during all of her sessions. She'll also write down homework for the upcoming week on this form. In addition, she can use this form to record questions and issues that arise during the week as she does homework. Explain that by the end of therapy, her filled-out copies of this form (which she will keep in her treatment binder) will provide a full record of the therapy.

Use your own *Therapist Session Form* (Form 6.1) to record what you and the patient do during each session.

Assess and Enhance Motivation

At this point, try to get a sense of how motivated your patient is for treatment. As the treatment progresses, you'll get a better sense of your patient's level of motivation.

Unless your patient clearly expresses willingness to make a significant effort toward resolving her BDD symptoms, directly explore her motivation for treatment. If she seems reluctant to engage fully in treatment, try to engage her with questions such as these:

"For how long have you been trying to solve your appearance problem with cosmetic treatments? . . . How useful has this been?"
"Have you ever tried another way of looking at your problem?"
"What could be the advantages of trying a new strategy?"
"Do you have anything to lose by trying a new approach?"

If your patient is fixated on a belief in her own ugliness, which she thinks you and CBT-BDD cannot fix, try focusing on the degree of her preoccupation and how much she is suffering (see Chapter 5). You can also suggest that after 22 sessions of CBT-BDD, the patient can always go back to her old strategies if those worked better. If these engagement strategies don't suffice and your patient has significant resistance to the idea of participating in treatment, begin to use strategies from Chapter 5 right away.

Regardless of how motivated your patient is, be optimistic about the likelihood that CBT-BDD will help her, if she is willing to give it a good try and make an effort. Don't be unrealistic, because improvement can't be guaranteed, but express optimism nonetheless. Remember, your most important goal for the introductory sessions is to give your patient hope that treatment will work.

Answer Your Patient's Questions

Ask your patient whether she has any questions at this point, and take the time to provide at least brief answers. You can also reiterate that the patient will learn much more about BDD and its treatment in the next few sessions.

Assign Homework

Remind your patient that she will get a homework assignment after each session. And remind her that later in the treatment, she will have input into her homework.

Assign your patient to read *What Is Body Dysmorphic Disorder?* (Handout 6.1) and *A Message to Current Patients from Past Patients* (Handout 6.2). Tell your patient that the second handout was prepared by patients from the Boston area for her and others like her.

Ask for Summary of/Feedback on the Session

Briefly summarize the major points covered during the session, emphasizing the positive points. Ask the patient to add any comments about what she has learned. (In later sessions, you will ask the patient herself to do this summary.)

Ask whether your patient has any concerns about the session or your behavior. Ask whether you didn't cover something she was hoping to talk about. Encourage her to comment both positively and negatively, even if she thinks that her reactions are minor. Respond thoughtfully to her concerns, apologizing if needed and/or explaining what occurred.

FORM 6.1

Therapist Session Form

Name: ______________________ Date: ________________ Session no.: _______

Mood and BDD symptom check:

Score on BID-II (or other depression measure):

Main points from previous session:

Agenda:

Homework review (also rate completion 0–100%):

Work on agenda/main points, difficulties:

(cont.)

Adapted with permission of the publisher from Wilhelm, S., & Steketee, G. (2006). *Cognitive Therapy for Obsessive-Compulsive Disorder.* Oakland, CA: New Harbinger Publications.

Therapist Session Form *(page 2 of 2)*

Summary of session:

New homework:

Feedback:

Points to discuss next time:

HANDOUT 6.1

What Is Body Dysmorphic Disorder?

Definition

Body dysmorphic disorder (BDD) is an excessive preoccupation with a nonexistent or slight defect in appearance. Most people with BDD spend more than an hour per day thinking about their perceived defect(s). Either they are concerned about something that others cannot see, or they worry excessively about a minor defect in their appearance, such as mild acne or scars. The preoccupation causes clinically significant distress and often interferes with daily functioning. The severity of BDD ranges from milder (i e., more manageable) to extremely severe.

Body Areas of Concern

Common complaints involve minor or nonexistent flaws of the head and face, but any body part can be the focus of concern. Individuals with BDD often complain about acne, wrinkles, pale skin, scars, excessive facial hair, hair thinning, or the shape or size of body parts such as the nose or teeth. Some people with BDD have concerns focusing on bodily asymmetry. "Muscle dysmorphia" is a variant of BDD in which individuals consider themselves as small or not muscular enough, when in fact they are quite normal or even muscular and large. Usually people with BDD are concerned with more than one body part.

Ritualistic Behaviors

Nearly all people with BDD perform repetitive behaviors to check, improve, or hide the perceived defect. These actions include checking the supposed flaw in mirrors or other reflecting surfaces, and trying to camouflage the perceived flaw with makeup, clothing, or special body positioning. Some people engage in excessive grooming, such as combing, cutting, or styling their hair. Others pick at their skin, trying to remove imperfections or to pluck/pull their hair. Many people with BDD ask for reassurance related to the imagined defect. They may also frequently compare their appearance with that of other people. The repetitive behaviors can take several hours per day and typically only provide temporary relief. BDD behaviors can vary from person to person and are not limited to those listed here.

(cont.)

Avoidance

Avoidance is common, especially avoidance of social situations or work/school situations. People with BDD usually have difficulty viewing their reflection in mirrors and often alternate between episodes of mirror avoidance and mirror checking.

Distress/Impairment

Most people suffering from BDD are very distressed by their supposed flaws and describe their preoccupations as "painful" or "tormenting." The preoccupations are difficult to control and time-consuming; most individuals spend at least several hours per day thinking about their perceived defects. BDD is also associated with difficulties in occupational, academic, and social functioning. Because of their appearance concerns, people with BDD may be late for work or school, may miss work or school, may be less productive, or may not work or go to school at all. BDD usually affects friendships, dating, relationships with family members, intimate relationships, and social interactions more generally. In its most severe form, it incapacitates persons with this illness and can keep them housebound for many years. Also, about a quarter of people with BDD attempt suicide.

Beliefs

People with BDD often believe that other people take special notice of the defect they perceive. For example, they may think that others stare at them or laugh about their problem. Often they believe that others will reject them because of it. These beliefs develop because of their negative body image and are rarely based on accurate observation.

Age of Onset/Sex Ratio

BDD usually begins during adolescence. BDD appears to be slightly more common in females, but it also affects males.

Rate of BDD

Preliminary estimates suggest that BDD may be common, with a rate of 1.7–2.4% in the general population.

(cont.)

Possible Causes of BDD

At this time, the cause of BDD remains largely unexplored, although a number of different theories have been proposed:

- Biological theories (e.g., genetic makeup and/or imbalance in serotonin, a natural brain chemical)
- Psychological theories (e.g., frequent teasing in childhood, importance of appearance when growing up)
- Sociocultural theories (e.g., influence of the mass media)

BDD and Cosmetic Treatment

About two-thirds of people with BDD receive cosmetic treatment for their BDD concerns. About 40% of patients receive dermatological treatment, and about 20–40% have cosmetic surgery. Many others receive dental treatments and other types of non-mental-health treatments. However, most patients are dissatisfied with the results of such treatment, which can actually worsen BDD symptoms.

HANDOUT 6.2

A Message to Current Patients from Past Patients

We have been where you are now, and we want you to know:

1. We care about you.
2. This disorder exists. Other people have it too. You aren't alone with this.
3. Be angry at the disorder, not yourself.
4. Drop the shame. The feelings you have are not your fault.
5. Allow, just allow, that your thoughts might be wrong. Remember that BDD is a disorder of thinking, not appearance.
6. Your old strategies focused on hiding or changing your appearance haven't worked. We are glad that you are trying something new and are here in treatment.
7. Stop the self-hatred and self-criticism. You are struggling with a disorder; treat yourself well.
8. It's the inside—how you feel and how you think—that needs attention, not the outside.
9. Comparing yourself to others is a waste of time. It is not a competition; it is about enjoying life.
10. You can't wait to feel good to do something. Sometimes you change how you feel by changing what you do.
11. Do not isolate yourself.
12. Pay attention to things you enjoy. Pay attention to your life, not your face, skin, hair, etc.
13. Give yourself credit for even the smallest effort.
14. Try to live in the present. It's all about creating pleasure and meaning in life, not dwelling on past regrets.
15. It's a progression. Listen, learn, and change your life.

Adapted with permission of the publisher from Wilhelm, S. (2006). *Feeling Good about the Way You Look: A Program for Overcoming Body Image Problems*. New York: Guilford Press.

CHAPTER 7

SESSION 2

Education and Case Formulation

SESSION SUMMARY

- ☐ Check mood and BDD symptoms.
- ☐ Briefly review the previous session.
- ☐ Set the agenda jointly with the patient.
- ☐ Review homework.
- ☐ Work on the agenda.
    - ☐ Explain features of BDD.
    - ☐ Discuss subjective and varying ideas about beauty.
    - ☐ Comment on the role of the media.
    - ☐ Clarify the big difference between appearance and body image.
    - ☐ Describe theories of how body image problems develop.
    - ☐ Develop a model for understanding the patient's BDD symptoms.
- ☐ Assign homework.
- ☐ Ask for summary of/feedback on the session.

SESSION FORMS AND HANDOUTS

BDI-II (or other depression inventory)

Personal Session Form (Form 2.1)

Therapist Session Form (Form 6.1)

Standard BDD Model (Handout 7.1)

Your Personal BDD Model (Form 7.1)

Sample Completed Your Personal BDD Model (Handout 7.2)

Introduction to This Session

This session will focus on educating the patient about BDD and its effects, as well as developing a model for understanding the patient's BDD. You will discuss BDD more comprehensively than you did in the first session. You will also discuss beauty and culture, appearance versus body image, and theories about how BDD develops. Some of the discussion points covered in this session have been informed by Thomas Cash's excellent body image research and books (e.g., Cash, 2008). During this stage of treatment, you are more like a teacher who is conveying essential knowledge to a student. Later, when you start applying CBT-BDD techniques, you will do less teaching and more collaborative guiding and coaching. However, even in the initial steps of treatment, you need to avoid long monologues. Make sure to elicit feedback from your patients.

Check Mood and BDD Symptoms

As you did at the start of Session 1 and will do at the beginning of every session, ask your patient for the BDI-II (or alternative depression measure) she has completed in the waiting room. Pay attention not only to the scale's total score, but also to the suicidality item, and ask further questions about suicidality if such questions are clinically indicated. Also briefly inquire about BDD symptoms over the course of the last week.

Hand out a copy of the *Personal Session Form* (Form 2.1) and remind the patient to record information she finds significant during the session.

Briefly Review the Previous Session

As at every session, briefly check in with the patient on his perception and understanding of the previous session.

Set the Agenda Jointly with the Patient

Convey the topics you would like to cover during the session. Remind the patient that this is more of an educational session, and that he will assume more of a role in setting the agenda as the treatment progresses. Nonetheless, ask the patient whether there are any issues he would like to cover in this session.

Review Homework

Discuss your patient's reactions to the two handouts from Session 1: *What Is Body Dysmorphic Disorder?* (Handout 6.1) and *A Message to Current Patients from Past Patients* (Handout 6.2). Your goal is to determine whether these handouts were helpful (and if so, how), and whether your patient had any negative reactions to the material.

WORK ON THE AGENDA

Explain Features of BDD

In Session 1, you have very briefly explained BDD and why you think the patient has it. In this session, you'll spend a little more time on this explanation. You can use some or all of the following points to explain BDD and help patients begin to consider an alternative view of their own symptoms. Whenever possible, incorporate each patient's own symptoms and experience in the discussion.

- Remind the patient that BDD is a preoccupation with a perceived defect in appearance (e.g., a large nose, large ears, thinning hair, facial scarring) that others believe is unimportant, nonexistent, or slight.
- Concerns typically involve the face and head—most often the skin (e.g., acne or scarring), hair (e.g., thinning), and nose (e.g., that it's too big). However, any body part can be the focus of concern.
- Most patients have multiple concerns. These concerns can change over time. However, some have just one unchanging concern; others dislike virtually everything about how they look.
- BDD affects both men and women. It affects people of all ages and from all ethnic groups and cultures.
- Most people with BDD spend at least several hours a day thinking about their perceived appearance defects.
- Nearly all people with BDD perform excessive, usually time-consuming behaviors. The goal is to check to see if they look or feel better about how they look. Usually, however, these behaviors don't help patients feel much better and end up taking lots of time. Here are several examples:
  - Checking or avoiding mirrors and other reflecting surfaces.
  - Excessive grooming (e.g., combing hair excessively, tweezing eyebrows, performing complicated skin regimens, applying makeup).
  - Using makeup or other camouflage (e.g., hats, clothing, body position) to cover up perceived defects.
  - Asking others for reassurance about their looks.
  - Comparing themselves to other people or to models in magazines or actors on TV or in movies.
  - Skin picking.
  - Hair plucking.
  - Tanning.
  - Excessive clothes changing.
  - Excessive shopping for clothes or beauty products.
  - Any other compulsive BDD behaviors that your patient engages in (mention these specifically).
- Nearly everyone with BDD has problems with daily functioning because of these concerns. Many avoid social situations, dating, friends, or sexual intimacy. Work or school are often affected; for example, patients may arrive late, get stuck in the bathroom checking mirrors, missing work or school, not having a job, or underperforming. Many function below their potential.

- People with BDD usually feel depressed and anxious because of how they look. Some even consider suicide. Others become angry and frustrated.
- Most people with BDD have clinical depression. Anxiety disorders (e.g., social phobia and OCD) are also common. Many abuse drugs or alcohol because of their appearance concerns.
- Many patients with BDD hide their symptoms because of embarrassment and shame. They often delay seeking help for BDD, or they seek help for other problems such as depression, even though BDD is their main problem.
- BDD usually begins during the teenage years (13 is the most common age). Without the right treatment, it is usually chronic.
- BDD usually gets better with the right treatment. The best treatments are CBT and the antidepressant medications known as SRIs (see Chapter 1 for details).

Discuss Subjective and Varying Ideas about Beauty

After describing BDD to your patient, engage your patient in a brief discussion about the subjective nature of beauty. You might begin by saying something like this:

> "What's considered beautiful changes a lot. It changes over time and varies across cultures. At one point, extremely thin models may be considered most attractive, but a few years later, magazines may be filled with more athletic-looking women. So what's considered attractive is subjective and changeable."

Remind the patient that, like clothing fashions, physical attributes go into and out of fashion—such as curly versus straight hair, large or small breast size, and tanned versus pale skin color. Give examples of historical changes in beauty images and fashions to illustrate that the "ideal" image of beauty fluctuates with the passage of time and the whims of the culture:

- Contrast the 1950s sex symbol Marilyn Monroe with anorexic-looking fashion models like Twiggy in the 1960s and with the lean, muscular look of Cindy Crawford and Christy Turlington in the 1980s.
- Note that female models and actresses have become noticeably thinner from the 1940s through the present day (e.g., Jennifer Aniston, Keira Knightley), while male models and actors have become more muscular across time (e.g., Hugh Jackman), making it harder and harder for ordinary women and men to match these unrealistic stereotypes.

In addition, comment on beauty attributes that differ by culture. Examples are non-Western ideals of very long necks in some African cultures, and obesity as a sign of wealth versus thinness as a sign of poverty in parts of India.

Comment on the Role of the Media

What we all see on TV or in magazines is unreal. Here you can refer to the use of airbrushing in magazine photos to erase defects. You can also briefly comment on how beautiful models, actors, and actresses represent only a tiny proportion of people in the world.

Clarify the Difference between Appearance and Body Image

Help patients learn the difference between "body image" (the mental pictures people have of themselves; their beliefs about how they look) and actual "appearance" (observable physical features). Appearance can differ greatly from how people think of themselves (their body image). People who are generally considered unattractive may feel fine about how they look, and people who are very attractive often don't see themselves that way. Here are a few examples of the difference between body image and actual appearance:

- Many people who are dissatisfied with their appearance are actually good-looking.
- People with anorexia nervosa are dangerously thin, but still believe that they're too fat. For some people with anorexia, the mismatch between their body image and how they actually look is so great that they might die from malnutrition. This is a good example of how poorly body image can reflect actual appearance.
- When people actually change their appearance through plastic surgery, their body image may not change (they may still hate the way they look).
- Patients with BDD often say that their areas of concern change over time, despite the fact that their appearance does not change.

You can say also something like the following, which focuses on the difference between body image and actual appearance:

> "For many people, there's a difference between what they actually look like and how they think they look (their body image). This is true for people in general, not just people with BDD. Some people who are very attractive think they look just average, or even unattractive. Many people who aren't very attractive objectively are happy with how they look.
>
> "This mismatch is even bigger in BDD. It's a lot like anorexia nervosa in this way. Are you familiar with anorexia, where people who are actually extremely thin think they're too fat? . . . In our treatment together, one of the things we'll work on is helping you develop a body image that's more accurate and helpful for you."

Explain that the mismatch between body image and actual appearance is very pronounced in BDD. It's important for your patient to learn in the early sessions that *BDD is a problem of body image, not appearance*, and that he needs help with his body image and how he *thinks* about his appearance, rather with his actual appearance. You can remind the patient that an important focus of CBT-BDD is on developing a more accurate and helpful body image.

If the patient keeps asking, "How can you help me? What I really need is surgery [or dermatological treatments, etc.]," remind her that CBT-BDD is only 22 sessions long and that she has little to lose by trying it. Moreover, the patient has probably seen dermatologists or plastic surgeons before, and this hasn't helped. It's time to try something new.

Describe Theories of How Body Image Problems Develop

There are three main theories about how BDD develops. These are biological (e.g., genetics, brain circuits, and the brain chemical serotonin), sociocultural (e.g., the media, cultural values) and psychological (e.g., teasing, parental values) (see Chapter 1). Explain that you will cover all of these but will focus primarily on psychological theories, since these are the basis of CBT-BDD. Discuss these ideas relatively briefly, including some or all of the information given below. You will develop these theories further when you and the patient together formulate a personal model of how the patient's BDD has developed.

Biological Theories

"We still don't really know what causes BDD. Scientists are trying to figure this out. But there's good reason to think that BDD results from a complex combination of biological, psychological, and sociocultural factors. The biological makeup you've inherited almost certainly plays a role, because it plays a role in all disorders—it's probably the same for BDD. For example, there are probably certain genes that increase the chance of getting BDD. Also, people with BDD may improve with medications known as serotonin reuptake inhibitors (SRIs or SSRIs for short). These medications regulate a natural chemical in the brain called serotonin. This suggests (although doesn't prove) that a chemical imbalance involving serotonin may play a role in bringing on BDD.

"Also, brain imaging and neuropsychological studies have shown that people with BDD tend to get caught up in details rather than to see the 'big picture' when they are processing visual information. This is important, because clinically we also see that people with BDD *selectively attend to flaws and often appear to ignore how the rest of their faces or bodies look*. It also seems that people with BDD have abnormal brain function when they are looking at pictures of their own faces, according to a study led by Dr. Jamie Feusner at UCLA. This study indicated that when viewing photographs of themselves, patients with BDD seem to underuse the parts of the brain most people use to see the face's overall shape and size. This tendency to overfocus on details of appearance, rather than to see the 'big picture,' is addressed in several parts of CBT-BDD."

Sociocultural Theories

THERAPIST: It's also likely that the society we live in contributes to getting BDD. It seems that today people expect more from their bodies than ever. We're inundated by TV ads and fashion magazines, telling us that there's a perfect look and we should try to achieve it by buying a certain beauty product, outfit, or exercise machine. The models that make it onto the magazine covers are so unusually beautiful that they represent under 1% of the people in the general population. And even the models that get on the covers really don't look that great in real life. Their pictures are taken only after they've spent many hours with professional makeup artists, hair stylists, and clothes designers. Many models have had plastic surgery, and most of them follow a rigidly controlled exercise and diet program. And even after the pictures are taken, the photos are often edited digitally. So these images are completely unreal, but we still end up assuming that they are what we should look like, because we're inundated with these pictures of impossibly beautiful people. What kind of an effect do you think the mass media have had on you?

PATIENT: I guess seeing those pictures over and over again distorts my views of what's normal. I compare myself and get dissatisfied with what nature has done to me.

THERAPIST: Yes, but are you really comparing yourself to a realistic standard?

PATIENT: Well, I'm not sure . . . maybe not. Maybe I have goals for my appearance that I could never reach, and this leaves me feeling defective.

Psychological Theories and the CBT Model of BDD

"A basic premise underlying the model of BDD is that how people feel about their bodies depends less on their *actual* appearance than on their personal *evaluation* of their appearance—that is, on their body image [see, e.g., Cash, 2008]. We've already talked about the mismatch that usually occurs between body image and actual appearance, and we've noted that this problem is even more pronounced for people with BDD. Body image becomes distorted when people misperceive their actual physical characteristics and also interpret them in a negative way. CBT-BDD is based on the assumption that people's perceptions, thoughts, and beliefs strongly influence their body image."

[For patients whose body concerns have changed over time, but for whom it isn't possible for the features to have changed, you can add:]

"In your case, the focus of your concerns about your body has changed several times over the past few years. Why would your concerns change so much? Your nose [or other focus of distress] has always looked the same, but you only started worrying about it a year ago. It seems unlikely that the actual appearance of your nose changed a year ago. It's more likely that your *view* of yourself—your body image—has changed for some reason."

[You can then continue, for all patients:]

"Even if our perceptions of our appearance are wrong, they can still make us miserable. Our thinking and beliefs can be quite mistaken, but they can still influence our emotions. A simple example of the effect of this thinking is that if we're hungry and imagine eating really good food, we're likely to salivate, even though no food is actually present.

"In a similar vein, factors in our context (such as stress) strongly influence our perceptions and thoughts. An example of how perception can be influenced by context is the type of music played during a movie. Music affects the audience's emotions and can convince people of danger, even if they know from the movie review that nothing dangerous will actually happen."

To help illustrate this with personal experience, ask the patient to observe her emotional reactions to music the next time she is watching a movie. Then continue to discuss the effect of word choice and context on her BDD symptoms as follows. In this passage, we continue to refer to the patient's nose as the focus of distress, but of course you should substitute a particular patient's own appearance concern(s) for the references to the nose.

"In your own case, let's look at your emotional reaction when you think, 'My nose has a bump on it,' compared to 'My nose looks hideous.' How do you think these two ideas affect your mood and what you think next?

"It's also possible that some of the personal experiences you've had in your life may have contributed to your getting BDD. For example, some people who've been teased a lot about their appearance can understandably become very self-conscious about how they look. Other people with BDD come from families that emphasized appearance a lot. Some (although not all) people from a minority culture may feel different because of how they look, worrying that they stand out in a negative way. Experiences such as these may make us *feel* there's something wrong with how we look, even when there really isn't. Have you had any experiences like these that you think may be related to how you feel about your appearance?"

Examples of the influence of cultural expectations are the concerns of some of our Asian patients about the shape of their eyes or about their short height. Hispanic patients or other patients from non-European racial or ethnic groups may be concerned that their skin is too dark.

Don't lecture your patient, and provide many opportunities for discussion. Also, ask the patient to summarize what she understands at this point. Invite questions and repeat information as often as necessary for the patient to remember it. A typical script might be as follows:

"We've just talked about body image problems and how they develop. Can you tell me what stood out for you? What seemed important to you? [Wait as the patient recounts the information.] Yes, it certainly seems like you have had some family and cultural experiences that have shaped your ideas of what a woman is supposed to look like. Did you have any additional questions or thoughts about this? [Respond to questions.] CBT-BDD should help you feel a lot less concerned about this."

Develop a Model for Understanding the Patient's BDD Symptoms

At this point, begin working on a model for understanding the patient's BDD symptoms from a CBT framework, using the patient's own symptoms and experiences. This model is a formulation of the case that incorporates a basic understanding of BDD and of the patient's own particular thoughts, feelings, and behaviors. It provides the foundation for the patient's understanding of her symptoms and for selecting treatment strategies. Try to have a general idea in your mind of what the final model might look like, so that you can offer suggestions as you are working on it with the patient, but be sure to develop it collaboratively with your patient. *You will later refer to the model at many points during the therapy* to help the patient understand why she is learning certain techniques and which aspects of the BDD problem the techniques are addressing. The model will also help the patient understand what is happening and why when the BDD symptoms flare up. *Thus this model becomes the basis for all of the subsequent components of therapy.* You will be able to revise the patient's model if new information comes to light during the treatment, but it is important to develop it fully at the outset, so that you and your patient have a shared understanding of how the patient's BDD developed and what currently maintains it. A standard model of BDD is shown in Handout 7.1. This model can be modified to suit each patient's particular situation, with the help of Form 7.1.

For the patient's initial BDD model, select the most common or most disturbing concerns if more than one symptom is problematic. Use Handout 7.1 to guide the discussion of the patient's experience and help the patient develop her own personal model on Form 7.1. Use the patient's own words to fill in the boxes of Form 7.1.

The following interactive dialogue illustrates how to ask questions and guide the patient to create a model that represents the BDD experience for her. Be sure to cover the highlighted points below to emphasize the links among thoughts, emotions, and behaviors, You will need to modify this dialogue slightly to fit each patient's situation (e.g., by substituting "hair" for "nose").

For this initial discussion, select one BDD concern from a recent situation. Others will be identified during homework assignments and in later therapy sessions. In this session, simply help the patient understand the various components of the model and see how it applies specifically to her own symptoms. Do not try to be overly comprehensive; just get the basic concepts of the model across clearly, so the patient can summarize the model as it applies to her by the end of the session.

Normalize Personal Physical Defects

Begin by mentioning a personal defect of your own. The purpose here is to normalize the patient's awareness of body defects and to begin to illustrate differences between ordinary appearance concerns and BDD symptoms. This point builds upon what was covered in Session 1, as it emphasizes that it isn't the body flaw itself, but the patient's negative body image that is problematic.

> "Of course, all of us have concerns about our bodies—that's very common. For example, this morning when I got ready for work, I looked in the mirror and noticed the scar under my left eye [select an actual minor body defect the patient can easily see], and I thought, 'Today my scar is a little red.' And naturally I didn't like the scar, but I also did not keep looking at it. It didn't bother me very much, and I didn't attach any special meaning to it. Then I let the thought go and went on with my day."

Determine the Patient's Triggers for Negative Thoughts about Appearance

THERAPIST: OK, now let's work out how the BDD process happens to you. Usually, it begins with some sort of trigger or cue for your concern about your nose [or other body part]. What are typical triggers for you? Let's take the recent situation you told me about. Do you recall what set your negative thinking off?

PATIENT: I was looking at my reflection in the store window.

THERAPIST: OK, so let's write this down in the box labeled "Triggers" [in Form 7.1].

Identify the Patient's Immediate ("Knee-Jerk") Thoughts about Appearance

THERAPIST: So what were the thoughts or ideas that went through your mind right then?

PATIENT: I was trying to see how my nose looked that day, and I thought it looked big.

THERAPIST: So let's write "My nose looks big" in the box labeled "Ordinary Appearance Concerns" [in Form 7.1].

Discuss the Patient's Interpretations of These Thoughts

THERAPIST: Now here's a very important part. What was your immediate interpretation of this idea? This would be your knee-jerk reaction.

PATIENT: I guess I was thinking, "Oh, how awful." You know, "It just looks ugly. People won't like me because of it."

THERAPIST: OK, your thought was "Oh, how ugly. People won't like me." Yes?

Repeat the patient's interpretation aloud, modifying it slightly if necessary to help the patient hear it clearly. Then have the patient write this interpretation down in the "Your Mind as a Filter" box under "Self-defeating interpretations" in Form 7.1.

At this point it's important simply to collect information about when and how the BDD symptoms occur, without trying to change the patient's interpretations or beliefs. You can respond as follows to comments like the patient's last one in the exchange above, which reflects maladaptive and erroneous beliefs about the overimportance of appearance in social interaction:

> "This is interesting what you say about your nose. I guess if I assumed that people won't like me because of my scar, I would feel pretty sad and anxious in social situations. So I guess while we both have negative thoughts about our appearance, what's different for you and for other people with BDD is that for you, those appearance flaws affect your thoughts about how likeable you are and your personal worth."

Point Out the Patient's Selective Attention to Flaws and Overfocusing

THERAPIST: What did you attend to in this situation? Did you pay attention to what was going on around you, or did you spend most of our time thinking about or looking at your nose?

PATIENT: Oh, I could care less what was going on around me. I was just staring at my nose and thinking about how bad it looked.

THERAPIST: OK, let's write down "Staring at and thinking about my nose" [in the "Your Mind as a Filter" box under "Selective attention, overfocusing" in Form 7.1]. It appears that you selectively attended to specific aspects of your appearance, rather than seeing the big picture that others would see when they look at you. What do you think would happen if I only paid attention to my scar whenever I look at myself? What do you think would happen if I were to stare at it for, let's say, 2 hours at a time?

PATIENT: I know what you mean. . . . I think your scar would look huge and distorted to you.

Identify the Patient's Emotional Reactions to the Interpretation

Now continue the model-building process by helping the patient identify the feelings that follow from these self-defeating beliefs and selective attention to the perceived appearance flaw.

THERAPIST: When you have these kinds of thoughts (*pointing to the relevant box in Form 7.1*), how do you feel?

PATIENT: Pretty awful, I guess.

THERAPIST: What kind of awful? Do you feel anxious?

PATIENT: Yes, anxious, but I mostly feel ashamed . . . and sad, I guess.

Ask specifically about other negative emotions if the patient doesn't mention ones that you suspect from your previous discussions. These include shame, anxiety, depression, hopelessness, disgust, anger, and possibly other negative feelings. Record these in the "Distressing Feelings" box in Form 7.1.

Determine What Influences the Thoughts, Interpretations, and Emotions

You have already talked to your patient about immediate triggers, but you have not actually identified other factors that might exacerbate appearance concerns. Next, work on identifying the more immediate factors that might influence negative thoughts about appearance, maladaptive interpretations, and negative emotional reactions. Later you might also inquire about more distant causes. This may require some additional education about possible causes, from which the patient can choose relevant ones. Questions you can ask (with patient responses) are illustrated in the exchanges below:

> THERAPIST: Your negative interpretation about your nose being ugly and then about people not wanting to talk to you could be influenced by various things. Let's consider carefully why you might be jumping so quickly to a negative body image of yourself and to the idea that people would reject you. Do stressors at work, at home, and in social situations play any role in how you think about your looks? For example, do they affect your mood, so you feel more anxious or more depressed?
>
> PATIENT: Well, if I just think about the last couple of days, I'd say that work is pretty stressful right now. I have a deadline to submit a really complicated report next week, and I'm pretty anxious about it. And whenever I'm anxious, I worry a lot about my nose.
>
> THERAPIST: Yes, I remember you've told me before that stress makes your appearance concerns worse. So let's write this down as one of your triggers as well.

> THERAPIST: Sometimes people interpret intrusive thoughts differently when they've heard or read something recently in a magazine or the media, or from someone they've talked to. Various sources of information can affect how you react to thoughts about your appearance. Does this apply to you?
>
> PATIENT: Oh, yeah. When I read a fashion magazine or watch a movie, I keep comparing myself to those beautiful models and actresses, and then I feel horrible afterwards.

As these examples indicate, ask specifically about stress, mood, and any other factors (such as reading a fashion magazine) that you suspect from your previous discussions. Record these in the "Triggers" box of Form 7.1.

> THERAPIST: As we discussed in our first treatment session, early life experiences often have strong effects on how people see themselves. Some examples are family experiences, childhood experiences with friends or other people, and your medical history (for example, having surgery). You've told me about being teased as a kid, and I suspect this is an important contributor. Let's talk about that and any other experiences you think might be related to your BDD.
>
> PATIENT: When I was a kid, I had bad acne and was overweight. I looked like a total dork. The other kids would tease me; they'd call me a loser. It got better as I got older and my skin and weight improved.
>
> THERAPIST: Sounds like you've been through a lot as a child, and even though your skin and weight have changed, and nobody teases you now, you're still struggling with your body image. So let's write "Teasing" in the box on "Life Experiences" [in Form 7.1].

Refer back to any ideas provided by the patient in the first treatment session or in last week's homework, and elicit any new thoughts about these. Family expectations about appearance sometimes play an important role. Be especially alert to negative social experiences (e.g., childhood teasing or feeling rejected by childhood peers, as in the dialogue just above) or traumatic events (e.g., a severe dog bit to the face or other physically damaging experiences).

> "What about biological factors? You told me that some of your family members have body image concerns and social anxiety. So it's possible that you might have a biological and genetic predisposition to develop anxiety in social situations. Possibly because of your teasing experiences, these might have been focused on your body. So let's record these on our form. Anything else you can think of?"

> "Another contributor is our own personality traits and our core beliefs about ourselves. These usually come from our early experiences. You and I have already spoken about your tendency to be perfectionistic. Do you think this is contributing to your harsh interpretation of your looks?"

Refer to any previous conversations with the patient indicating personality traits and/or core beliefs that might belong in the model. Patients' common core beliefs about themselves and others include "I'm a freak," "I'm unlovable," and "Others will reject me." Record such traits or beliefs in the "Personality Traits and Core Beliefs" box in Form 7.1.

Patients are often unaware of their core beliefs at this early stage in treatment. If this is the case, do not push the patient to complete this box, simply leave it blank or only fill in personality traits.

Although this discussion of the possible causes of negative thoughts about appearance for each patient is important, it's best to accomplish this relatively briefly, usually in about 15 minutes. Some patients (especially those who have had psychodynamic therapy in the past) may want to discuss these issues at length and in great detail. However, this is not a focus of CBT-BDD treatment and is generally not productive, as it takes time away from learning strategies for change. Again, the purpose of developing this understanding is to create a model of the patient's BDD, which will then inform the treatment.

Identify the Patient's Self-Defeating Coping Strategies

Now turn to filling in the "Self-Defeating Coping Strategies" box in Form 7.1, with the patient's help.

> THERAPIST: OK, now let's fill in this part about coping strategies. We've figured out that after you're reminded of your nose, your interpretation makes you feel very anxious and ashamed. [Refer back to the previously filled-in boxes of Form 7.1 here.] As I understand it, you then avoid social situations, and you also avoid bright lights and making eye contact. Let's write down these avoidance methods here.
>
> PATIENT: OK.
>
> THERAPIST: When you can't avoid these situations, you then do things like checking your nose in your car mirror and in the pocket mirror you carry with you. You also ask your

mother for reassurance that you look OK, and you've told me you spend time comparing yourself to other people on TV. Also, you've made several doctors' appointments in the past few months to see about cosmetic surgery. Is there anything else?

PATIENT: Nothing I can think of at the moment.

THERAPIST: Let's write these behaviors, which are also called "rituals" or "compulsive behaviors," in this box. Rituals are behaviors people feel a strong urge to do over and over to try to reduce unpleasant feelings. In BDD, these are things like checking mirrors and asking for reassurance about how you look.

PATIENT: Oh, I didn't know that.

THERAPIST: The other thing I think we want to be aware of is that negative interpretations and emotions often cause people with BDD to further narrow their attention to the flaws, so they actually focus on them more than they might otherwise do. So selective attention can show up at various points in this model.

Handout 7.2 is an example of what a completed version of Form 7.1 might look like and what you should be working toward with your patient. Your patient might benefit from seeing this as an example.

Now discuss the (negative) effects of these coping strategies on the patient's thoughts and beliefs.

"Let's look at the effect of your coping methods on your thoughts about your nose. Avoiding social situations helps you temporarily avoid feeling bad when you're around people, but the problem is that it also reinforces the notion that your nose is really ugly. What I mean is that if you avoid socializing, you never get to see whether people actually react badly to you. In fact, when you're with people and feeling bad about your appearance, you avoid looking at them—so you might be missing positive or negative reactions. You don't really pay attention to their reaction, because you're so focused on your appearance. Does this make sense? [After confirming:] So what we're saying is that by avoiding social situations your discomfort is relieved in the short term, but it really leaves you feeling more anxious in the long run, because you don't have the chance to disconfirm your fears.

"The same problem occurs with the compulsive behaviors you do to try to reduce your discomfort. Every time you check the mirror or compare yourself with other people, you end up caught in a vicious cycle. Initially you sometimes might feel better, but sometimes only very briefly. This leads you to do the action again because it worked, even if only a little. But in fact, all the checking and comparing and reassurance seeking just reinforce the idea that something is wrong with you and give you no opportunity to challenge this idea. They don't give you a chance to see how you'd feel if you didn't do these things. These behaviors also keep you focused on the BDD rather than on other things in your life, and in this way they just feed the BDD.

"What about the effects of focusing so much on your nose?"

Let your patient respond. If appropriate, you could say something like this:

"It seems like the selective attention to your nose might trigger your anxiety, and then you might end up in a vicious cycle where the increase in anxiety leads to an increase in selective attention on your nose, which in turn makes your anxiety even worse."

At this point, many patients can see for themselves that this doesn't help them reduce their discomfort, but in fact makes it worse. You can use an analogy to help emphasize the point:

> "Focusing closely on anything often makes it seem distorted or unpleasant. Have you ever had the experience of staring at a word long enough that it begins to look odd or misspelled? Another example is paying close attention to a feeling in your body, like the pressure of your backpack strap on your shoulder. If you pay close attention to this for just a little while, it can feel as if the strap is cutting into your shoulder very painfully, even though this is not true. It is just an effect of focusing your attention."

Next, discuss the difference between attending to what is happening in a particular situation versus attending to one's perceived flaws. Help the patient consider whether the selective focus on the perceived appearance flaw and the negative thoughts and feelings associated with it might prevent her from observing external information that might disconfirm her concerns. Some or all of the questions below might be helpful during this discussion:

> "How often does it happen to you that your attention is just focused on yourself—in particular, your nose, and all the negative thoughts and feelings that go along with your appearance dissatisfaction?"
>
> "Do you think there might be some things to gain from paying attention to other aspects of yourself?"
>
> "Is it possible that you sometimes miss out on important things or information in your environment because you're so focused on what's going on inside your own mind?"
>
> "What would be the advantages of paying more attention to the world around you and less attention to your nose?"

In addition, help the patient consider how different her reaction would be if her interpretation of her thoughts about her appearance were benign, rather than negative:

> "Imagine for a moment that instead of thinking, 'My nose is ugly; people won't like me because of my nose,' you thought, 'Maybe my nose is not as perfect as I would like it to be. But that's OK. Most people aren't perfect anyway and they still have friends. In fact, my friends don't seem to care about my nose at all.' Would that change how you feel emotionally? [After reply:] Would it change what you do?"

The aim here is to point out the powerful effect of interpretations about the body (body image) and to distinguish these from actual appearance. A person can have actual physical flaws but *not* develop a negative body image and the negative emotions and behaviors that follow, whereas people with BDD usually look normal (or have very minor flaws) but experience very negative emotions and problematic behaviors as a result of their negative body image.

Ask the Patient to Summarize and Explain the Model

Ask the patient for a summary of what she now understands about the model and her own BDD symptoms. Fill in any gaps to make sure that the summary links thoughts about appearance to interpretations, negative emotions, and coping behaviors (avoidance, rituals). Tell the patient that the model is probably not yet complete, and that as treatment progresses, you will both be making changes and additions whenever new information emerges. Add that you will both refer back to this model throughout the treatment. Give the patient the copy of Form 7.1 you have completed together during the session for her notebook.

Assign Homework

Ask the patient to complete a blank copy of *Your Personal BDD Model* (Form 7.1) for typical intrusive appearance-related thoughts that occur during the coming week. Give your patient the *Sample Completed Your Personal BDD Model* (Handout 7.2) as an example. Encourage the patient to observe the triggers for BDD thinking, her immediate interpretations, her negative emotions, and her subsequent maladaptive coping and its effect on interpretations and emotions. Ask her to consider what factors might have contributed to that particular experience of BDD symptoms, and to record these in Form 7.1. Explain that this is an opportunity for the patient to think more about the model you have developed together in this session and to apply it to a different (but typical) BDD thought. The model the patient works on for homework will be discussed in the next session.

Ask for Summary of/Feedback on the Session

Briefly summarize the major points covered during the session, emphasizing positive points. Ask the patient to add any comments about what she has learned. Ask for feedback about any concerns the patient has about the session or your behavior, and respond accordingly.

FORM 7.1

Your Personal BDD Model

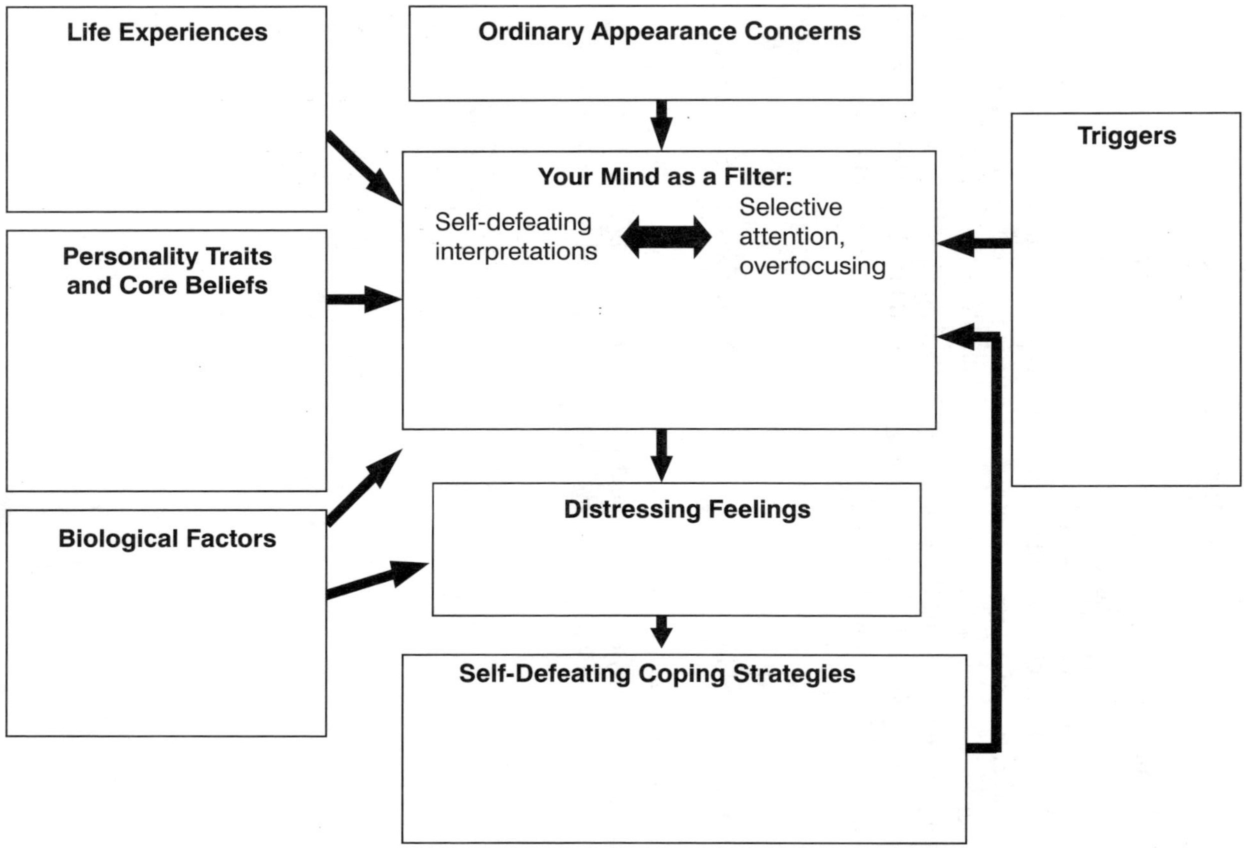

Adapted with permission of the publisher from Wilhelm, S. (2006). *Feeling Good about the Way You Look: A Program for Overcoming Body Image Problems*. New York: Guilford Press.

HANDOUT 7.1

Standard BDD Model

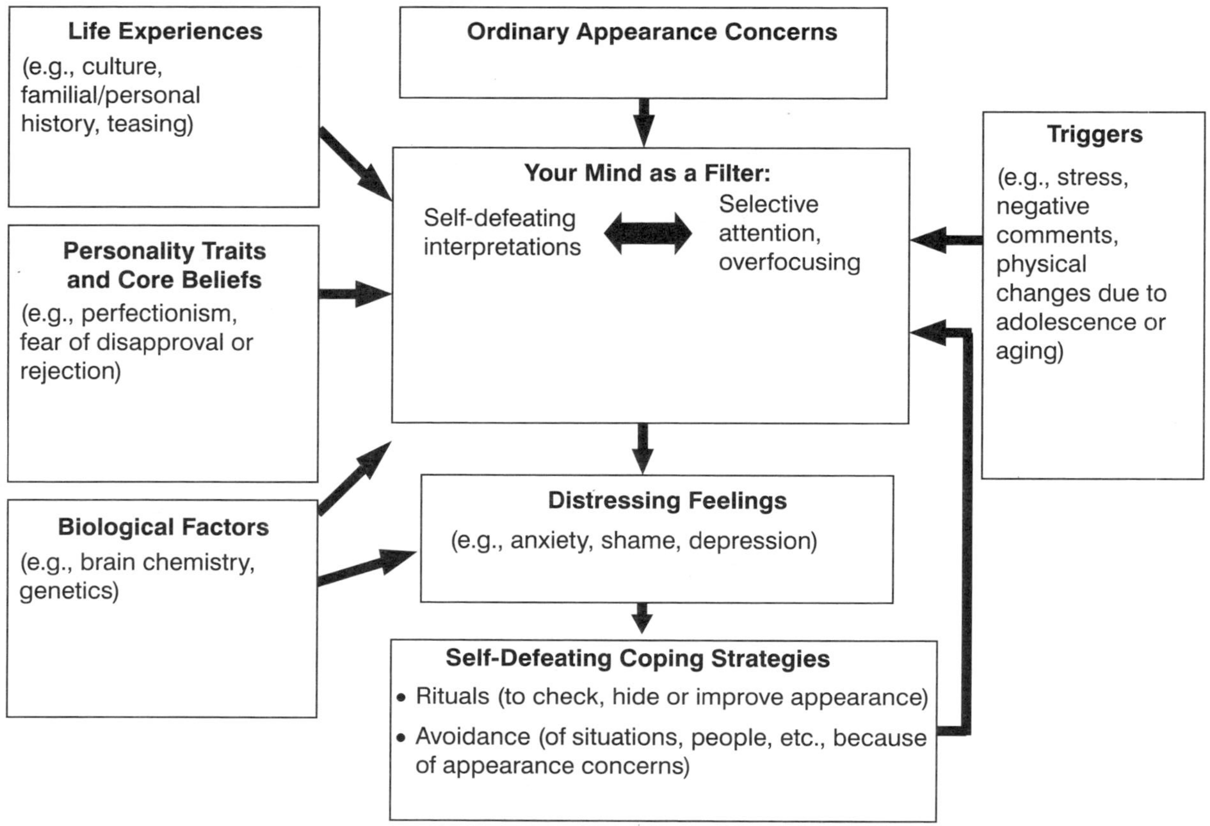

Adapted with permission of the publisher from Wilhelm, S. (2006). *Feeling Good about the Way You Look: A Program for Overcoming Body Image Problems*. New York: Guilford Press.

HANDOUT 7.2

Sample Completed Your Personal BDD Model

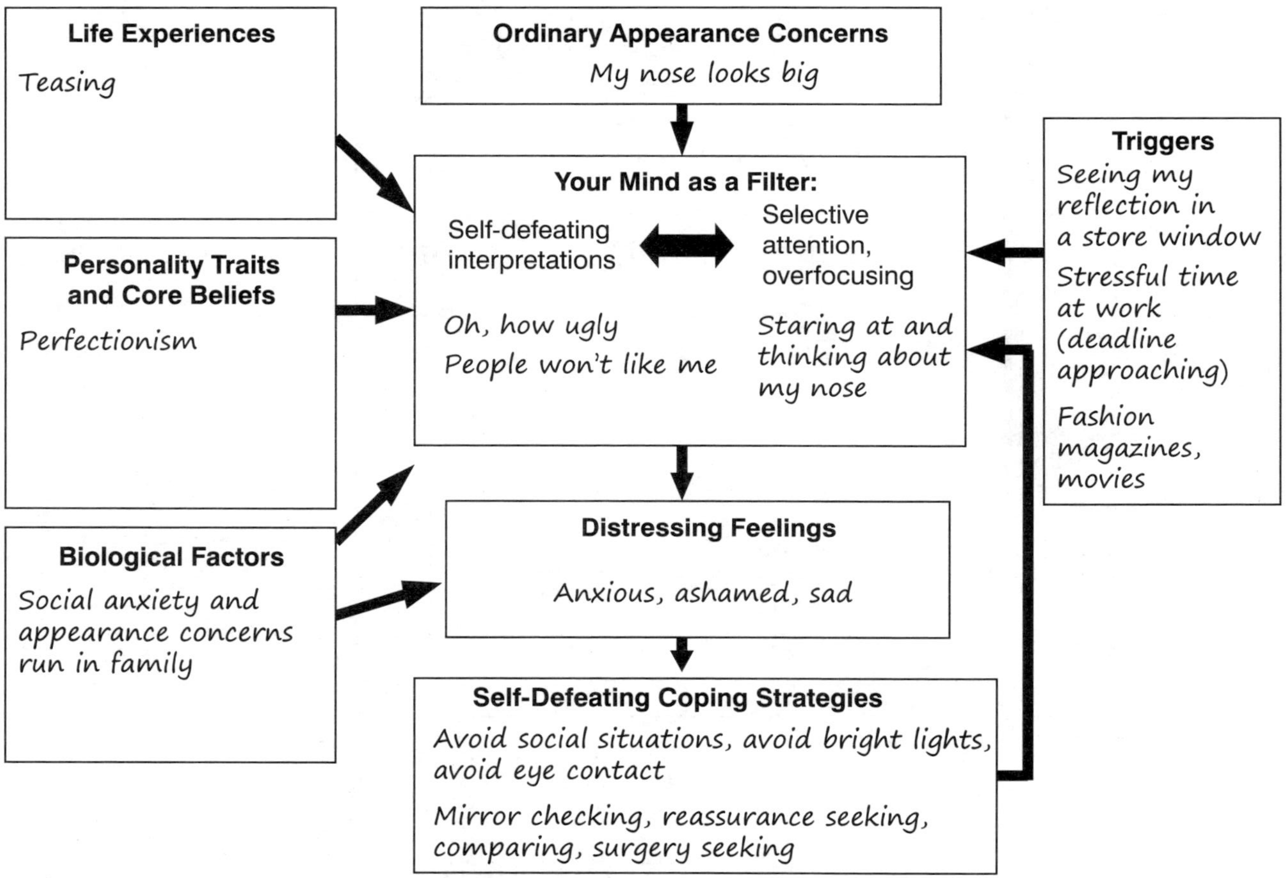

CHAPTER 8

SESSION 3

Setting Goals, Describing CBT-BDD, and Assessing Thoughts

SESSION SUMMARY

- ☐ Check mood and BDD symptoms.
- ☐ Briefly review the previous session.
- ☐ Set the agenda jointly with the patient.
- ☐ Review homework.
- ☐ Work on the agenda.
  - ☐ Discuss the patient's values and therapy goals.
  - ☐ Explain how CBT-BDD will help the patient.
  - ☐ Discuss the patient's therapy expectations.
  - ☐ Discuss expected progress.
  - ☐ Review the *Therapy Agreement* (Handout 8.3).
  - ☐ Offer a family session.
  - ☐ Discuss how to assess thoughts and beliefs.
- ☐ Assign homework.
- ☐ Ask for summary of feedback on the session.

SESSION FORMS AND HANDOUTS

BDI-II (or other depression inventory)

Personal Session Form (Form 2.1)

Therapist Session Form (Form 6.1)

Your Personal BDD Model (completed copy, plus several extra blank copies for homework) (Form 7.1)

BDD Model with Treatment Techniques (Handout 8.1)
Graph of Progress in Therapy (Handout 8.2)
Therapy Agreement (Handout 8.3)
Keeping Track of Your Thoughts (plus seven extra copies for homework) (Form 8.1)
Examples of Thoughts and Feelings (Handout 8.4)

Introduction to This Session

This chapter describes the third treatment session, which begins with an assessment of what your patient values and wants to accomplish in treatment. Your patient will get an overview of the treatment techniques to be covered, and you and your patient will work on setting realistic treatment expectations. You will also summarize what is expected from the patient, as well as what the patient can expect from you, during treatment. At this point in therapy, it is often helpful to discuss whether it would be helpful for a family member to come in for a session or part of a session. The session will end with a discussion of assessing thoughts and beliefs.

Check Mood and BDD Symptoms

Check the *BDI-II* (or other depression questionnaire) the patient has completed in the waiting room, and check the score on the suicidality item as you did in Session 2, responding as appropriate. Briefly explore the patient's general mood, and discuss BDD symptoms since the last session. Hand out a copy of the *Personal Session Form* (Form 2.1) so that the patient can record information he finds significant during the session.

Briefly Review the Previous Session

Briefly check in with the patient regarding his perception and understanding of the previous session.

Set the Agenda Jointly with the Patient

Convey the topics you'd like to cover during the session, including values and what the patient wants to accomplish in therapy, as well as how CBT-BDD will help the patient. You will discuss expectations, expected progress, and the *Therapy Agreement* (Handout 8.3; see below). You will end with an introduction on how to assess thoughts and beliefs.

Review Homework

Discuss your patient's homework from the previous session, including his observations of the link between thoughts and feelings during the week, and relate this to the patient's BDD model.

Ask to see his completed *Your Personal BDD Model* form (Form 7.1) and discuss the details of what he was able to identify as relevant factors and symptom sequences.

WORK ON THE AGENDA

Discuss the Patient's Values and Therapy Goals

Patients with BDD often say that their lives are dominated by their appearance concerns. Their efforts to avoid or control their negative thoughts or perceived flaws often only serve to perpetuate their distress. For example, a man who wishes to be in a relationship may never put himself in a situation where he could actually meet a woman, for fear of getting rejected because of his looks. Although he may be aware of the pain associated with his loneliness, he may not be fully aware of everything he does to perpetuate it. Thus one of the aims of CBT-BDD is to help patients to become less dominated by their appearance concerns, and to fully engage more in other things they may value in life (Hayes, Strosahl, & Wilson, 1999).

Thus your job as a therapist is not only to help your patients reduce their BDD symptoms, but also explicitly to enhance their quality of life by encouraging them to participate in valued activities. Engage a patient in a discussion about his values by asking about what, other than his appearance, might be important in his life. Typical topics we have discussed with our patients include romantic or family relationships (e.g., you might ask, "What kind of a parent do you want to be?"), social relationships (e.g., "How do you want to be in your friendships?"), work (e.g., "How important is your career to you?") or volunteerism (e.g., "Is there anything you want to do for your community?"), education (e.g., "What is important to you with respect to your training?"), and self-nurturance (e.g., "What do you want to do to enjoy yourself? Are you taking good care of yourself in terms of nutrition and exercise?"). Keep careful notes of the patient's values, as they are the general compass that will guide the process of therapy. Values will often make goals motivating, so you and your patient will refer to them frequently over the course of your treatment.

After reviewing your patient's values, you need to discuss what obstacles stand in the way of living consistently with his values. Encourage your patients to provide specific examples of how his BDD might get in the way of engaging in meaningful activities. This discussion often directly informs the specific goals you and your patient set jointly for treatment. Values differ from goals, in that values are ways of being that are important to your patient (e.g., leading a healthy lifestyle), and goals are focused on the future and on specific outcomes (e.g., taking a class).

After the discussion about values, have a brief discussion of what your patient wants to accomplish in therapy, and set long-term goals you both agree on. Record these on a piece of paper and copy this, so that each of you has a copy to refer to. Encourage the patient to think of *specific* goals that pertain to reducing BDD symptoms (negative thoughts and emotions, compulsive behaviors). In addition, help the patient consider increasing some behaviors that are now missing from his daily experiences (e.g., attending social events, taking a class). The goal of modifying body parts (e.g., with surgery) that the patient dislikes should not be included here, and you can suggest that if the patient still feels strongly about this later in the treatment, this can be a topic for discussion. (You can also address this issue later in treatment with the cosmetic treatment module; see Chapter 17.)

The following are examples of specific and potentially attainable long-term goals that might be appropriate for a man who worries excessively about his thinning hair. They reflect changes in thinking, emotions, and behaviors pertinent to the patient's BDD symptoms:

- Spend less than 10 minutes per day checking my hair in the mirror.
- Be able to take off my hat in public.
- Reduce my negative thoughts about myself.
- Attend more social events (even when I feel self-conscious).
- Focus more on preparing to get a (better) job.
- Take steps to begin dating.

The following are examples of the types of goals to avoid because they are unrealistic and probably unattainable, because they focus on attractiveness rather than on feeling and functioning better, or because they are too vague and nonspecific:

- Be the handsomest guy at work.
- Get any pretty girl to go out with me.
- Be the life of the party.
- Get a hair transplant.
- Be happy all the time.
- Never feel anxious.

You and the patient can prioritize his goals in a general way—for example, by working to reduce BDD symptoms first, and then focusing on things such as employment and dating. *You will want to refer back to the goals frequently during this treatment program*, to be sure that you and your patient are focusing on the same things and that the patient is making progress toward achieving his goals.

Explain How CBT-BDD Will Help the Patient

Now proceed to discuss how CBT-BDD will address the problems evident in the patient's model and will help him meet his goals for therapy. Illustrate with the *BDD Model with Treatment Techniques* handout (Handout 8.1). Make sure that this does not become a lecture, and encourage the patient to respond periodically or ask questions. You can say something like this:

> "Treatment will focus on helping you learn skills and strategies to overcome your BDD symptoms.
>
> "The first strategy is using cognitive therapy methods [point to "Cognitive Restructuring" in Handout 8.1]. Remember, 'cognitive' refers to 'thinking,'—as opposed to feelings or behaviors. Cognitive methods are designed to help you evaluate your interpretations and beliefs, even your basic beliefs about yourself. We have already seen that your beliefs about your appearance provoke a lot of negative emotions and rituals and avoidance, so it makes sense that changing beliefs can change emotions and also your behaviors.
>
> "You might have personal experience with this in the past. Did you smoke in the past but gave it up, or perhaps do something else that is good for your health? Public health information about the harmful effects of smoking and other practices have led lots of people to conclude that smoking wasn't good for them personally, and in a short time,

many people quit smoking. Because they changed their thoughts about smoking, they then changed their behavior. Can you think of any changes you've made in your own behavior because of changes in your beliefs?"

Modify the example below to best reflect the patient's specific symptoms.

"To help you with changing your self-defeating thoughts and beliefs, you might learn to ask yourself, 'What evidence do I have for my prediction that nobody will talk to me at the party? Has this happened before? Is it possible that I'm exaggerating my fears? If it's happened before, are there other possible interpretations for what happened besides my appearance? For example, if I don't make eye contact and only stand in a corner to make sure that nobody notices me, could this explain why others don't speak to me?'

"So, if we can evaluate your thinking about your appearance, this will go a long way toward changing your negative feelings and reducing your avoidance and rituals. [Point out this cycle on Handout 8.1 to reinforce this very important assertion]. We have a variety of methods for doing this, and I will explain them as we get further along in treatment.

"To help you with thoughts about your appearance and your tendency to overfocus on your flaws, we will also use mindfulness skills. [Point to "Mindfulness Skills" in Handout 8.1.] These are ways of using your mind, a little like simple meditation techniques, to enable you to tolerate negative thoughts about your appearance for longer and longer periods. You will learn simply to observe your thoughts without jumping to fight them or fix them. So, in other words, you will learn to just let your thoughts come and go naturally, without doing anything about them.

"Another part of therapy focuses on managing your strong negative emotional reactions. We call it emotion regulation or emotion management training. [Point to "Emotion Regulation Skills" in Handout 8.1.] For example, we might work on your depressed feelings by helping you become more active in what you do. Right now you tend to stay home a lot, and from what you've told me, this is not having a good effect on your mood. Often more activity and exercise can improve mood greatly. We can talk about this a little later on.

"We'll also work directly on helping you become more comfortable with your physical appearance through gradual exposure to situations you've been avoiding. You and I will work out a list of situations that you want to feel more comfortable in, and we'll develop homework assignments to help you do this."

Provide your patient with examples (e.g., going to a party, wearing an outfit that reveals a scar, etc.) that are consistent with his particular fears and fit with his goals. In some cases, brief exposures will be used to test whether the patient's beliefs are accurate. Since the prospect of doing exposure may frighten some patients—perhaps because people pushed them hard in the past—explain that you will work with them to make exposure manageable. Explain to each patient that this will be challenging, but that you will design the exposures together, and that the patient will have considerable input into the process.

Next, explain to the patient that therapy will gradually help him reduce the rituals that seem to be feeding his BDD. (Point to "Response Prevention" in Handout 8.1.) Provide your patient with examples from his model that fit his specific problem (e.g., decreasing mirror checking). When the patient has tried to cut down on his rituals without success, explain that he will learn these skills over time and will try to accomplish this gradually.

Then continue:

"We will also work on helping you redirect your attention—a kind of attentional or perceptual retraining, so you don't focus so exclusively on specific body parts that your perception becomes distorted. [Point to "Perceptual Retraining" in Handout 8.1.] As part of attentional retraining, you will learn again to see your entire face [body], rather than just focusing on the parts you don't like. Part of this will also be that you'll learn to take a nonjudgmental and more holistic stance. You will just look at yourself, and describe your appearance, without judging it.

"A related issue is that you might have noticed your attention shifting inward in many social situations. Instead of paying attention to whatever is going on around you (e.g., when you are talking to a friend) your attention might shift inward and you might be thinking about how anxious you feel or might be concerned whether others notice your perceived appearance flaw.

"Together, we will try to retrain your attention toward whatever is required in a particular situation, which typically means that you need to shift your attention outward (e.g., towards the story your friend might be telling you) instead of inward (i.e., towards your anxiety provoking thoughts and feelings)."

An important goal of CBT-BDD is to help patients learn skills so that they can retrain their own thinking and their behavior, as well as reduce their discomfort. Your discussion of treatment should impart confidence that the patient can work very effectively to relieve his body concerns. Use the research findings described in Chapter 1 of this manual to enhance the patient's expectations of success with CBT-BDD.

You can conclude by briefly summarizing the treatment approach:

"So, to summarize, our work in CBT-BDD will include helping you learn how to do these things:

- Evaluate unhelpful thinking and mistaken beliefs.
- Just tolerate negative thoughts without jumping to fight them or fix them.
- Do gradual exposures to feared situations.
- Cut back on rituals and avoidance behaviors that interfere with your life.
- Retrain your attention so that you don't just focus on your appearance concerns.
- Develop skills to prevent this problem in the future, especially under stress.

"Treatment requires work on thoughts and beliefs, emotions, and behavior. Therapy is a skill-building process. [Pause to give the patient time for reflection.] This is a lot to take in at once, and we'll work on these treatment components step by step over the next few months. What are your thoughts about all of this?"

Discuss the Patient's Therapy Expectations

Discuss the patient's therapy expectations and methods, to make sure that the patient is comfortable with what he will do in therapy. Early in this session, you can provide the following reassurance about his problem and treatment:

"You have a treatable condition. Treatment aims to help you feel much better, much less preoccupied, and much less anxious about your appearance. You aren't to blame for this problem. BDD is an illness, and there are specific things you can learn during therapy to manage your symptoms. You may have periods of feeling upset during treatment as you struggle with your fears, but these are temporary. If you stay in treatment, it is likely that your BDD symptoms will improve.

"Our goal is to substantially reduce your BDD, but we will probably won't eliminate it completely. Nevertheless, you'll learn many skills to enable you to reduce your fears and manage your tendencies to worry about your body."

Reassure the patient that while you'll encourage him to do his best and make progress, you won't force him to do anything he really doesn't want to do. Emphasize in these early sessions and throughout treatment that you will work as a team and that you will always want feedback from him:

"You're the one who will always decide what you do in this treatment. I'm here to make recommendations about what to do and to give you guidance. We'll work as a team, and you can give me feedback about what is and isn't working for you. If we need to make some changes in the treatment, we can do that."

If the patient expresses ambivalence about engaging in treatment, use the strategies from Chapter 5 to resolve the ambivalence and strengthen the patient's commitment to therapy. If necessary, you can add:

"I'll be asking you to take a 'wait and see' approach by trying out new ways of thinking before you decide what you'd like to do about your body image concerns."

Discuss Expected Progress

Be sure to prepare your patient for times when symptoms might worsen during treatment. This prevents a lot of anxiety and feelings of inadequacy later, at times when progress is slow or moving in the wrong direction. You can say something like the following:

"Most people expect that their progress in therapy will be very smooth, and that they will just steadily improve from the first day of treatment on. [Draw the graph shown in Figure 8.1.] But for most people it doesn't work like that. Most likely, your progress won't always be as fast as you'd like, and there will be some ups and downs. Here's an example of the pattern of progress that occurs for most people during treatment. [Draw the graph shown in Figure 8.2.] See those bumps? These are little lapses—some backsliding—that everyone has from time to time. In some ways it's good when they occur during treatment, because this way I can teach you problem-solving skills. Learning how to manage setbacks prevents relapse (getting worse) after treatment ends. [Give Handout 8.2 (*Graph of Progress in Therapy*) to the patient.] We'll work at a pace you can manage, and we both have to remember that patience is a virtue!"

Therapy Agreement

At this point, you can ask the patient whether he has any questions about the therapy. Once you have answered any such questions, the two of you can then draw up a formal therapy agreement. If it seems helpful, provide the patient with the *Therapy Agreement* (Handout 8.3) to help

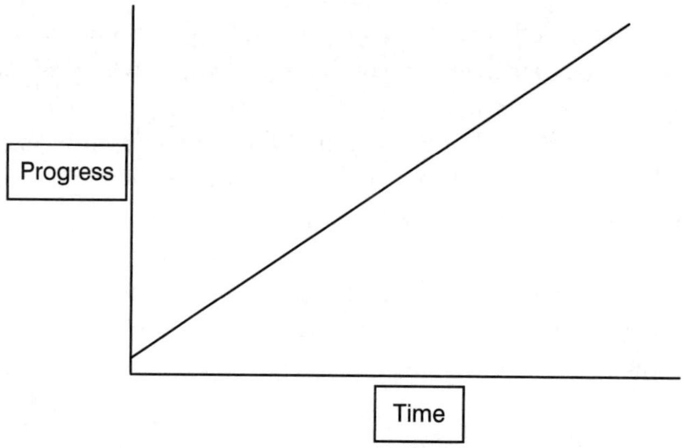

FIGURE 8.1. Graph of unrealistic progress in therapy. Adapted with permission of the publisher from Beck, J. S. (2011). *Cognitive Behavior Therapy: Basics and Beyond* (2nd ed.). New York: Guilford Press.

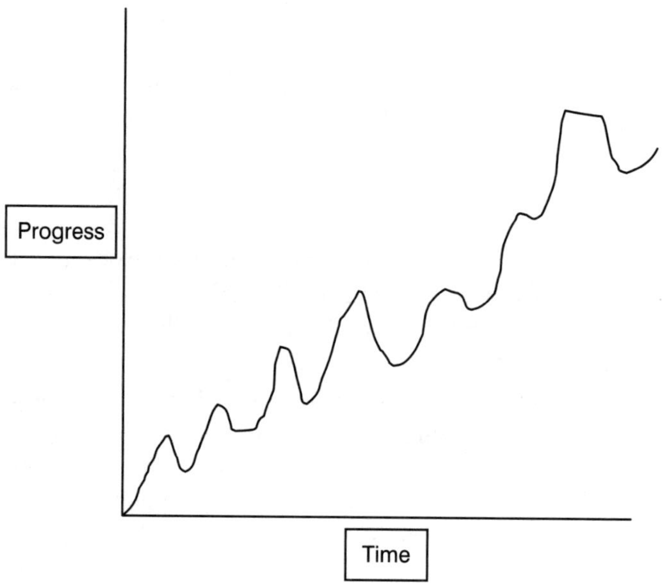

FIGURE 8.2. Graph of realistic progress in therapy. Adapted with permission of the publisher from Beck, J. S. (2011). *Cognitive Behavior Therapy: Basics and Beyond* (2nd ed.). New York: Guilford Press.

enhance his commitment to treatment and to helping himself. Ask the patient whether he has any questions about the agreement or would like to discuss it.

Offer a Family Session

Consider arranging a family session with the patient's parents and/or partner, to describe the treatment plan for them and to explain their potential role in therapy. If the patient refuses to have the parents or partner involved, you can explain that it's usually helpful to have family members attend one meeting, but you should also honor the patient's decision. A family meeting may enhance the parents' or partner's support of the patient, demystify the treatment, and help them stop any behaviors (e.g., participating in rituals) that may unwittingly be reinforcing the patient's BDD. From your perspective as the clinician, it can be helpful to have family members as "allies," especially with suicidal patients.

However, many patients keep their BDD a secret from family members because of embarrassment and shame and will not want to reveal their concerns at this time. In such a case, you can explore whether the patient has ever thought about telling family members and what the patient is afraid will happen if he reveals his symptoms. You can also explore the advantages and disadvantages of having the patient reveal the symptoms to a family member/partner. Again, whether to do so is ultimately the patient's choice.

If a family session takes place, we recommend that the patient be present for this meeting. In fact, family members may simply join the patient for a regularly scheduled session. Usually, the part of the session when the family is present will take about 30 minutes, but this is flexible. The purposes of the meeting with the family are as follows:

- Educate family members about BDD.
- Suggest reading materials for learning more about the disorder.
- Ask for the family members' observations about the patient's symptoms.
- Explain what the treatment will involve.
- Offer hope that BDD is very treatable.
- Advise family members that at some point during treatment, the patient and you will probably agree that family members' reassurance and accommodation is no longer in the patient's best interest. At this time, the patient will ask them to curtail these behaviors, but they should wait until they are requested to do so. Radically and immediately altering their behavior toward the patient will probably only produce resentment that won't help the BDD symptoms.
- Answer any questions that may arise.

If patient safety (i.e., suicidality) is a concern, the patient's parents or partner can be very helpful. Let the family members know of your concern, and develop a safety plan that involves the family. For example, let them know how to reach you in an emergency, including after hours, and emphasize that you welcome hearing from them if they have concerns for the patient's safety.

If the patient views a family meeting skeptically or negatively, ask the patient why, and determine whether there's anything he might like to accomplish in such a meeting. Some patients will want to think over the option of a family meeting, and you can ask them about it at the next session. The family meeting can be held at any point in the treatment, although it may be more helpful earlier in the treatment. It may also be helpful to invite family members back later in treatment—perhaps when you and the patient are addressing reassurance seeking, accommodation, and other issues that directly involve the family. However, this treatment is intended as an individual treatment for adults, not as couple or family treatment. Thus the focus of any meetings that involve the family should always be on the patient. However, in work with younger patients, family members will typically have to be much more directly involved in the treatment.

Discuss How to Assess Thoughts and Beliefs

All patients with BDD have maladaptive thoughts and negative beliefs that need to be addressed in treatment. The work you do during this part of this session will introduce the ideas contained in Chapter 9 on cognitive techniques. At this point, you simply want the patient to *learn to identify negative thoughts about appearance and the interpretations that follow these thoughts.* This is the first step of cognitive restructuring (you have already laid some groundwork for this when you and the patient developed his BDD model). In the next sessions, the patient will learn to critically evaluate his thoughts.

Remember that many patients with BDD believe that they have a physical problem, rather than a psychological one. Do *not* reject such patients' appearance-related beliefs outright, or get into battles about whether their perceived defects are real or not. On the other hand, do *not* reinforce their belief that there's something wrong with how they look. Don't agree with them if they try to convince you that they're right.

Also, do *not* agree even partially by saying something like "Well your nose is a little big, but it's not that bad," or "Well your nose isn't perfect, but you have beautiful eyes." Statements like these can be devastating to patients, who may even drop out of treatment as a result. Simply acknowledge the patients' perception of their appearance and explore further how they interpret this (i.e., the meaning of the defects they perceive). For example, you might say, "Even though your sideburns aren't as symmetrical as you'd like them to be, does this really mean that you can't leave the house?" More details on how to identify, evaluate, and modify the meaning of the perceived defects are provided below.

You can begin eliciting such thoughts directly in the session as follows:

THERAPIST: Let's spend a few minutes talking about the connection between thoughts and feelings and behavior. Tell me about the most recent occasion when you felt anxious or ashamed because of the way you look.

PATIENT: Just on my way here today . . . I felt pretty anxious.

THERAPIST: Can you describe what happened?

PATIENT: There was a woman walking on the sidewalk, actually walking straight toward me . . . and as soon as she was right in front of me, she started looking down!

THERAPIST: What was running through your mind just then?

PATIENT: She must have noticed my scars and was thinking how bad they look! That's why she looked down! So I immediately went to the other side of the road.

THERAPIST: OK, this is a good example of the kind of negative thoughts we want to work on in treatment. These kinds of thoughts determine how you feel and even what you do. You had the thought 'She must have noticed my scars.' How were you feeling when you had this thought?

PATIENT: Awful! Really embarrassed . . . sort of ashamed.

THERAPIST: So your thought produced an emotional reaction—a feeling—and then you crossed the road, so it also influenced what you did—your behavior. You avoided the person. Whenever you feel anxious, discouraged, or self-conscious about your looks, and do things to protect yourself, it's the result of your negative thinking. We'll be talking about this a lot in the next few sessions.

Introduce the Patient to Evaluating Thoughts and Interpretations

Notice how the therapist in the exchange above points out the *impact of interpretations on the patient's feelings and behavior.* This is a central part of the standard cognitive-behavioral model of BDD and is illustrated in the personalized model you and the patient have already developed. In the exchange below, pay attention to how the therapist introduces the idea that the patient's interpretation of the situation may be false:

THERAPIST: Just because you think that the woman looked down because of your scars doesn't mean that this was actually the reason she looked down. Do you ever evaluate your thoughts? I mean, do you ever ask yourself if there are any other possible interpretations of the situations that bother you?

PATIENT: No, I don't. What else could it be?

THERAPIST: It's possible that your negative interpretation of this situation is true, but it's also possible that it's wrong. Of course, even if your interpretation was wrong, it would still make you feel upset!

PATIENT: Hmm . . .

THERAPIST: What I'm trying to say it that you aren't reacting with anxiety to this particular situation. Rather, you're reacting with anxiety to your *interpretation* of this situation. And I am also saying that *it's possible that your interpretation is just one viewpoint, and there might be others.* Let's imagine for a moment that she did just what you saw. She looked down, but you knew it wasn't because of you or your appearance. How do you think you'd feel if you saw her look down but didn't think it was because of you? [After patient's reply:] How does this fit into our model of your BDD?

PATIENT: I suppose I'd feel a lot better, less ashamed.

THERAPIST: So if you thought that the only reason the woman looked down is because she's a little shy, and looking down is what she always does, you'd feel better, less ashamed?

PATIENT: Yes.

THERAPIST: So it's actually not the woman's behavior that's causing a problem, but the meaning you attached to her behavior—your interpretation of her behavior.

PATIENT: Maybe . . .

THERAPIST: I wonder if you don't usually consider other explanations, but just assume your interpretation is correct?

PATIENT: I guess I do.

THERAPIST: In therapy, we'll go through a number of different steps. First, we'll pay attention to when your mood gets worse. We'll try to notice when you suddenly start feeling anxious, ashamed, or sad. Then we'll identify what caused that change in the way you felt. *Usually changes in your feelings are caused by a thought.* Next, we'll evaluate whether your interpretation of that thought is really helpful and correct. If it's unhelpful or not reasonable, we'll try to change it. Does this make sense?

PATIENT: Yes, it does.

THERAPIST: Let me show you how this fits with the cognitive-behavioral model we discussed last week. (*Points to various parts of Handout 8.1 while talking.*) Here you can see the trigger, your thought, and your interpretation—in other words, the meaning you attach to it. And here is how this makes you feel. And here, in the box right next to the interpretation, you can see "Cognitive Restructuring." So this is just a fancy way of saying that we are going to check out your thoughts to see if they are useful or not. Can you summarize for me what we have talked about so far?

PATIENT: Well, I think we said that I usually just assume that my negative thoughts related to my appearance are true . . . and so I often feel anxious. But I actually never evaluate whether my thoughts are right. So in therapy I will learn to consider other ideas, maybe change my thinking.

THERAPIST: That's exactly right. Great.

Figure 8.3 is a summary of the strategies you can use to help your patients identify negative thoughts.

Introduce the Patient to Monitoring Negative Thoughts

After a general discussion with the patient about the relationship among thoughts, feelings, and behaviors and the fact that thoughts might be false, turn your focus to *thought monitoring*. Provide the patients with several copies of the form titled *Keeping Track of Your Thoughts* (Form 8.1). Alternatively, the patient may prefer to buy a small notebook and create his own thought record. That's fine as long as he follows the format recommended below.

In the first section of Form 8.1, ask the patient to fill in the date and time of the situation that triggered the negative thought. In the next section, the patient will briefly describe the situation itself. After this comes the immediate negative thought, followed by how the thought

STRATEGIES TO HELP PATIENTS IDENTIFY NEGATIVE THOUGHTS

1. Ask patients to describe a recent situation when they noticed a mood shift or felt especially upset.
2. If you notice mood shifts in the session, ask patients what they were just thinking. Use questions like these:
   "What were you thinking in that situation?"
   "What was running through your mind?"
   "What did this situation mean to you?"

FIGURE 8.3. Strategies to help patients identify negative thoughts.

makes the patient feel. In the exchange below, the therapist describes the use of thought records to a patient who believed that everyone was staring at his nose when he entered a friend's apartment for a party.

THERAPIST: Next, I'd like to show you a form that will help you keep track of your negative thoughts. This type of form is called a "thought record." I'd like you to use it during the coming week when you feel upset about your appearance. At the top I'd like you to describe the situation that made you feel anxious. So when did you have the thought?

PATIENT: Last night around 7:30, as soon as I walked through the door of my friend's apartment where the party was.

THERAPIST: OK. So let's put "October 8, 7:30 P.M., entering friend's apartment" in the first section. Now, in the second section, write down the actual thought that bothered you. What were you thinking just then?

PATIENT: I was thinking, "Everyone is looking at me! They must be thinking, 'Look how big his nose is!' I look like a freak!"

THERAPIST: OK, let's write that down in the next section. In the last section, describe how the thought made you feel.

PATIENT: Anxious, really terrified.

THERAPIST: And how anxious were you? Let's use a scale from 0, which is no discomfort at all, to 100, which means as anxious as you have ever felt in your life. How anxious were you then?

PATIENT: 110.

THERAPIST: That's not on our scale, so do you mean 100? That was truly the worst you ever felt? Are you sure?

PATIENT: Maybe not the worst, but really bad. Say 90.

Ask your patient to try to fill in as many thoughts as possible in each blank copy of Form 8.1 (or other thought record) he completes. An example of a completed Form 8.1 can be found in Figure 8.4.

Date/time: *October 8, 7:30 P.M.*
Situation: *Entering friend's apartment*
Thoughts: *Everyone is looking at me! They must be thinking, "Look how big his nose is!" I look like a freak!*
Feelings and intensity (0–100): *Anxious (90)*

FIGURE 8.4. Sample completed *Keeping Track of Your Thoughts.*

Help the Patient Differentiate Thoughts from Feelings

Some patients have difficulty differentiating thoughts from feelings. They may benefit from *Examples of Thoughts and Feelings* (Handout 8.4). Even patients who are fairly good at this may find the handout useful. You can spend a little time looking at Handout 8.4 and helping your patient understand these concepts. If there isn't time to do this in this session, you could review it at the next session while reviewing the homework. It may also be helpful to refer back to this handout later in the treatment if the patient seems to be struggling with identifying thoughts and feelings. It's important for the patient to grasp this difference in order to learn cognitive restructuring.

Assign Thought Records for Homework

After introducing thought monitoring in the session, ask your patient to complete one or more copies of Form 8.1 (or other thought records) per day for homework.

THERAPIST: The goal of thought monitoring is to make you aware when your negative thoughts pop up. These thoughts can happen so fast you're hardly aware of them. You'll get the most out of this exercise if you fill out thought records on a daily basis, writing down at least a few thoughts a day. It's best to write these thoughts down right after they occur, but if this isn't possible, record them as soon as you can find the time.

PATIENT: But I usually try to distract myself from this stuff because it upsets me. Now you're asking me to do just the opposite. I really don't like focusing on this stuff. What if writing down the thoughts makes me feel worse?

THERAPIST: It's possible that writing down the thoughts will make you feel worse at first, because you haven't learned skills yet to cope with the thoughts. But raising your awareness of the thoughts is an important step in our treatment that we can't skip. I've done these thought records many times with my patients, and I think you'll find that the discomfort is temporary. Could you consider the discomfort you feel while filling out thought records as an investment in your future?

PATIENT: What if I don't have any negative thoughts about my appearance before the next session?

THERAPIST: If you don't have any, we'll talk next time about what to do. But, meanwhile, keep on the lookout for any situation in which thoughts or concerns about your appearance come up.

ASSIGN HOMEWORK

As just discussed, explain *Keeping Track of Your Thoughts* (Form 8.1) and assign this to be completed several times in the coming week.

Also, ask the patient to complete one or more additional blank copies of *Your Personal BDD Model* (Form 7.1) immediately after specific experiences during the week that are typical of their BDD experiences. This will require the patient to observe the cues for the BDD fears, as well as current thoughts, interpretations, behaviors (or avoidance), and past events he believes are contributing. The patient should bring these completed forms to the next session for discussion.

Be sure that the patient feels comfortable with, and is prepared to follow through with, homework. Check to verify that he believes he can complete the homework just assigned. The easiest way to do this is to ask the patient, "How likely do you think you are to be able to do this? Do you think you are 80% likely, or just 60%, or some other number?" If the number is below 80%, discuss changing the homework to something that the patient is sure he can complete. You'll want to do this in every session when you assign homework.

Ask for Summary of/Feedback on the Session

Ask the patient to briefly summarize the major points covered during the session. Also ask whether the patient had any concerns about the session or your behavior, and respond appropriately.

FORM 8.1

Keeping Track of Your Thoughts

Date/time:
Situation:
Thoughts:
Feelings and intensity (0–100):

HANDOUT 8.1

BDD Model with Treatment Techniques

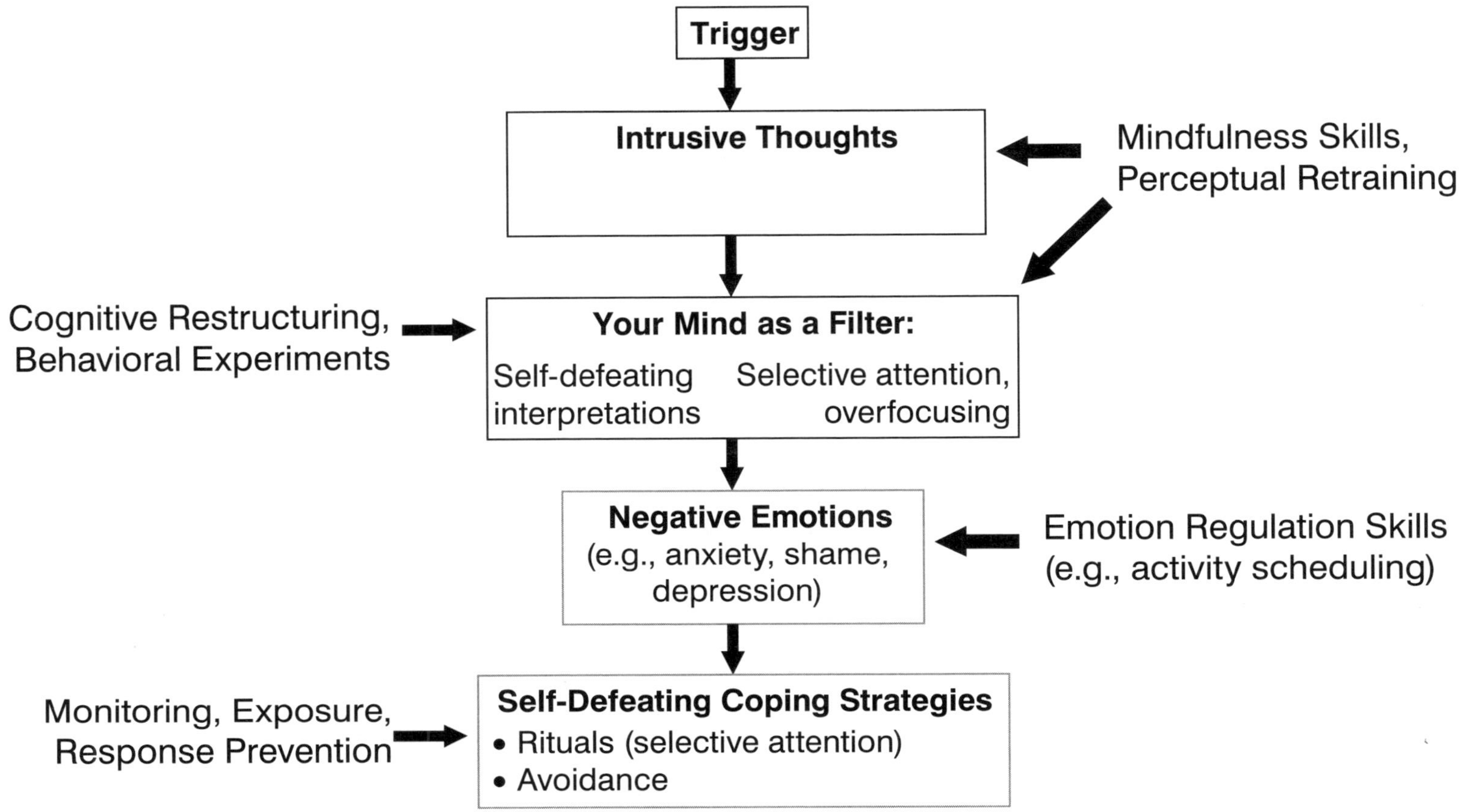

HANDOUT 8.2

Graph of Progress in Therapy

Unrealistic Progress in Therapy

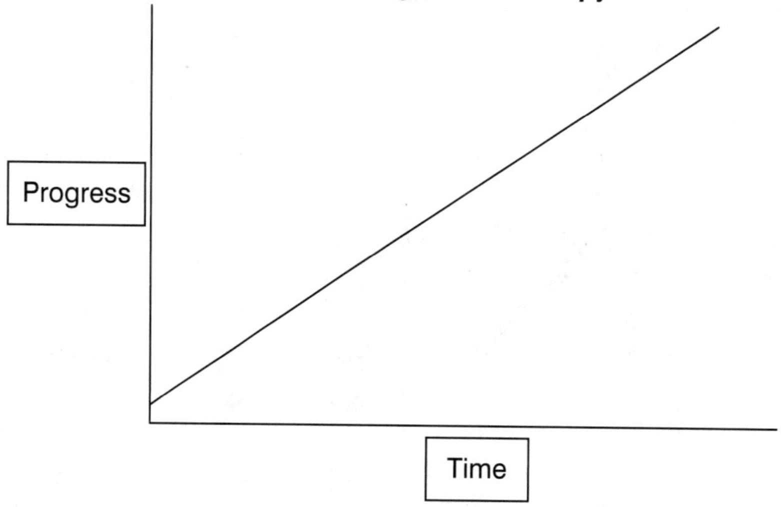

Realistic Progress in Therapy

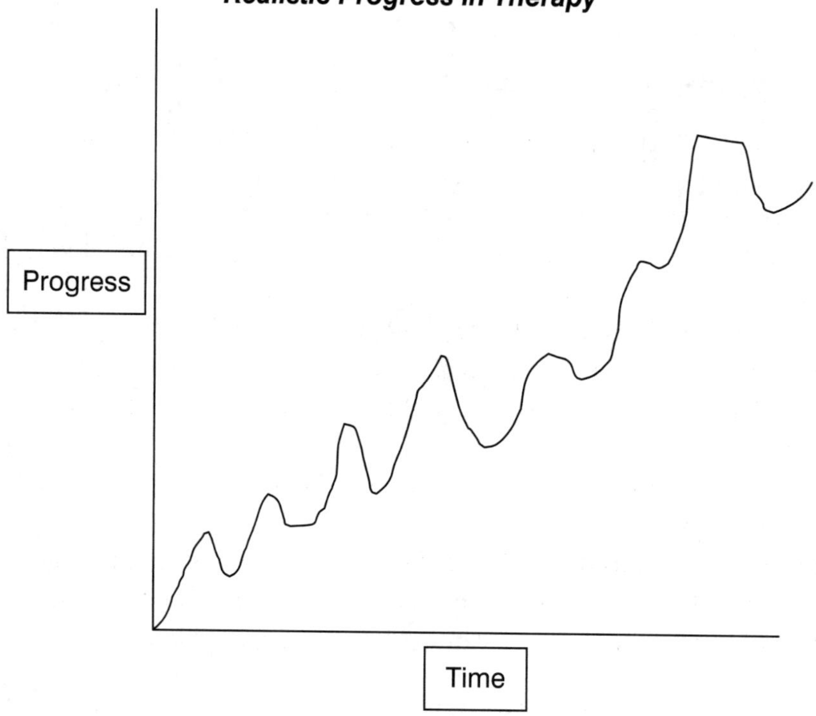

Adapted with permission of the publisher from Beck, J. S. (2011). *Cognitive Behavior Therapy: Basics and Beyond* (2nd ed.). New York: Guilford Press.

HANDOUT 8.3

Therapy Agreement

The patient agrees to:

1. Attend all scheduled therapy sessions or call in advance to change the appointment.
2. Help set the agenda for sessions.
3. Understand personal BDD symptoms in the context of family, cultural, and personal experiences
4. Complete assessments of BDD and related symptoms.
5. Learn cognitive strategies to deal with thoughts and beliefs.
6. Complete exposures to reduce discomfort about body perceptions.
7. Work on reducing and stopping rituals and avoidance behaviors related to BDD symptoms.
8. Design and complete homework; report on any problems with homework assignments.
9. Give the therapist feedback about the treatment.
10. Plan strategies for maintaining the benefits of therapy.

The therapist agrees to:

1. Attend all scheduled therapy sessions or call in advance to change the appointment.
2. Set the agenda for each session in consultation with the patient.
3. Help identify specific symptoms of BDD.
4. Provide education about BDD symptoms in the context of family and cultural experiences.
5. Teach cognitive strategies to deal with thoughts and beliefs.
6. Plan and guide exposures to reduce discomfort about body perceptions.
7. Help the patient reduce and eventually stop rituals and avoidance behaviors related to BDD symptoms.
8. Review assigned homework from the previous session.
9. Design homework with the patient.
10. Review progress and help the patient determine the next steps in treatment.
11. Listen to any feedback and take appropriate action to correct problems.
12. Plan strategies with the patient to maintain the benefits of therapy.

Adapted with permission of the publisher from Wilhelm, S., and Steketee, G. (2006). *Cognitive Therapy for Obsessive-Compulsive Disorder.* Oakland, CA: New Harbinger Publications.

HANDOUT 8.4

Examples of Thoughts and Feelings

Examples of Thoughts

"Everyone's staring at my skin! They must be thinking, 'Look how red his face is!' I look like a freak!"

"My skin looks terrible today—it's a total disaster."

"I'll look totally ugly for the rest of my life."

"No girl will ever want to go out with me because I'm not big enough."

"No one will talk with me at the party because my hair looks so bad."

"Everyone in here must be thinking I look really ugly."

"I look like such a freak—I'll never have any friends."

"I'll be the only one at the meeting who'll look really bad."

"Everyone's going to stare at me in math class."

"I'll never look as good as that model."

Examples of Feelings

Anxious

Annoyed

Irritated

Upset

Nervous

Sad

Depressed

Down

Frustrated

Hopeless

Ashamed

Self-conscious

Angry

Enraged

Disappointed

Gloomy

PART III

CORE TREATMENT COMPONENTS

This third part of the manual focuses on *core treatment components* that are typically used with all patients. Those core components include the evaluation of self-defeating thoughts (cognitive restructuring); exposure to avoided situations, along with ritual prevention; perceptual and attentional retraining to help the patients shift their attention, attend to things other than the perceived appearance flaws; and advanced cognitive strategies that focus on distorted deeper-level beliefs.

Patients vary in the speed at which they learn the core treatment components, but new strategies are typically introduced until the end of Session 11, often even later. As treatment progresses, your patients will need to combine the core treatment strategies they have already learned within treatment sessions and in homework assignments. They will also engage in increasingly challenging exercises. For example, exposures done later in the treatment will be more difficult than those done earlier in the treatment. Typically, patients continue to practice all of the core strategies until Session 20, although individual treatment needs will vary.

Because patients may suffer from symptoms that require specialized treatment approaches (such as skin picking), you can supplement the core treatment components with the optional treatment modules that address specialized problems. These optional modules are introduced in Part IV of the manual.

No treatment would be complete without a proper focus on termination, relapse prevention, and booster sessions, and therefore the content of those sessions is covered at the end of Part III.

CHAPTER 9

SESSIONS 4–5

Evaluating Self-Defeating Thoughts

SESSION SUMMARY

- ☐ Check mood and BDD symptoms.
- ☐ Briefly review the previous session.
- ☐ Set the agenda jointly with the patient.
- ☐ Review homework.
- ☐ Work on the agenda.
  - ☐ Discuss types of cognitive errors.
  - ☐ Help the patient identify her common thinking errors.
  - ☐ Help the patient begin to evaluate automatic negative thoughts.
  - ☐ Help the patient select thoughts to work on.
  - ☐ Help the patient begin to answer negative thoughts with rational responses.
- ☐ Assign homework.
- ☐ Ask for summary of/feedback on the session.

SESSION FORMS AND HANDOUTS

BDI-II (or other depression inventory)

Personal Session Form (Form 2.1)

Therapist Session Form (Form 6.1)

Types of Maladaptive Thinking (Handout 9.1)

Questions to Evaluate Negative Thoughts (Handout 9.2)

Sample Completed Thought Record (Handout 9.3)

Thought Record (plus several extra copies for homework) (Form 9.1)

Introduction to This Session

All patients with BDD have negative thoughts that contribute significantly to their symptoms. In fact, these thoughts play a central role in maintaining BDD symptoms. This chapter focuses on evaluating self-defeating thoughts and developing more rational and helpful thoughts. This process is also known as "cognitive restructuring" and is of fundamental importance. It builds upon the groundwork on identifying thoughts that was laid in Session 3 (Chapter 8).

Usually you will start cognitive restructuring in Session 4. However, as described earlier, you need to use your own judgment in deciding how quickly you can move with a particular patient. Most of the interventions described in this chapter can be covered in one session. However, in our experience, it is usually helpful to use all of Session 5 to review the homework for Session 4 and fill out new thought records to practice the skills described in this chapter. This is especially the case for patients with poorer insight and those who are delusional (i.e., completely convinced that their appearance beliefs are true and undistorted). It can take a fair amount of practice for such patients to grasp the basics of cognitive restructuring.

After two sessions on cognitive restructuring, you can move on to exposure and response (ritual) prevention. We have found it helpful to train patients in cognitive restructuring before introducing exposure and response prevention, because cognitive restructuring helps them gain a new perspective on anxiety-provoking situations. In this way, their willingness to reenter those situations and decrease rituals is often enhanced. Cognitive restructuring will later be integrated into the exposure and ritual prevention exercises that are learned in Chapters 10 and 11, and it will continue to be used and practiced throughout the treatment. More advanced cognitive strategies are described in Chapter 13.

As in previous sessions, first briefly check on BDD symptoms and mood since the last session. In the previous session, your patient has learned to identify thoughts about her appearance. You have discussed that thoughts can be false. This message is important and can be repeated as necessary over the course of this session. For homework, your patient has attempted to record thoughts related to her appearance. As you review the homework, ensure that the patient has written thoughts (not feelings or descriptions of the situation) in the appropriate section. If she is unable to identify thoughts or to distinguish them from other experiences, keep working on this critical step before you move on, using *Examples of Thoughts and Feelings* (Handout 8.4).

Check Mood and BDD Symptoms

Check the *BDI-II* (or other depression inventory) the patient has completed in the waiting room, and check the score on the suicidality item, responding as appropriate. Briefly explore the patient's general mood, and discuss BDD symptoms since the last session. Hand out the *Personal Session Form* (Form 2.1) so that the patient can record information she finds significant during the session.

Briefly Review the Previous Session

Briefly check in with the patient regarding her perception and understanding of the previous session.

SET THE AGENDA JOINTLY WITH THE PATIENT

Convey the topics you'd like to cover during the session, and get the patient's feedback on these.

REVIEW HOMEWORK

Discuss your patient's homework from the previous session, including the copies she has filled out of *Keeping Track of Your Thoughts* (Form 8.1) and *Your Personal BDD Model* (Form 7.1).

WORK ON THE AGENDA

Discuss Types of Cognitive Errors

Now that you have taught the patient to identify maladaptive thoughts, help her learn how to evaluate these thoughts. This requires her to take a step back and determine whether her thoughts are true and useful, or instead are unhelpful and may contain errors. A first technique is to evaluate whether the thoughts contain any cognitive errors. These cognitive errors are based on Judith Beck's (2011) work and have been informed by Thomas Cash's (2008) work.

Be careful to introduce thinking errors as *normal* as you show the *Types of Maladaptive Thinking* handout (Handout 9.1) and give it to your patient:

> "Here is a handout on various types of thinking. [Give the patient Handout 9.1.] Our task is to figure out whether you might be making any of those errors. Many people do, myself included. Also be aware that your negative thoughts can contain more than one thinking error."

It's helpful to read this handout together with the patient and ask which errors she thinks she sometimes has in her thoughts. When a thinking error seems to be particularly relevant, engage the patient in a discussion about how this particular error makes her feel and how the error affects her behavior.

Below are suggestions for introducing the various thinking errors. Have the patient look at the handout as you go through this material.

All-or-Nothing Thinking: Model or Monster?

> "Let's take a look at the all-or-nothing thinking error. It means that you see things as either black or white. There are beauties and beasts, fashion models and monsters . . . and nothing else. Since very few people really look perfect, the model category is difficult to get into, but it's really easy to end up in the monster category. If you have a minor imperfection, you'd consider yourself absolutely hideous, because there's no such thing as just looking average or OK. You're either stunning or revolting. All-or-nothing thinking can also be reflected in thoughts that include words such as 'always,' 'never,' or 'I'm the only one.' In other words, it involves thinking in extremes. Here are a few BDD examples: 'With skin like this, I'll always look *totally* ugly.' Or 'I'm the only one in the store who looks like such a freak.' "Do you engage in all-or-nothing thinking? [If yes:] Can you give me an example?"

Unfair Comparisons

"People with all-or-nothing thinking often have a tendency to make unfair comparisons, too. In other words, you might be more likely to compare yourself with the picture from an airbrushed supermodel who has spent several hours doing her makeup than with the girl next door. Do you think you ever struggle with unfair comparisons? [If yes:] Can you give me an example?"

"Should" Statements

"If you have an issue with 'should' statements, you have overly rigid rules about the way things 'should be,' and you're very bothered if something doesn't quite meet your expectations. For example, if your rule is 'I should never have a blemish on my skin,' then you're holding yourself to a standard that's so high you can't live up to it. Do you engage in 'should' statements? [If yes:] Can you give me an example?"

Mind Reading

"If you engage in mind reading, you assume you know what other people are thinking, and usually you think that they're thinking negative things about you. Because you don't like the way you look, you assume that other people don't like your looks either, and that they're thinking about your appearance. But, you know, how you look might not be that important to them, and it's quite possible that they're thinking about something completely unrelated to your looks. Have you done any mind reading lately? [If yes:] Could you give me an example?"

Fortune Telling

THERAPIST: Fortune telling is similar to mind reading. With both of these, you jump to a conclusion without having all the facts. The main difference is that in fortune telling, you're predicting that things will turn out badly in the future. A typical example would be to expect that you'll have a bad time at a party, because nobody will want to talk to you because of your appearance. Do you sometimes engage in fortune telling?

PATIENT: I guess so. I think I'll gross people out because of my scars. So, even if a guy seems nice to me, I won't talk to him at a party because I think he'll put me down.

THERAPIST: So what kind of an effect does this have on your feelings?

PATIENT: It makes me anxious in social situations, and hopeless.

THERAPIST: And in this case, what kind of an effect does the fortune telling have on your behavior?

PATIENT: Well . . . I won't talk to anyone at parties.

THERAPIST: So you just predict that things will turn out badly, and you don't allow the opportunity to find out how things would have turned out if you hadn't tried to predict the future, but had just talked to the guy to see for yourself how he would react.

In the exchange above, the therapist suspects that fortune telling is a major problem for this patient (as it is for many patients with BDD). Therefore, right after introducing this type of error, the therapist follows with questions about the impact of the error on thoughts and behaviors. This is something you should do every time you believe a particular error is highly relevant for a patient.

Catastrophizing

"The next error on the handout, catastrophizing, is an extreme form of fortune telling. It means that you predict that things will turn out horribly, without having any real evidence for this. So, for example, if you notice a minor blemish on your face, you predict that it will turn into this huge, disgusting zit covering half of your face, and that your boyfriend will be so disgusted he'll break up with you. Or you predict that because of how you look, you'll always be alone."

Personalization (Self-Absorption)

THERAPIST: The next error on the handout is personalization or self-absorption. This means that you interpret all kind of events as having something *negative* to do with *you*. So, for example, when you buy groceries, and the cashier is rude, you think "If I didn't have those freckles, he would've been nice to me." On the other hand, if the cashier had smiled, you'd have thought that he was laughing about your freckles. Do you think you might have an issue with personalization?

PATIENT: Yes, I think I do this all the time. When people smile at me, I think they're laughing about my freckles. When they look away, I assume that they're disgusted about my freckles and can't stand looking at them. I can't win. No matter what other people do, I always think it has to do with my freckles.

Emotional Reasoning

THERAPIST: Emotional reasoning is an error I encounter all the time when working with my patients. Basically, it means that you believe that something *is* true just because it *feels* true. So feelings have become the evidence for the truth, in the absence of any objective evidence. Other people may be telling you that you look good, but you just won't believe it. This error explains why your body image can change, even though your appearance hasn't changed. For example, after we hear a negative comment about our appearance or after we eat a pint of ice cream, our actual looks haven't really changed, but we may feel less attractive. Does this make sense?

PATIENT: Yes, it's like "I feel hideous, therefore I am."

THERAPIST: Exactly. Another important aspect of emotional reasoning is the impact of your mood on your thinking. On a day when you're already anxious and unhappy because your boss dumped way more work on you than you can possibly handle before your next deadline, it's a lot easier to get anxious about your bumpy nose than on a day when everything has gone fine. In this case, the stress that's related to your job just spreads to your appearance. [Here the therapist can refer back to the portion of the *Standard BDD Model* (Handout 7.1) that shows the influence of stress and other triggers (on the right side of the handout) on thoughts.]

Labeling

"If you label yourself, basically you're calling yourself names. For example, you might be calling yourself 'pig nose,' 'freak,' or 'ugly.' Obviously, these labels aren't really helpful. In reality, you might actually only dislike your nose, but when you call yourself 'pig nose,' it's like nothing else matters but your nose. The other aspects of your appearance, your personality, and everything else about you are just being disregarded. Do you think you engage in labeling? [If yes:] Can you give me an example?"

Selective Attention and Magnification

THERAPIST: Selective attention means that you focus more on certain things than on others. So, for example, you might focus more on the wrinkles on your forehead than on your pretty eyes, your nice voice, or your accomplishments as a working mother. Because you're so caught up with your wrinkles, you miss the big picture. Other examples are "All that matters is my hair. My nice shoulders and skin don't count." Or "This pimple is huge and disgusting—it's the only thing anyone sees on my face!" How relevant is the selective attention error for you?

PATIENT: It's pretty relevant. Actually, I seem to be beating myself up for my flaws all the time . . . and you're right: I never seem to notice anything good.

THERAPIST: Selective attention might also be at work when you stand in front of the mirror. You are just busy hunting for flaws, rather than seeing the big picture. So if you see a wrinkle or an enlarged pore, you might just keep staring at it. And if you do this for a while, eventually it appears huge and obvious. So it's like your perception changes because you keep looking at it for such a long time. Magnification means that you not only pay attention to your shortcomings, but you blow them out of proportion. It's like looking at them through a magnifying glass. Let me ask you this: When you look at other people, do you think you get a realistic image of what they are like? Can you see the big picture there?

PATIENT: No, I only notice the features that are better than mine.

Or, if the patient says that she does see the big picture when she looks at others, you can comment that it's interesting that the patient does this when looking at others but not at herself.

Discounting the Positives

THERAPIST: It's only human to pay attention to things that are in line with your beliefs, and to disregard the rest. Many people with BDD don't pay any attention to their positive traits—it's as if they didn't have any. They only focus on the negatives. For example, they may say things like "It doesn't matter if I'm smart and nice to other people. All that matters is how big my thighs are." Do you think you ever do this?

PATIENT: Oh, yeah. All the time!

THERAPIST: Since you're convinced you look unattractive, it's probably also a lot easier for you to remember times when you got teased than times when someone gave you a compliment. How do you respond when someone tells you something nice about yourself?

PATIENT: Well, my brother's friend recently said I had a beautiful smile. But that only made me feel bad . . . I made an excuse and left the room.

THERAPIST: How come? What was running through your mind just then?

PATIENT: He probably just felt sorry for me. After all, he's known our family for a long time. He must know that I never date and always sit at home. I know he meant well; he just said it to cheer me up. But I just felt pathetic. I don't want his sympathy.

Patients with BDD often feel that others are just nice because they feel sorry for them. If a patient mentions this in session, you can ask the patient whether there are other possible explanations why the other person might have been nice (see the section below on evaluation of thoughts). Another avenue is to explore the consequences of minimizing compliments with your patient. For example, you could discuss that this prevents her from enjoying compliments and using them as a foundation for improved self-esteem. Discounting a compliment (e.g., "You really like this old sweater? I always thought it was pretty ratty") might actually make the person who originally made the compliment feel awkward. Also, ask your patient how she would feel if she gave someone a compliment and it was rejected. You can also ask for an example of this. Most importantly, discounting compliments disqualifies evidence showing that the negative appearance-related beliefs are wrong.

Help the Patient Identify Her Common Thinking Errors

After you have reviewed all of the thinking errors with your patient, help her start to identify the types of errors that are common in her automatic thoughts. She can use the *Thought Readers* (Form 8.1) she completed at home for this purpose. The *Thought Record* (Form 9.1), which is an extended version of *Keeping Track of Your Thoughts* (Form 8.1), is used for this purpose. As soon as your patient finds a particular error, have her write the error in Form 8.1 under the thought. If one type of error occurs more often than others, point this out and discuss the impact of this particular error on feelings and behavior. Especially earlier in the treatment, patients will find it much easier to identify cognitive errors if they actually look at *Types of Maladaptive Thinking* (Handout 9.1) and select the one(s) they think apply to a particular thought. (Keep in mind that many thoughts contain more than one type of error.)

It's important that patients thoughtfully select the errors that apply to each thought. Some patients write down the same errors for all thoughts, without really thinking this through. When reviewing a *Thought Record* with a patient, you can ask, "How do you think this error applies to the thought you have here?"

Help the Patient Begin to Evaluate Automatic Negative Thoughts

After your patient has gained some skill in identifying maladaptive thoughts and thinking errors, begin working on the core skill of cognitive therapy: evaluating thoughts. The patient will learn to examine the usefulness and validity of her negative thinking about her appearance and herself. If the thoughts are not useful or are invalid, you can help the patient replace them with more helpful and accurate ones.

As you're introducing this technique, be sure not to imply that you believe everything your patient thinks is distorted. Acknowledge that many of her thoughts are valid and that some thoughts contain some truth. For example, the distress patients express in response to their negative thoughts is always real, and many patients do have some minor physical defect, giving a small kernel of truth to their (overly) negative interpretations. But also introduce the idea that sometimes it may be useful to consider a different perspective:

THERAPIST: As we agreed earlier, not all thoughts are true, and many contain thinking errors that make you feel bad. So next I'd like to show you a way to evaluate thoughts. This will help determine if your thoughts are useful or not, and if they're true or distorted. If they're not helpful or if they're distorted, we'll want to come up with new thoughts and beliefs that may be more accurate and more helpful for you.

PATIENT: (*Laughs.*) Sounds like brainwashing.

THERAPIST: Well, the idea isn't to just replace a bad thought with a good thought—it's not simply positive thinking or brainwashing. What we'll try to accomplish is very much like what a scientist or a detective would do. We'll just treat your thoughts like theories or assumptions to be tested, rather than facts. Here, why don't you take a look at these questions? (*Shows patient Handout 9.2,* Questions to Evaluate Negative Thoughts.) They'll help us with evaluating your thoughts. (*Patient and therapist read through questions.*) Not all of those questions will be helpful for all of your thoughts, so these are really just guidelines. The number and type of questions we can ask is limited only by our creativity, and we'll make up our own questions as we go through treatment.

Help the Patient Select Thoughts to Work On

Most likely, your patient will tell you about many negative thoughts over the course of each session and in her homework. How do you select which thought(s) to focus on in treatment? There are several criteria you should apply.

First of all, the target thoughts should *apply to the goals* the patient has set for therapy. So if the thoughts pertain to a problem that is not BDD-related or relates to only some minor BDD problem, it may not be worth focusing on it (although later in the treatment it will be fruitful to do cognitive restructuring of core beliefs, such as "I'm worthless").

Ask your patient to rate any thoughts in terms of how much *distress* they cause, on a scale from 0 to 100. The most distressing thoughts should be addressed first. However, if this is too overwhelming for the patient, you could focus on less distressing thoughts first.

If your patient has certain thoughts *frequently*, try to focus on these, rather than on thoughts that are unusual or less common.

It is usually more productive to focus on thoughts that address the *meaning*, or the patient's *interpretation*, of the perceived defect (e.g., "I'll never get a date because my nose is so ugly"), rather than thoughts that just describe what the defect looks like (e.g., "My nose is too bumpy" or "I'm ugly"). As another example, it's more profitable to do cognitive restructuring for the thoughts "No one will want to talk with me at the party because I look so ugly," or "Everyone is thinking how strange I look," rather than "I have red spots on my face." This is because the first two statements include clear cognitive errors that can be identified (e.g., fortune telling, mind reading). The statement about the red spots does not lend itself to cognitive restructuring. It's harder to identify cognitive errors in such a statement, and the patient will often discount attempts to find cognitive errors with "This is what I see when I look in the mirror." However, if the patient can agree that she was also thinking something like "These big red spots make me look really ugly," or "These red spots are totally disgusting," you can more easily help her identify cognitive errors such as labeling, emotional reasoning, and all-or-nothing thinking. The thoughts provided in *Examples of Thoughts and Feelings* (Handout 8.4) in Chapter 8 exemplify the types of thoughts common in BDD that contain cognitive errors and are fruitful to focus on in treatment.

Similarly, avoid focusing on thoughts that express feelings about the defect (e.g., "I hate my nose"). Feelings do not contain cognitive errors and are therefore not amenable to cognitive restructuring. Those thoughts should be reframed (e.g., "I know your nose isn't as straight as you'd like it to be, but does this really mean that . . . ?").

It also isn't helpful to focus on wishes—for example, "I wish I looked better." Wishes generally do not involve cognitive errors. Instead, focus on negative thoughts.

Early in treatment, as the patient is still practicing her cognitive skills, it's usually better to focus on beliefs that are easily accessible to her and are triggered by specific situations. As the patient becomes more skilled, you can focus on deeper, more global beliefs (core beliefs) that usually start with "I am . . . " and are very brief (e.g., "I'm not good enough," "I'm unlovable"). Working with core beliefs is discussed in Chapter 13.

It can be more difficult to do cognitive restructuring with patients who are delusional (i.e., those who are completely convinced that they look abnormal and don't have any doubt about this). When you begin working on thoughts with such a patient, *work on less firmly held beliefs first*. You can develop a hierarchy of negative thoughts and ask the patient to rate these according to how strongly she believes them. You can then work with the less firmly held thoughts/beliefs first and then work up to the more firmly held beliefs. (Chapter 10 contains a lengthier discussion of working with delusional patients, with a focus on doing exposures with these patients.)

After you have introduced *Questions to Evaluate Negative Thoughts* (Handout 9.2) to your patient, apply these questions to some relevant thoughts and fill out a *Thought Record* (Form 9.1) with the patient. This *Thought Record* is an extended version of *Keeping Track of Your Thoughts* (Form 8.1), introduced in the previous session. Give the patient the *Sample Completed Thought Record* (Handout 9.3) to use as a guide. You can work on thoughts the patient has mentioned during that session, or you can select some thoughts from the homework assignment.

The following exchange illustrates how a therapist and patient would have completed the sample *Thought Record* shown in Handout 9.3:

THERAPIST: So let's take a look at the thoughts you had right when you and your sister entered the restaurant: "They'll think my sister looks better than me," and "Everyone is staring at my skin! They must be thinking, 'Look how red her face is!' " It seems like the thought about your sister didn't bother you much—you rated it pretty low. So let's look at the other thought about your skin. You rated this one 90 on the distress scale. Do you think there are any cognitive errors in your thinking?

PATIENT: I'm not sure. They probably *were* thinking that.

THERAPIST: OK, what you just said now—"They probably were thinking that"—let's write it down. Is there any cognitive error in this statement? Let's look at the list [i.e., Handout 9.1].

PATIENT: (*Looks at the list.*) Well, maybe it's mind reading—but, you know, they could be thinking that.

THERAPIST: Nice job on this. Mind reading does seem to fit, because you were guessing at what they thought. Did they actually say to you or your sister that your face looked red?

PATIENT: No, I suppose not, but I thought they were all focusing on me.

THERAPIST: So maybe another cognitive error was personalization? You thought they were all focused on *you* rather than on their food or the conversation they were having. What do you think?

PATIENT: Yeah, probably.

THERAPIST: Let's also see if any of the questions on the other list [i.e., Handout 9.2] would help you figure out whether your thought was correct or not. Take a look at the questions. Would any be useful?

PATIENT: Let me look. Maybe "What is the evidence . . . ?"

THERAPIST: I agree. So let's try to answer this question. What is the evidence that people were thinking about your face?

PATIENT: Well, in this case there wasn't really any, but other times I do see people looking at me funny.

THERAPIST: OK. For the moment, let's stick to this situation. You didn't have evidence that people were staring at or thinking about your face. Is there an alternative point of view? What else might they be thinking about?

PATIENT: Hmm, could be anything. Maybe other stuff that's more important to them, I guess.

THERAPIST: Like what?

PATIENT: Maybe their own appearance. Or, actually, since they're in a restaurant, I suppose they might be thinking about dinner, or about the conversations they're having.

THERAPIST: Do you think it's more likely that they think about your looks, or about other stuff?

PATIENT: Their own stuff, I guess.

THERAPIST: OK, let's summarize this and write it on your *Thought Record* [Form 9.1]: "There's no evidence they're thinking about my appearance. It's more likely they're thinking about things that are more important for them, like their dinner or their conversation." Got that down?

Help the Patient Begin to Answer Negative Thoughts with Rational Responses

As you can see in the dialogue presented above, and in Handout 9.3, a therapist uses a patient's answers to the questions to generate a rational response. This is basically a summary of the patient's ideas about alternative explanations. The rational response represents a new, more likely, and more helpful perspective on the original thought. It incorporates what the patient has learned by identifying cognitive errors.

A rational response needs to be *at least somewhat believable* to be helpful. If the rational response is not at all believable, the patient is unlikely to accept it or to change her thinking as a result. If it's not believable at all, try to help the patient come up with something that's at least a little bit believable (the more believable the better). Especially early in treatment, including words like "maybe" or "possibly" may work better than more definitive statements that the patient won't believe at all. For example, a delusional patient is more likely to accept a rational response such as the following if it includes the word "maybe": "Maybe they were talking about something else, like the baseball game they were watching, not my nose." Keep in mind that patients are very unlikely to consider the rational response to be *completely* believable, especially early in treatment. Insight in BDD tends to be very poor, and lots of practice with cognitive restructuring is usually required before this is achieved.

If a patient has trouble coming up with a rational response, suggest responding or "talking back" to the cognitive errors. For example, if the patient has identified mind reading as a cognitive error, a rational response could start with "I really can't read people's minds," or "I really don't know what they are thinking." Sometimes we do a brief exercise in a session where we have a patient try to guess what we are thinking, or we try to guess what the patient is thinking. Usually the guess is wildly wrong, which illustrates that no one—not even a therapist—can do this. A rational response to a fortune-telling error could include "I really can't predict the future and don't know for sure what will happen."

If the patient balks, saying that there's no actual evidence that the rational response is true, you can agree with this and emphasize that the point of this exercise is to *consider* whether there may be an alternative thought, rather than simply to accept her thoughts as true. You can note that later in the treatment the patient will conduct experiments (during exposure) to collect actual evidence as to whether her negative thoughts are true. If the patient continues to have a lot of difficulty generating a rational response that is more accurate, you can shift to putting more focus on generating a rational response that is more *helpful* (i.e., less distressing) to the patient.

Sometimes patients suggest rational responses that reflect unrealistic positive thinking. These responses, too, are not very believable and therefore not very helpful. For example, a patient whose coworker didn't pay attention to her might think, "Everyone rejects me because of my hideous nose." A rational response would *not* be "My coworkers love me," because this is not very convincing. A more appropriate, realistic, and believable alternative response might be "He's very busy with our upcoming deadline, and that's probably why he didn't stop by and chat like he usually does."

It is generally more helpful to put the rational response in terms of what *is* likely to be true than only in terms of what *isn't* likely to be true. For example, notice in the dialogue above and in Handout 9.3 that the therapist helps the patient to conclude not only "There's no evidence they are thinking about my appearance," but also "It's more likely they're thinking about things that are more important for them, like their dinner, or their conversation." This helps the patient think more broadly about the situation and about possible alternative and helpful perspectives. As another example, rather than having the patient write simply "I am ignoring my positive traits," it would be helpful to have her note also that she has some and what a few of them are. To help the patient take this step, you can say something like this:

> "So you've written down here that there's no evidence they were thinking about your appearance. That's very good. So what do you think they might have been thinking about? . . . Good. Why don't you write that down too?"

Here you'll want to be careful that the patient doesn't come up with too definitive a statement, such as "I'm sure they were thinking about their dinner." First, this may not be believable. Also, it involves the kind of cognitive error (mind reading) you are trying to help the patient avoid! Instead, the idea is to help the patient open her mind to other possibilities, or likelihoods, that she can consider.

When a patient feels she has developed a particularly helpful rational response, you can suggest writing it down on a small piece of paper or a note card to carry with her (e.g., in her wallet) so that she can look at it from time to time—whenever it might be helpful. It may be more helpful to suggest this a little later in the treatment, after the patient has had more experience with cognitive restructuring and is more likely to have developed helpful responses that she more fully believes.

ASSIGN HOMEWORK

The homework assignment for Session 3 (see Chapter 8) was to have the patient record her thoughts on the preliminary thought record described there (*Keeping Track of Your Thoughts*, Form 8.1). Now that the patient has begun to identify erroneous thinking and generate alternative thoughts, the following assignment would be appropriate:

THERAPIST: For homework, I'd like you to try to come up with rational responses to the negative thoughts you're struggling with this week. Can you summarize for me how you'd go about this?

PATIENT: First, I'd record the situation that makes me feel upset on my *Thought Record* form. Then I'd identify the upsetting thoughts and how they made me feel. Then I ask myself some questions. The answers to the questions will help me develop a rational response. Then I'll write down a rational response.

THERAPIST: Great.

PATIENT: But I have one question: What if all of my thoughts are basically the same? Should I write the same thought more than once?

THERAPIST: It's fine to write the same thought down more than once, but it would be good to try to capture as many different thoughts as possible.

PATIENT: OK.

THERAPIST: For homework, please fill out your own copies of the *Thought Record* (*hands patient blank copies of Form 9.1*) for new situations that come up. Don't be disappointed if you can't come up with great rational responses at first. It's like learning any new skill, sort of like learning to figure-skate or become a good baseball player [or any other example that is meaningful to the patient].

ASK FOR SUMMARY OF/FEEDBACK ON THE SESSION

As in Session 3, ask the patient to briefly summarize the major points covered during the session. Also ask whether the patient had any concerns about the session or your behavior, and respond appropriately.

GOING FORWARD

As described above, different patients learn at different paces. Although most of the cognitive skills described in this chapter can be introduced in just one session, you are likely to need a second session (and perhaps even more time than this) to review what was learned in the first session on cognitive restructuring, review the homework, and have the patient fill out new copies of the *Thought Record*.

During the second session, you can follow the same general session structure used throughout this manual (start with checking mood and BDD symptoms, etc.) and pick up where you left off with the content of this chapter. Below is a session outline you can follow, should you decide that your patient would benefit from a second session entirely devoted to the evaluation and modification of self-defeating thoughts.

SESSION SUMMARY FOR THE SECOND SESSION ON SELF-DEFEATING THOUGHTS

- ☐ Check mood and BDD symptoms.
- ☐ Briefly review the previous session.
- ☐ Set the agenda jointly with the patient.
- ☐ Review homework (the copies of the *Thought Record* [Form 9.1] the patient has completed at home). This can sometimes be rather time-consuming, as the patient may still be having difficulties completing the *Thought Record*.
- ☐ Work on the agenda.
  - ☐ Complete one or more copies of the *Thought Record* in session (e.g., based on experiences the patient had over the course of the week or on the way to the session).
- ☐ Assign homework: Have the patient complete further copies of the *Thought Record* (Form 9.1) and apply the methods learned during treatment to generate rational responses.
- ☐ Ask for summary of/feedback on the session.

As noted above, once you have finished introducing the patient to cognitive restructuring, this skill should be integrated into future sessions and practiced as part of homework assignments for the rest of the treatment. Because you will keep practicing cognitive skills over the course of the treatment, your patient does not need to master the cognitive strategies perfectly before you move on to the exposure exercises described in Chapter 10.

FORM 9.1

Thought Record

Date/time:
Situation:
Thoughts:
Believability of thoughts (0–100):
Feelings and intensity (0–100):
Cognitive errors:
Questions:
Rational response:
Believability of rational response (0–100%):
Feelings and intensity (0–100):

Adapted with permission of the publisher from Beck, J. S. (2011). *Cognitive Behavior Therapy: Basics and Beyond.* New York: Guilford Press.

HANDOUT 9.1

Types of Maladaptive Thinking

All-or-Nothing Thinking: Model or Monster?

You see things as either black or white. There are only beauties and beasts, models and monsters. Average-looking people do not exist. All-or-nothing thinking can also be reflected in thoughts that include words such as "always," "never," or "I'm the only one." In other words, it involves thinking in extremes.

BDD examples:

"With skin like this, I'll always look *totally* ugly."

"I'm the only one in the store who looks like such a freak."

Unfair Comparisons

If you have unrealistically high standards and focus primarily on the few people who meet those standards, you'll find yourself inferior in comparison. For example, you compare yourself with airbrushed models in magazines and feel upset that you don't look as good as they do. Thus, all-or-nothing thinking is often related to "unfair comparisons."

BDD examples:

"I'll never look as perfect as that model on the cover of *Cosmo*."

"I look like a wimp compared to those guys in *GQ*."

"Should" Statements

You have overly rigid rules about the way things "should be," and you're extremely bothered if something doesn't quite meet your expectations. Thoughts with "must" and "have to" and "ought" fall in the same category.

BDD examples:

"My hair has to be perfect."

"I should never have a pimple."

(cont.)

Adapted with permission of the publisher from Beck, J. S. (2011). *Cognitive Behavior Therapy: Basics and Beyond*. New York: Guilford Press.

Mind Reading

Mind reading is a form of jumping to conclusions without having all the evidence. You assume that *other people* are thinking badly about your appearance, because *you* don't like the way you look.

BDD examples:

"I know she's thinking I look bad."

"People in my class will think I look ugly."

Fortune Telling

Fortune telling is similar to mind reading, in that you are jumping to a conclusion without having all the facts. The main difference is that in fortune telling you are predicting that things will turn out badly in the future. It's as if you have a crystal ball.

BDD examples:

"I know I'll have a terrible time at the party; no one will want to talk to me because I look strange."

"I know she's going to smirk at me when she sees I'm losing my hair."

Catastrophizing

Catastrophizing is an extreme form of fortune telling. You predict that things will turn out absolutely horribly, without having evidence for this.

BDD examples:

"I'll always be alone."

"No girl/guy will ever want to go out with me."

Personalization (Self-Absorption)

You interpret all kind of events as having something negative to do with you, even if they actually don't.

BDD examples:

"Everyone on the subway must be thinking how bad I look today."

"I know people in the mall are judging me and staring at me."

(cont.)

Emotional Reasoning

You believe that something *is* true just because it *feels* true. Feelings have become the evidence for the truth, in the absence of any objective evidence.

BDD examples:

"I feel so fat after eating this donut; I must look like an elephant."

"I'm ugly. Period!"

Labeling

You call yourself bad names. For example, you might be calling yourself "pig nose" or "freak." These are labels that discount and put down yourself as a whole person.

BDD examples:

"I look like a freak."

"I'm so ugly."

Selective Attention and Magnification

You focus more on certain negative parts of your appearance than on other parts. Because you are so caught up with those negative aspects, you miss the big picture. In magnification, you not only pay attention to your shortcomings, but you also blow them out of proportion. This is like looking at them through a magnifying glass. Also, when you look at others, you only notice the body parts you consider more attractive than your own.

BDD examples:

"All that matters is my hair. My nice shoulders and skin don't count."

"This pimple is huge and disgusting—it's the only thing anyone sees on my face!"

Discounting the Positives

You disregard the good things you have going for yourself.

BDD examples:

"It doesn't matter if I'm smart and nice to people. All that matters is how big my thighs are."

"All people are noticing is how tiny my breasts are."

HANDOUT 9.2

Questions to Evaluate Negative Thoughts

1. Is this thought helpful right now? What are the advantages and disadvantages of this type of thinking?
2. Is there an alternative/more advantageous point of view?
3. What is the evidence for my thought? What is the evidence against it? Which is more convincing?
4. Is my thought logical? Is there another—perhaps more rational—way of looking at that? Is there another explanation for . . . ?
5. Am I really 100% certain that . . . , or is this just one out of many possibilities?
6. So what if . . . ?
7. What's the worst that could happen if my fears came true? Could I live through it? Would it really change the big picture? Would I still care about it a few years down the road?
8. What's the best that could happen?
9. Does . . . really mean that . . .
10. What would I tell a friend in this situation?
11. What would a friend say to me about this? What would my friend advise me to do?
12. What can I do now?

Adapted with permission of the publisher from Beck, J. S. (2011). *Cognitive Behavior Therapy: Basics and Beyond*. New York: Guilford Press.

HANDOUT 9.3

Sample Completed Thought Record

Date/time: *September 12, 7:30 P.M.*	
Situation: *Entering restaurant with my sister*	
Thoughts: *They'll think my sister looks better than me.* *Everyone is staring at my skin! They must think, "Look how red her face is!"*	
Feelings and intensity (0–100): *Anxious, frustrated (90)*	
Believability of thoughts (0–100): *25 for first one, 90 for second*	
Cognitive errors: *Mind reading, personalization*	
Questions: *1. What is the evidence for (and against) my prediction that they think all of this stuff about me?* *I don't have any evidence that people were starting at or thinking about my face.* *2. Is there an alternative point of view?* *Yes, they might be thinking about stuff that's more important to them, like their dinner, or about the conversations they're having.*	
Rational response: *There's no evidence they are thinking about my appearance. It's more likely they're thinking about things that are more important for them, like their dinner, or their conversation.*	
Believability of rational response (0–100): *70*	
Feelings and intensity (0–100): *Anxious (20), Frustrated (0)*	

CHAPTER 10

SESSION 6

Introducing Exposure

SESSION SUMMARY

- ☐ Check mood and BDD symptoms.
- ☐ Briefly review the previous session.
- ☐ Set the agenda jointly with the patient.
- ☐ Review homework.
- ☐ Work on the agenda.
  - ☐ Motivate your patient to reduce avoidance behaviors.
  - ☐ Address doubts directly.
  - ☐ Explain how exposure works.
  - ☐ Identify distressing situations and organize them into an exposure hierarchy.
  - ☐ Select a situation with a moderate anxiety level for the first exposure.
  - ☐ Help the patient anticipate negative thoughts, evaluate them, and formulate rational responses.
  - ☐ Set specific, achievable goals for the exposure.
  - ☐ Complete an exposure in session (if time permits).
  - ☐ Encourage the patient to shift attention toward the exposure task.
  - ☐ Evaluate and reward the exposure.
- ☐ Assign homework.
- ☐ Ask for summary of/feedback on the session.

SESSION FORMS AND HANDOUTS

BDI-II (or other depression inventory)

Personal Session Form (Form 2.1)

Therapist Session Form (Form 6.1)

Exposure Worksheet (plus several extra copies for homework) (Form 10.1)

Distressing Situations Worksheet (Form 10.2)

Sample Completed Distressing Situations Worksheet (Handout 10.1)

Henry's Sample Completed Exposure Worksheet (Handout 10.2)

Thought Record (plus several extra copies for homework) (Form 9.1)

Completed *Your Personal BDD Model* (to illustrate the impact of avoidance) (Form 7.1)

Completed BDD-SS (plus a blank copy) (Form 4.3)

Completed *BDD Information-Gathering Form* (Form 4.4)

INTRODUCTION TO THIS SESSION

In this chapter, you will learn how to help your patients identify the situations they have been avoiding and replace their maladaptive behaviors with healthier ones by gradually entering feared and avoided situations. Exposure is usually introduced in Session 6, but it is important to be flexible about the timing of this. With some patients (e.g., those with milder symptoms), you might start exposure a little earlier in the treatment. For more severely ill patients, who will find exposure more difficult, you might want to start exposure a little later in the treatment, after they have had more time to master cognitive skills. Exposure helps patients feel more comfortable in anxiety-provoking situations and helps them enter situations they avoid. Often these are social situations.

Our exposure exercises incorporate the cognitive restructuring a patient has just learned in Sessions 4–5. Our exposures also involve testing beliefs or hypotheses that the patient has about the situation he will enter (e.g., that everyone will laugh at him because of how he looks). Thus our exposures are designed as "behavioral experiments." We have incorporated these cognitive elements into exposure exercises because they increase the exercises' effectiveness, as they enhance the learning that occurs during exposure.

In our experience, it is helpful to spend one to two full sessions on cognitive restructuring before moving on to exposure. This is especially the case for patients with poorer insight and those who are delusional. It's all right to move on to exposure even if your patient still needs a lot of work on the cognitive skills, as he will continue to practice his cognitive skills throughout the treatment. Ultimately, your patient will benefit most if he learns to combine cognitive with behavioral exercises.

Exposure can be difficult and will cause your patient some anxiety. Below are some suggestions for how you can approach this. Many additional strategies that can help the patient reach exposure goals can be found in Chapter 5 on MI. Further discussion of exposure (including strategies for working with delusional patients) is presented at the end of this chapter.

- *Provide a rationale and agree to a plan.* Exposure can be challenging; therefore, it is important for your patient to understand how exposure works. Do not begin exposure until you and your patient agree on the details of the exposure practice.
- *Strike a balance between validating your patient's anxiety and guiding him toward change.*

> "I know it makes you anxious to go to parties, but people who are really brave get anxious, too. You can go out even though you're anxious. Our goal is not to avoid anxiety; the goal is to do things *despite* the anxiety. This is what makes people brave: They do things even though they're anxious! You and I will work on methods to help you tolerate the discomfort and make it more manageable."

- *Be both challenging and encouraging.*

  "I know that this is difficult, but I wonder if you've done difficult things before? [Give the patient a chance to think about this.] I suspect strongly that you can do it. Just give it a shot!"

- *Be patient.* It's OK to expect a lot, but don't push any of your patients to do something they are not ready for. They may get discouraged and drop out of treatment. Some patients are able to tackle their problems head on, but others can only very gradually work themselves up to do more difficult tasks. Expect all patients to do their best, but recognize that the pace will be different for different patients. Be careful to assign exposures your patients can complete successfully.
- *Be a cheerleader.* Show each patient how excited you are when he masters a situation that he has been avoiding or has never tried before. Compliment the patient on his courage.
- *Combine cognitive with behavioral interventions.* When you ask your patient to complete the *Exposure Worksheet* (Form 10.1, discussed in more detail later), be sure that he fills out the section focusing on predictions about what will happen during the exposure. Identifying and evaluating maladaptive beliefs, and developing more realistic predictions regarding the outcome of exposures, will help the patient keep the anxiety more manageable. After each exposure exercise, discuss what your patient has learned from it. Did the feared consequences occur? If not, why not? What does this mean for your patient's beliefs? Should they be revised? Can the patient come up with a more rational alternative thought?
- *Encourage your patient to fill out and complete the Exposure Worksheet* (Form 10.1 for each exposure exercise he engages in). Some patients will try to avoid actually filling out the form. Emphasize the importance of actually filling out the *Exposure Worksheet* before entering each avoided situation. Filling out this form (and all other forms) is a very important and powerful part of CBT-BDD. Later in the treatment, once the patient has had lots of practice with exposure and with filling out the *Exposure Worksheet*, you want to encourage him to start preparing for and processing exposures "in his head," so that the process becomes second nature. However, even after the patient has mastered this technique, he may benefit from sometimes filling out the form before and after exposures.
- *Move on quickly to ritual prevention.* Although we discuss exposure and ritual prevention in separate chapters of this manual, so that we can explain both sets of skills in sufficient detail, it is important for your patient not to ritualize or engage in any other safety behaviors during exposure. So it is important to combine these treatment elements as soon as possible. In other words, you might introduce exposure by working on a few exercises where appearance-related rituals are not an issue. However, given that most patients have rituals in many different situations, you then have to move on to combining exposure with ritual prevention. The reason is that if the patient ritualizes during exposure (e.g., asks for reassurance or applies makeup), this will compromise the effectiveness of the exposure.
- *Encourage your patient to practice exposure daily.* It is really important for you to encourage your patient to practice every day. Once the patient has mastered a certain exposure situation once in treatment (e.g., making eye contact with a receptionist), make

sure that he does not avoid the situation in the future, and that he keeps practicing exposure to this particular situation (or variations of the situation) over and over again.

Check Mood and BDD Symptoms

Ask your patient for the BDI-II (or other depression inventory) he has completed in the waiting room. Pay attention not only to the scale's total score, but also to the suicidality item, and ask further questions about suicidality if clinically indicated (see Chapter 2). Also briefly inquire about BDD symptoms over the course of the last week.

Hand out the *Personal Session Form* (Form 2.1), and remind the patient to record information he finds significant during the session.

Briefly Review the Previous Session

Briefly check in with the patient on his perception and understanding of the previous session.

Set the Agenda Jointly with the Patient

Convey the topics you'd like to cover during the session. Tell the patient that he will learn a new set of skills called "exposure." Also ask the patient whether there are any issues he would like to cover in this session that you could try to weave into the session.

Review Homework

Discuss your patient's homework from the last week—the copies of the *Thought Record* (Form 9.1) he has completed.

Work on the Agenda

Motivate Your Patient to Reduce Avoidance Behaviors

Giving up avoidance behaviors is not easy. Therefore, it is important to provide your patient with a rationale for why he should be doing something that scares him. As you talk, have the patient take out his completed *Your Personal BDD Model* (Form 7.1) and point out the relevant sections of this model.

THERAPIST: Today we'll start working on some of the behaviors that feed your appearance concerns. You've told me that if someone invites you to get together during the day, you get very anxious, because you think that they might notice how small your chin is.

PATIENT: Yes, I feel really scared and ashamed. I hate feeling this way. That's why I don't go anywhere.

THERAPIST: Yes, it's certainly not pleasant to feel this way. So to stop feeling bad, you've told me that you avoid situations by turning down invitations. You've also mentioned that you turn your face away from other people so they can't see how small your chin is. What are the short-term consequences of this?

PATIENT: In the short term, I feel relieved. At least I don't have to go anywhere. So I won't have to feel embarrassed.

THERAPIST: OK, so in the short term, the avoidance makes you feel better. What about the long-term consequences?

PATIENT: Well, I'm pretty miserable. I never do anything spontaneous or fun. I've lost friends because they didn't understand why I never want to go anywhere.

THERAPIST: Sounds like there's a cost to your avoidance behavior. It really steals the fun from your life. Also, if you always avoid going places, like parties, you don't know what would have happened if you'd just gone. Maybe nothing bad would have happened after all, but you'll never know. So you're losing out on opportunities to learn that your fears may not be justified. What does avoidance do to your confidence when a situation comes up in the future?

PATIENT: Well, the next time around I'm even more anxious, because now I've really convinced myself that I can't deal with the situation.

Notice how the therapist in the exchange above elicits several important points from the patient. First, the therapist reviews the role of avoidance behavior in the context of the patient's BDD model with the patient, and points out how avoidance actually feeds BDD thoughts and beliefs. The therapist also discusses both the short-term and the long-term consequences of avoidance, as well as reinforcement circuits as shown in the patient's BDD model. The most important point in this discussion is the therapist's focus on the costs as well as the benefits of the avoidance behaviors. Although a patient is usually very aware of the benefits, raising the awareness of the costs (e.g., how avoidance robs the patient of enjoying or achieving things) will motivate your patient to tolerate the anxiety that comes along with reducing avoidance.

Address Doubts Directly

At this point in treatment, your patient usually has a vague idea of what exposure is. As the patient gets getting closer to conducting his first exposure, he may express more ambivalence about the need to change his avoidance behavior. Most likely, he is somewhat scared of starting the exposure exercises. Below, we give you some guidance for how to have an honest discussion with your patient.

THERAPIST: To ensure that you're not missing out on so many aspects of your life, we have to reduce your avoidance behavior. The treatment strategy that we'll use to reduce your avoidance and related anxiety is called "exposure." In exposure practice, you'll face situations that make you anxious.

PATIENT: To be honest, I'm pretty anxious just listening to you.

THERAPIST: Yes, this can sound a little scary. But don't worry—we'll decide on the exposure exercises together, so you won't get overwhelmed. We'll use a step-by-step approach to help you get comfortable gradually with the situations you currently avoid. And we'll only go as fast as you can.

PATIENT: So I won't be anxious?

THERAPIST: It would be nice if you could just go into the situations you've been avoiding without experiencing any anxiety or discomfort, but this is probably not possible. In fact, feeling some anxiety is a sign that you're doing a challenging exposure, and this means that you're more likely to make progress than if you do an exposure that's too easy. Nonetheless, you'll learn to tolerate and manage your anxiety as you try to overcome your appearance concerns.

What if your patient is not convinced that exposure treatment is right for him? In this case, you'll have to address some doubts regarding exposure treatment before your patient will be convinced to get on board. It's very important to understand what your patient's concerns are and to address them. For example, your patient might tell you that he has tried to reduce avoidance behavior on his own, and it didn't work.

PATIENT: There are things that I've tried on my own. Like some parties, or going to temple. I've actually tried to force myself to do this, but I'm still really anxious. Just recently I went to a wedding, but I would still be afraid to go to another one. So how is the treatment we're doing here different?

THERAPIST: It must have been really challenging for you to go to these events, and it's great that you are trying so hard to work on them yourself. [Note how the therapist reinforces the patient's efforts.] I'm also really glad that you're asking about the difference between CBT-BDD and your own efforts. Let's look more closely together at the situations you've described. For how long did you stay in these situations, and at what point did you decide to leave?

PATIENT: Well, I never stayed long at all . . . maybe I stayed for 30 minutes or 45 minutes at the most . . . and I always left before anyone else did. Actually, I usually left when I got really anxious, because I thought that something disastrous would happen if I stayed longer.

THERAPIST: I wonder if the reason why you didn't benefit from these exercises a whole lot might have been that you left the situation too early, before you really had a chance to see that nothing bad would have happened even if you'd stayed longer.

PATIENT: That's definitely true. I always left early. I never took a chance to see what would happen . . .

THERAPIST: OK. How would you feel about trying something new in treatment, then? Maybe you could try to stay in the situation even if you get anxious. This will allow us to observe what happens over time and help us find out if your fears really come true or not.

PATIENT: Sounds a little scary, but I think it makes sense to give it a try.

THERAPIST: Great. I'm glad that you are willing to try to see if this would work for you. Do you remember what you did when you went to the wedding or to the parties? Do you remember if you engaged in a subtle avoidance behavior, such as [the therapist gives an example for this particular patient—e.g., hiding the body part of concern]?

PATIENT: Oh, yes, I remember very well what I did. I definitely avoided eye contact; I never showed the "bad side" of my face; and when things got really bad, I first went into a darker part of the room, and finally, I just left.

THERAPIST: Well, it's great that you went to all of these events in the first place, despite the fact that they were pretty challenging for you! Over the course of our treatment, we will work on the avoidance behaviors that you just described, because they are actually keeping your fears alive. We will keep practicing exposures to parties and other social events over and over again, because if you do an exposure just once, it's is hard to get used to the new behaviors. And if an exposure isn't as successful as we'd like it to be, we can usually figure out why, and we can try to make the next one go better. Another difference between your old approach to these situations and the new approach we will use in treatment is that we will work on your negative thinking before you do the exposure. This might help you see some of those situations in a less anxiety-provoking way. Do you have any other questions about how the treatment is different from what you have tried on your own?

Sometimes patients *have* been successful doing exposures or other treatment strategies on their own. If this is the case, praise their successes, and liken the upcoming exposures to things they have already done. For patients who have not been successful doing exposures for BDD, ask whether they've ever gotten over other fears and how exposure may have played a role in this. Reinforce the patients' previous courage in the face of fear, and express optimism that they can do it again in the present treatment.

Explain How Exposure Works

It's important to explain how exposure will help your patient enter avoided situations, because the patient will find exposure challenging and may be reluctant to try it.

> Exposure will help you go into situations you currently avoid or tend to escape from, like . . . [give examples]. You might be anxious at first, but after prolonged and regular exposure to those situations, you'll get accustomed to them and will feel more comfortable in them. You won't respond to them with anxiety any longer; in other words, your fear will 'habituate,' and your impulse to escape from the situation will 'extinguish.'"

You can use the example below to explain this further:

> Extinction might be easier to understand if you think of someone with OCD who washes his hands over and over again, because he is afraid that he might get very sick if he does not wash. If he ate a meal, for example, without washing his hands first, he would be really terrified. But if he eats a meal over and over again, without washing his hands and without getting sick, his anxiety will eventually decrease. He would learn that he doesn't need to wash his hands as much. So, in other words, extinction is based on a learning process. In this case, the patient with OCD learned that he was safe even if he doesn't wash his hands excessively all the time.

To motivate your patient to do exposure, it's also helpful to discuss how learning to enter feared and avoided situations will help him meet some of his treatment goals, which you can briefly review.

As the sample explanations above illustrate, it's important to caution your patient that he will be anxious when first entering a situation he would normally avoid. This way he won't be caught off guard when it happens. Emphasize the need to work on a particular situation more than once and to stay in the situation for an extended period of time, so that the patient has a chance to get used to it. How long the patient stays depends on how long it takes him to get comfortable. Stopping too early, when the anxiety is still high, actually makes it *harder* to approach that situation later. A general rule of thumb is to stay in the exposure situation until the initial discomfort is reduced by 30–50%, so that the patient can really feel the difference. In other words, he should stay until it's clear that he feels better than he did initially. A well-arranged exposure practice also gives the patient the chance to compare his unrealistic fears to real-life experience and determine whether the fears actually come true and are realistic or not:

> During the exposure practices, you can find out if the outcomes you fear really occur. Once you get first-hand experience that your fears aren't confirmed, your anxiety will fade. You'll probably have to repeat the exposures (and related learning experiences) a number of times until you become comfortable in the situation.

Let your patient know that anxiety is a normal and expected part of exposure practice. Ask him about situations in the past when he became anxious, and discuss whether the anxiety decreased over time (e.g., when he first learned to swim, ride a bike, or drive). Now many of those situations that used to be scary are actually fun.

If doing so is applicable to your patient, evaluate whether he might be engaging in emotional reasoning, which is a cognitive error discussed in Chapter 9. Emotional reasoning is the belief that if a thought *feels* true, then it is true. Discuss whether anxiety always means that negative thoughts will come true. Tell your patient that usually the moments right before the exposure starts are the most anxiety-provoking, and after that anxiety usually decreases over the course of the exposure. After your patient has repeated a particular exposure several times, it will become easier.

Identify Distressing Situations and Organize Them into an Exposure Hierarchy

From the information you have obtained with the BDD-SS (Form 4.3) and the *BDD Information-Gathering Form* (Form 4.4), as well as your initial meeting with the patient, you probably have a general idea of the kinds of situations your patient avoids and how distressing they are. You need to administer the BDD-SS again at the beginning of exposure treatment, so that your information regarding your patient's avoidance behavior is up to date. In addition, your discussion of treatment goals will give you a general idea of where you and your patient need to go with exposure. Now determine the short-term steps that will help your patient reach those treatment goals.

Begin by asking your patient to write down 10–15 situations he avoids that pertain to his most important treatment goals. Next, transform those situations into exposure tasks, and create a list of these exposures. For example, if your patient's goal is to be comfortable in more social situations, you can develop a list of exposures that pertain to this goal. Keep in mind that avoidance behaviors can be subtle (e.g., covering the perceived flaw with body position, hands, clothing, or hair, or avoiding eye contact), and that each of these behaviors will need to be reduced or stopped if the planned exposures are to be successful.

Below are some general examples, to give you some ideas of exposure situations you can help your patient work on.

- Go to a family gathering or party.
- Get a haircut.
- Go to church or temple.
- Sit across from someone.
- Sit in the front row in a concert.
- Go to a doctor's office and get a physical checkup that will reveal the body part(s) of concern.
- Engage in an activity that makes it impossible to hide the perceived flaws (e.g., go swimming, which messes up your hair, or go to a sauna, where you can't wear clothing or makeup to protect your flaws).
- Get your picture taken.
- Go for a short walk without your hat, without having your hair styled, and without sunglasses.
- Have close physical contact that permits someone to touch the flaw.
- Make eye contact with a stranger.
- Sit close to a person to expose the body part of concern.
- Sit/stand under a bright light.
- Go outside on a sunny day without avoiding the bright light.
- Deliberately show your flaws (e.g., smile to expose crooked teeth or facial wrinkles, wear clothing that doesn't cover imperfections).
- Keep the light on when undressing in front of your partner.
- Engage in sexual positions that expose your flaws.
- Go to places where appearance is emphasized (e.g., a gym or dance studio with mirrors on the wall, a singles' gathering, a dressy occasion, expensive stores or makeup counters).

The list should include only specific situations that are actually feasible for future exposure practice. Instead of "Meet all classmates," for example, a suitable goal would be "Go to the beach with Larry on Saturday afternoon for 1 hour; wear bathing suit." After you and your patient have identified several situations to work on, organize them into a hierarchy of increasing difficulty, using the *Distressing Situations Worksheet* (Form 10.2). A copy of this form, which has been completed by a patient with concerns about blemishes, is provided as Handout 10.1; your patient can use this handout as a guide for developing a personal hierarchy.

To develop the hierarchy, ask your patient how distressing each situation is on a scale from 0 to 100. A rating of 0 means that the situation is not distressing at all. A rating of 100 means that the situation is extremely distressing, the most fearful or uncomfortable the person has ever felt. For example, if the situation is only mildly uncomfortable, your patient might rate it a 20. A situation that causes moderate distress might be rated about 50. Situations that cause your patient to feel highly distressed would be rated 75 or more.

Next, ask your patient to rate how much he avoids each situation, using the *Sample Completed Distressing Situations Worksheet* (Handout 10.1) as an example. Have the patient use the same 0–100 scale; in this case, 0 means never avoiding, 50 means avoiding about 50% of the time, and 100 means always avoiding it. Encourage your patient to use the full range of the scale.

Select a Situation with a Moderate Anxiety Level for the First Exposure

Note that the *Sample Completed Distressing Situations Worksheet* (Handout 10.1) omits very mildly disturbing situations and instead begins with situations that provoke moderate discomfort. This is deliberate, since you will want to begin with exposure to situations that provoke distress and avoidance ratings near 40. This degree of discomfort is tolerable for most patients and enables them to observe the reduction in anxiety that occurs with prolonged exposure. Exposure to situations that cause very little anxiety makes it more difficult for patients to notice that their distress is reducing. Also, it may not be the best use of their time to work on such situations, since the situation is already tolerable. On the other hand, exposure to situations that cause more distress (e.g., levels of 75 or more) might be too difficult for most patients to tolerate at this stage, and they may refuse to complete the homework.

To begin the exposure process, select a moderate-level item (e.g., distress of about 40) on the hierarchy that you can actually observe during the session, if possible. For example, you could ask your patient to make eye contact with someone in your waiting room, or ask the receptionist a question while revealing the perceived flaw. Observing the patient enables you to spot additional compulsive or avoidance behavior your patient is unaware of; such behavior will interfere with the success of the exposure. Moreover, you are right on site to encourage your patient to keep going, to cheerlead, and to praise his efforts.

If you aren't sure a patient can really master the selected situation, select an easier one to make sure the first exposure is a success and to minimize the likelihood of dropout from the treatment. To be sure, we usually ask patients how confident (0–100%) they feel about actually doing the exercise, and we only assign it if patients rate themselves as at least 70% confident.

For example, Henry was preoccupied with his height. He believed that he looked like a midget or a freak, and that others were talking about his looks and wouldn't take him seriously because of his height. Because of these concerns, he avoided any interactions with tall people. He also always wore elevated shoes. We planned to conduct his first exposure on site. We asked Henry to wear sneakers to the session and to talk to one of our receptionists, who is very tall. We also planned that the receptionist would stand up while Henry was right next to her.

Ask your patient to fill in the *Exposure Worksheet* (Form 10.1) before doing the planned exposure you will observe. Your patient should describe the most unpleasant aspects of the situation and identify the subtle avoidance behaviors (such as avoiding eye contact) he is going to stop using. As you can see, this form also included an abbreviated version of the *Thought Record* (Form 9.1) that the patient has recently learned to complete. Feel free to add a section for cognitive errors to the exposure forms you use; this may be helpful if your patient has trouble identifying them. *Henry's Sample Completed Exposure Worksheet* (Handout 10.2) can be given to patients to guide them as they learn to complete their own *Exposure Worksheets*.

Help the Patient Anticipate Negative Thoughts, Evaluate Them, and Formulate Rational Responses

Exposure exercises provide opportunities to collect evidence for or against maladaptive beliefs. In planning the first exposure situation, help your patient predict his negative thoughts and counter them ahead of time by filling out the *Exposure Worksheet*. To do this, encourage your patient to imagine being in the exposure situation or to engage with you in a role play of the situation. For example, Henry could play himself and the therapist could play the tall receptionist (the therapist could even stand on a chair or on tiptoe). Usually these imaginary exercises or role plays are much easier than a real exposure, and are therefore very useful in helping the patient anticipate his thinking during the exposure.

When your patient is filling out the *Exposure Worksheet* (Form 10.1), ask him to write his negative thoughts in the space provided. Now encourage your patient to apply the cognitive strategies he has learned so far. Start by looking for thinking errors. Ask the patient questions to evaluate the thoughts ("Is there any evidence against this thought?"). Then formulate a rational response to each thought. Again, this process is the same as the one the patient has learned for completing the *Thought Record* (Form 9.1). Evaluating negative thoughts ahead of time will assist your patient during challenging exposures, when anxiety is high and it is more difficult to recall cognitive therapy strategies. As described in Chapter 9, your patient can write down the alternative thoughts (rational responses) on an index card to take with him into the situation and to help him recall the alternative thoughts when needed.

Using this method, Henry generated a number of rational responses/alternative thoughts on his *Exposure Worksheet* before the exposure. Handout 10.2 (which, again, can be given to patients for guidance) presents Henry's automatic negative thoughts and the rational alternatives he generated.

Set Specific, Achievable Goals for the Exposure

Patients often set unrealistic and global goals early in treatment. Teach your patients to *set specific and realistic behavioral goals* before they start any exposure, so they can easily determine what goals to work toward and whether the exposure was successful. Many patients with BDD are perfectionists. If their goals aren't clearly defined, they may discount the entire exposure exercise simply because they felt anxious or because the exposure wasn't flawless.

For example, patients often suggest that they can do a planned exposure without feeling anxious. Although the long-term aim of treatment is to make your patients more comfortable in a broad range of situations, it isn't possible for them to avoid feeling anxious in any specific situation. Indeed, early in treatment most goals will require your patients to do things despite their anxiety. Thus goals that involve controlling feelings are not desirable or achievable. So if a patient writes down a goal such as "I will feel comfortable at the mall," explain that it is very hard for anyone to control feelings. Here you can remind the patient that CBT-BDD focuses primarily on modifying thoughts and behaviors, rather than feelings. Then encourage the patient to change this goal to something objective and behavioral, such as "I will stay at the mall for 1 hour and won't hide in the bathroom while I'm there."

As this example illustrates, appropriate goals include *objective, specific, measurable behaviors*. Other examples include "I will talk to the tall receptionist for 2 minutes," or "I will stay in the waiting room for 10 minutes no matter what happens." These are better than a vague goal like "I will go out in public." Make sure that the goals you and the patient set don't depend on other people's behavior and are within your patient's control. For example, your patient may not be able to arrange a date, but he can invite a friend to go out.

As Handout 10.2 shows, Henry set four specific, attainable goals for his exposure:

1. Stand 2–3 feet from the receptionist.
2. Maintain eye contact.
3. Ask at least one question.
4. Stay for at least 3 minutes.

Complete an Exposure in Session (If Time Permits)

Conducting the first exposure during the office visit may take extra time, depending on your patient's initial discomfort and on how quickly this discomfort decreases. If there isn't enough time, you can plan to do the first exposure in the next session. Delaying the first exposure to the next session will definitely be necessary if you need to make special arrangements for an exposure (e.g., asking the patient to wear certain clothing or not to put on makeup; arranging for a receptionist or colleague to be present).

Encourage the Patient to Shift Attention toward the Exposure Task

When your BDD patient gets anxious, he might scrutinize his environment for possible signs of danger (e.g., a frown, which he could interpret to mean that others are reacting negatively to his appearance). Moreover, he might get excessively self-focused (e.g., he might think about his appearance, and the way others might judge his perceived flaws). As the human brain is limited in its capacity to process information, these processes can easily interfere with the exposure exercise, as your patient may not be able to attend to information that may actually disconfirm his self-defeating beliefs (e.g., that most people around him are actually friendly). Furthermore, given that your patient's attention is focused inward, he might not be able to fully concentrate on whatever is happening in a particular situation (e.g., a conversation), which could interfere with his social performance. Therefore, it is important that you encourage your patient to actively direct his attention away from maladaptive targets (e.g., from scanning the environment for frowns, or from thinking about his appearance flaws) and toward the task at hand (e.g., the conversation). Similar efforts to retain attention have yielded beneficial results in social anxiety disorder and fear of blushing (e.g., Bögels, Sijbers, Voncken, 2006; Mulkens, Bögels, & deJong, 1999). Research on task attention training in BDD is currently being conducted by Dr. Sandra Mulkens in the Netherlands. Thus, prior to conducting an exposure exercise, it can be helpful to ask your patient to estimate the percentage of their attention that he would typically devote in such a situation to himself, threatening cues in the environment, and the task at hand, and (if applicable) encourage an attentional shift toward the task at hand. After the exposure exercise, review with your patient what he actually attended to and how this affected his discomfort during the exposure exercise. You can find more information on shifting attentional processes (and thus helping your patients see the big picture) when we discuss ritual prevention (especially prevention of comparison rituals) in Chapter 11 and in the chapter on perceptual retraining (Chapter 12).

Evaluate and Reward the Exposure

After your patient has completed an exposure, praise him for having tried it and then collaboratively evaluate how it went. It's helpful to convey open-minded curiosity about the results of the exposure, such as "I'm interested to hear what happened." The next sections on the *Exposure Worksheet* will help you structure those evaluations.

Ask the Patient to Rate Distress

After each exposure, ask your patient to evaluate his distress, using the 0–100 scale. How distressed was the patient right before he started? Did his distress increase or decrease during the exposure exercise? Most likely, he was more comfortable at the end than at the beginning of the exposure. (As you can see in Handout 10.2, this was certainly true for Henry.) The ratings help you track your patient's improvement over the course of this treatment program. It's unrealistic to think that after just one exposure, anxiety ratings will fall to as low as a 10 or 20 after the exposure. Convey to the patient that a smaller drop is adequate and is a sign of success.

If the patient's anxiety increased over the course of the exposure, determine why, and discuss possible coping strategies with your patient. For example, if the patient is bombarded by unexpected maladaptive thoughts or interpretations of the situation, consider having him use some of the skills described in Chapter 9 during role plays or imagined exposures before assigning more exposure as homework. Alternatively, the patient may have underestimated how hard the exposure would be, and in this case would probably benefit from trying an easier exposure.

After completing an exposure exercise, patients often tend to focus selectively on the anxiety they felt and what went wrong. When Henry was asked right after the exposure how he thought it went, the first thing he said was "Well, I was anxious and I blushed." Although such aspects need to be discussed, be sure to counteract selective attention to imperfect aspects of exposures. Focus mainly on whether your patient met his goals for the exposure. Henry, for example, actually exceeded his goal by staying in the situation longer than he had originally planned (see Handout 10.2). Be sure to point out when patients meet their goals and praise them accordingly.

When Exposure Goals Are Not Met, Discuss Why and Provide Support

When the patient does not meet the goals, convey curiosity about what happened (as you would with any other experimental results that didn't turn out as planned), rather than disappointment or criticism. Determine what went wrong, but if at all possible, find something positive about the exercise. Perhaps you picked a situation that was too difficult, and your patient left before the exercise was complete. Next time, select an easier one and ensure that your patient moves up the hierarchy step by step, so that the most feared situations are completed in the latter part of the treatment program. If the patient has difficulty with a specific exposure exercise, try breaking it down into smaller, more manageable steps. You could also role-play the exposure before the patient does it. You could play the patient, and the patient could play the therapist and coach you through it.

Sometimes patients' anxiety does not decrease during an exposure because they engage in subtle avoidance behaviors or rituals while doing the exercise. For example, a woman who was afraid that other people might react negatively to her skin continued to feel anxious despite a prolonged exposure that consisted of walking around in a crowded shopping mall. Her anxiety did not decrease because she kept checking and reapplying her makeup. Thus she didn't have the opportunity to see what would happen if she didn't keep reapplying her makeup; this undermined what she learned from the exposure. She also avoided eye contact during the exposure. Patients with BDD commonly avoid eye contact with—or even looking directly at—other people. It can be very upsetting for them to look at other people, because they are so sure they're being laughed at or mocked because of how they look. The problem with not looking at other people is that this prevents the patients from collecting evidence about their negative thoughts/predictions and determining whether their predictions are true or not. Usually it's necessary to look around while collecting evidence for and against their predictions. If patients do not look around and just look at the floor while in the exposure situation, they'll just *assume* that their negative thoughts/

predictions are true, and the exposures will not be helpful. For instance, if he hadn't looked at the receptionist, Henry would have just assumed that she looked really unfriendly and arrogant, and he wouldn't have seen that the receptionist actually had a friendly expression on her face.

The worst possible outcome for an exposure is that the feared consequences actually occur. When this happens, the exposure was often set up poorly. Exposures should not include situations that would upset most people. For example, exposure to teasing from a highly critical family member is not likely to be successful. In this case, training in assertive communication is likely to be more productive.

Review Thoughts: What Did the Patient Learn?

Be sure your patient records whether his anxiety-provoking predictions came true. These predictions are often wrong. If any unexpected negative thoughts came up, ask the patient to write them down on a copy of the *Thought Record* (Form 9.1) and evaluate them, to determine whether these thoughts might have involved cognitive errors. You can also examine whether the patient's learning might have been undermined by subtle avoidance behavior. For example, if the patient didn't actually collect any evidence, or engaged in avoidance behavior while in the exposure situation (e.g., hid in the bathroom at a party), he probably just assumed that the negative consequence occurred.

It's very important to focus on what the patient learned from the exposure and to have him fill out this part of the *Exposure Worksheet*. Learning from the exposure—specifically, learning that the feared prediction didn't occur—is one of the main ways in which exposure helps patients change. Have the patient write down what he learned from his observations during the exposure; it can be helpful if this incorporates components of his alternative thoughts.

If the patient needs help with figuring out what they learned, assist him in thinking this through. It's important for the patient to write down something that is *relevant to his progress and his beliefs about his appearance*. As an example, a helpful response to "What did I learn?" is "Maybe people in the store are more interested in what they're buying than what my jaw looks like." An unhelpful response is something like "The store isn't very busy at midnight." *Henry's Sample Completed Exposure Worksheet* (Handout 10.2) shows what Henry wrote about his predictions and his learning experience during the exposure practice.

Encourage Rewards

Encourage your patients to reward themselves after exposures, especially if the exposures were difficult. Patients might take time to watch a favorite show, or buy themselves something as a small reward. Patients may not be used to being nice to themselves, and you may really have to encourage them to do this.

ASSIGN HOMEWORK

Homework assignments often build directly on the exposures that were conducted during sessions. Often your patient will just repeat the same exposure (or a minor variation thereof) for homework. In other cases, especially if the in-session exposure went very well, you might just decide that the patient can use the homework to move on to the next item in the hierarchy of distressing situations.

For example, in collaboration with his therapist, Henry decided to keep moving up his hierarchy. His homework included going on a 45-minute walk with a tall friend and shopping for 10 items at a grocery store on Wednesday night, while he was wearing flat shoes. In addition he kept completing copies of the *Thought Record* (Form 9.1). Keep in mind that homework assignments should be chosen jointly by the patient and you. This is especially important, given the anxiety-provoking nature of exposures. Eliciting your patient's input when deciding on homework increases the probability that your patient will be successful. Remind your patient to complete the top half of the *Exposure Worksheet* prior to each exercise, and the lower half after the exposure exercise.

Ask for Summary of/Feedback on the Session

At the end of Session 6 and each exposure session thereafter, ask your patient for a session summary and feedback. The summary will help you and your patient gain a clear understanding of what you have accomplished, and your request for feedback will give you a sense of your patient's reaction to the exposure session. Indeed, patients often react strongly to exposures; for example, they may be bothered by a certain aspect of an exposure exercise they have just completed. Thus asking for feedback will give you the opportunity to resolve any maladaptive interpretations of what may have occurred during the treatment sessions.

Next Steps for Exposures

If your patient is very anxious, he may need to repeat the first exposure or a variation thereof in another session or at home a couple of times until he becomes more comfortable with the feared situation. As the treatment progresses, you can do additional exposures during your treatment sessions. For example, Henry walked down a busy street near his therapist's office wearing flat shoes, and he asked tall people for directions. He also went to a local restaurant or cafeteria to do a similar exposure exercise. Easier exposures could have involved walking near the therapist's office in a less busy area.

It may take you one or two sessions to introduce the exposure concept. However, when you are designing exposure exercises, keep in mind that most patients with BDD engage in BDD-related rituals in many situations. Therefore, as soon as possible, you will need to incorporate strategies into exposure exercises that focus on reducing rituals (see Chapter 11 for a detailed description of these strategies). Exposures to avoided situations and ritual prevention usually need to be done in combination. We only describe exposure and response prevention separately in this manual because this enables us to describe each treatment strategy in sufficient detail.

Keep Working on Exposure throughout the Treatment

It is very important to keep working on exposure throughout the entire CBT-BDD program. Be sure that exposure is part of your patient's homework every week. *Ideally, your patient will complete at least one exposure every day for the rest of the treatment.* This will enable him to continue to make progress. The initial exposures will get easier over time, and he can move on to more difficult exposure situations. Have your patient gradually try increasingly challenging assignments by moving up the hierarchy. As noted above and described in Chapter 11, you will also begin to incorporate response prevention into the exposures.

In addition, you can have your patient do exposures that aren't based on the initial hierarchy, to increase his ability to enter a variety of situations. You can augment exposures with tasks such as having your patient start a conversation with someone if he currently avoids talking to people, even if having a conversation isn't on his initial hierarchy. The key is to design doable and yet challenging exposures of increasing difficulty that will help improve the patient's functioning.

It's good for exposures to gradually incorporate more meaningful and necessary activities in a patient's life, such as social interactions. This will increase the patient's productivity and, ideally, increase the pleasure he gets from life. In our experience, staying busy with meaningful or enjoyable activities can be very helpful in overcoming BDD. Patients often tell us that the busier they are, the better their BDD seems to get.

Once a patient masters a particular exposure, there is "no going back." In other words, he needs to keep entering this situation in the future. For example, if a patient successfully does an exposure by attending a meeting at work that he often avoids, he needs to continue to attend the meeting each week.

You can work on exposures during later treatment sessions in several ways:

1. *In the process of reviewing the previous week's homework.* In earlier sessions, while the patient is still learning exposure, you'll want to spend more time on this to help him improve his skills. Later in the treatment, you can review the exposures more briefly to see how they went and to congratulate the patient for his hard work and progress.
2. *As part of the session agenda, if your patient would benefit from additional work on exposures.* This may be especially helpful for delusional patients, who may have more difficulty designing the exposure, doing the cognitive portion of the exposure, setting reasonable behavioral goals, or processing what they learned. Any time a patient has a particularly hard time with an exposure or feels it didn't go well, try to take some time to review and process it.
3. *While coming up with each week's exposure homework assignment with your patient.* As the treatment progresses, you'll want your patient to increasingly take the lead in designing the exposures, but your input can be helpful, especially earlier in the treatment.

Help the Patient Decide How Many Situations to Work on at One Time

For some people, working on one exposure situation per day is sufficient. Other patients may benefit more from working on several situations at once, especially if these exposures are tied to events that don't necessarily occur daily (e.g., going to a holiday party or other dressy occasion).

Help the Patient Examine Unplanned Exposures

Patients sometimes do "unplanned exposures." If this is something a patient initiated (e.g., going to a store on a crowded day because there was a sale), be sure to congratulate him for making the effort, especially if it was very challenging for him. Ask whether the patient completed an *Exposure Worksheet* (Form 10.1) for the unplanned exposure; if so, you can review it in the session. If the patient didn't do this, you can still ask how the exposure went and what he learned from it.

If the unplanned exposure didn't go well, you'll want to figure out why not and determine how it might go better in the future. Filling out a *Thought Record* (Form 9.1) or an *Exposure Worksheet* during your session can help the patient process how the exposure went and whether he might think about what happened in a more accurate and helpful way.

Keep in mind that it can be very hard for a more severely ill or housebound patients even to attend a therapy session, as getting to your office involves exposure. For this reason, the patient may be upset upon arrival, because he believes he was stared at or laughed at on the way. In this case, it may be helpful to have the patient fill out a *Thought Record* (Form 9.1) for the upsetting event during the session.

Keep Track of the Patient's Progress

We recommend that your patient save each copy of the *Exposure Worksheet* (Form 10.1) he completes. You'll want to review these at the next session when going over the homework. In addition, this will help you and the patient keep track of his progress. Progress will be evident in the following:

- Lower initial discomfort level during the exposure situation.
- Less time required to reduce discomfort during the exposure situation.
- Ability to do more difficult exposures on the hierarchy.

As noted above, exposure to feared situations will continue throughout the therapy. It will stop only when the patient is no longer significantly afraid of situations that used to bother him and when he no longer avoids situations that most people engage in easily.

Encourage the Patient to Practice Exposures Daily

After beginning exposure exercises, your patient should invest about 45–60 minutes per day in CBT-BDD. About half of this time should be spent completing copies of the *Thought Record* (Form 9.1) and preparing for exposures. The rest of the time should be focused on entering previously avoided situations—that is, doing actual exposures. Once again, daily exposure practice should continue for the rest of the treatment.

For homework assignments, you and your patient will have to agree on specific exposures based on the *Distressing Situations Worksheet* (Form 10.2). It can be helpful to fill out the top half of the *Exposure Worksheet* (Form 10.1) in the session to get your patient started. If there isn't enough time to do this in the session, you can have the patient refer to *Henry's Sample Completed Exposure Worksheet* (Handout 10.2). In assigning exposure homework, remember to select situations that are rated at least 40 on the *Distressing Situations Worksheet* (Form 10.2). Over time your patient will need to engage in increasingly difficult exposures, and you might want to encourage your patients to try them as long as they are at least 60% confident that they can complete the task.

EXPOSURE WITH DELUSIONAL PATIENTS

For many patients with BDD, the techniques described above—with lots of practice during the course of the treatment—will be sufficient to diminish their avoidance substantially and to change their appearance beliefs. However, for more delusional patients, whose beliefs are more entrenched and rigid, you may also need to try some of the adapted exposure techniques described below.

When you are working with a delusional patient, it's important first to get a sense of how firmly convinced the patient is that his beliefs are true. Is the patient 100% certain he is ugly? Is he 100% convinced that people stare or laugh at him? Has anything ever happened that made the patient doubt his beliefs, even a little? If so, what was that? Has the patient ever wondered whether people weren't focused on his nose (or other body part of concern)? Or did he first think people were focusing on his nose, but as he got to know the other persons, he realized they weren't? Affirmative answers may be useful in designing exposures, as you can try to build upon any doubt the patient expresses about his beliefs.

Patients who are delusional (i.e., those who are completely convinced that their beliefs are true and undistorted) may find it hard to come up with an alternative thought that's even a little bit believable. Or they may misinterpret what happens during an exposure and conclude that their prediction was true. They may say things like "My prediction *was* right. I *saw* that guy laughing at me!" Or "People *did* look away from me; I *know* they were thinking I was ugly." Delusional patients may also have particularly prominent and distressing delusions of reference; that is, they may believe that other people are staring at them, laughing at them, mocking them, or otherwise reacting to their appearance. It can be helpful to focus on ideas or delusions of reference when such patients are completing *Thought Records* and doing exposures, as these delusions involve clear cognitive errors, such as personalization and mindreading. However, delusional patients may have great difficulty in correctly interpreting the behavior of other people.

As is always the case when you are doing cognitive restructuring with any patient, it is crucial to use Socratic methods and help a delusional patient come to his own, more rational conclusions about the accuracy and helpfulness of his thoughts. It's very important for the patient not to view you as one more person who is going to try to talk him out of his beliefs. Trying to strong-arm the patient into agreeing with you simply won't work. As one such patient said to us, "I'm as convinced that what I see in the mirror is correct as you are that the box on that table is rectangular and not round!" However, you may need to offer a delusional patient more suggestions for designing exposures, considering alternative ways of thinking, and processing what he has learned.

Techniques for Negative Thoughts and Predictions

Make a Prediction Very Specific

If you don't encourage the patient to make a prediction very specific, the patient may find a way to conclude that the prediction came true, even if it really didn't. By contrast, if the prediction is very specific, it will be easier to determine whether it did come true. This will also make misinterpretation less likely. For example, you can have the patient make predictions about quantities, percentages, time, the exact looks that people will have on their faces, and so forth. These techniques are described below.

Incorporate Quantities and Percentages into the Prediction

For example, rather than simply predicting that people will look away from, or look at, the patient because he looks so frightening, the patient can specify what percentage of people will look away from him or at him. If he really looks frightening, presumably most people would do this (perhaps 80% or 90%). This way, if 5 or 10 out of 50 people look away or at the patient—which could happen for reasons that are completely unrelated to the patient—he won't be able to conclude that his prediction came true. Avoid a prediction such as "When I walk down the sidewalk, people will cross the street to the other side because I look so awful." Again, at least a few people are likely to cross the street for reasons that have nothing to do with the patient, and the patient may misinterpret this as proof that he is ugly. Instead, have the patient specify the percentage of people who will cross the street and when this will happen—for example, "Because I look so ugly, when I walk down the sidewalk 70% of people will cross the street to the other side after they look directly at me and before they pass by me."

Incorporate Time into the Prediction

Encourage the patient to incorporate time into the prediction if it's relevant to the exposure being planned. For example, rather than vaguely predicting that people will walk away from him in the video store because he's so ugly, the patient can specify what percentage of people will walk away from him (as discussed above) and in what period of time. For example, the prediction might be "Because I look so ugly, 75% of people in the video store will walk away from me within 5 seconds."

Educate the Patient That There Are Many Possible Explanations for People's Behavior

Help the patient develop more of an awareness that there are various possible explanations for other people's behavior, many or most of which have nothing to do with how the patient looks. This can be useful while the two of you are developing the prediction, and also after the experiment, when you are processing whether the prediction came true. For example, encourage the patient to consider all the possible reasons why other people may glance in our direction. Perhaps it's because we walked toward them, and they want to be aware of their surroundings and see who is approaching them. Perhaps they were looking in our direction but focusing on something other than us. As we walk by other people, it's pretty normal for them to look in our direction so they don't crash into us. If they didn't look at us at all, this could happen. Try to discuss these possibilities via Socratic questioning and to elicit possibilities such as these from the patient, rather than simply telling the patient. Similarly, you could ask:

> "When people are driving, should they only look perfectly straight ahead and not notice people on the side of the road or the sidewalk? What do you think might happen if they never looked around them at all or at people on the side of the road?"

It can also be helpful to discuss personal space. For example, it's normal for other people to move away from us if we get too close to them. People in our society tend to feel uncomfortable when strangers get close to them, and they like to have a big personal space around themselves. Thus they may move away from the patient for this reason, not because of how the patient looks.

It may be helpful to have the patient make a pie chart that includes all of the possible reasons a person may have looked at him. Make the size of each slice of the pie correspond to the likelihood that this was why the patient was looked at. Have the patient put his appearance into the pie last.

Techniques for Alternative Thoughts

Delusional patients are likely to need more help from you than other patients in coming up with more rational, alternative thoughts. As noted previously, making an alternative thought more tentative initially, by using words such as "possibly" and "maybe," may make this thought at least somewhat believable and more acceptable to a patient. Later in treatment, as the patient makes progress, the thoughts can be stated more definitely. Once again, always let the patient try to formulate the alternative thought himself, with you as a guide; avoid "telling" him what it should be. Especially early in the treatment, if the patient isn't able to come up with more *accurate* alternative thoughts, it may work better to focus on developing more *helpful* thoughts (i.e., thoughts that cause less distress). Later in the treatment, you may be able to return gradually to a focus on developing more accurate beliefs.

Precautions during the Behavioral Experiment

Be sure that the patient actually observes the situation to collect evidence and doesn't simply assume that the prediction is coming true. This is a common pitfall and we discussed the importance of shifting attention from an internal to an external focus earlier in this chapter. After the exposure, the patient may say that his prediction came true—but when you ask him what happened, you learn that he ran into the exposure situation, looked down the entire time, ran out, and just assumed that bad things happened (e.g., that people laughed at him). Emphasize the importance of looking around and looking at people to collect evidence for and against his prediction. Your patient has to be a good scientist and collect evidence about his negative thoughts/predictions while doing the exposure, so that he can see what actually happens.

The second precaution you need to take is to make sure that the patient doesn't take this advice to an extreme by staring at other people or following them around to collect evidence. This may frighten the other people, who may in turn take special notice of the patient or react in a fearful way in response to the patient's behavior. Similarly, have the patient avoid other potentially provocative behavior that could induce a fearful or angry response from others. For example, one of our patients came to the realization that he was so sure other people were mocking him that he automatically gave other people a dirty look. He was able to recognize that this behavior sometimes elicited dirty looks from the other people.

Techniques after the Experiment

A delusional patient may have a harder time than other patients with processing the exposure and identifying something useful that he learned from it. Thus it is especially important to focus adequately on this aspect of the exposure. If the patient believes his predictions came true, express curiosity and wonder about this. What is the basis for his conclusion? Try to determine whether this faulty conclusion reflects a problem with the prediction. Maybe it wasn't specific enough. If your patient says something like "People *did* look at me," you can ask, "How many of them looked at you with expressions of horror on their faces?" You can also ask the patient to quantify his experience. For example, how many people were there, and how many looked at the patient with disgust? Sometimes if even one person looks at your patient in a "negative" way, he may conclude that his beliefs must be true. Ask him:

> "If only 1 out of 300 people did this, does this mean your thought is true? If it is, why didn't the other 299 people take special notice of you? What were the other 299 people doing, and what did they seem to be focusing on?"

If you think that the patient misinterpreted the exposure experience because of cognitive errors, you can have him fill out a *Thought Record* in the session to explore his interpretation further and determine whether any cognitive errors were involved. If someone actually made a comment to your patient, ask what was said, and help the patient think through alternative explanations for what the person meant.

A delusional patient may be particularly likely to cast what he learned in terms of some concrete aspect of the exposure situation, rather than in terms of the implications for his BDD beliefs. Help such a patient devise helpful responses about himself or how others react to him, such as those shown in Handout 10.2. Responses such as "There aren't too many people who drive around here at night" aren't helpful, because they don't shift the patient's beliefs about himself in a more realistic or helpful direction.

If the patient can't come up with something useful that he learned, you can suggest some possibilities. If the experiment had a major flaw and failed, you can still try to see whether he learned anything helpful in the process, although you won't want to reinforce faulty conclusions that are based on a flawed experiment.

For a further example of a successful and productively processed exposure exercise, see Lorenzo's sample completed *Exposure Worksheet* (Figure 10.1). Lorenzo was completely convinced that he looked abnormal, and that as a result people took special notice of him in a negative way. Note how Lorenzo's worksheet incorporates some of the specific suggestions discussed above.

FILL OUT THIS PART *BEFORE* THE EXPOSURE

My Exposure Situation (Be specific)

Going to the grocery store at 3:00 on a Saturday afternoon when it's busy, to buy groceries with Juanita.

What aspect of the situation causes me the most distress?

Being around other people and thinking they're noticing how ugly I am.

What subtle ways of avoiding do I need to watch out for?

Not looking around the grocery store to see what people are doing.

Preparing My Thoughts

Negative thoughts/predictions

Because I look so bad, 80% of people will look at me with disgust and think I'm a freak. They'll move away from me within 5 seconds.

Alternative thoughts

1. *I'm doing fortune telling and personalization. Maybe people will be more interested in their shopping than in me. I can't predict the future anyway.*
2. *I'm labeling myself negatively and using emotional reasoning. Just because I feel like a freak doesn't mean I really am a freak.*

Goals for the Exposure (How will I know I did well?)

1. *Buy all the groceries on my list without shopping really fast. This should take at least 45 minutes.*
2. *Look around me while I'm in the store so I can see what people are doing.*

FILL OUT THIS PART *AFTER* THE EXPOSURE

Distress Rating: Beginning *50* Half-time *40* Ending *30*

Evaluating My Efforts

Did I reach my goal?

Yes, I bought all of my groceries without rushing. I stayed in the store for 1 hour. And I looked around me while I was shopping.

(cont.)

FIGURE 10.1. Lorenzo's sample completed *Exposure Worksheet.*

Did my negative thoughts/predictions come true?
No, they didn't. About 30% of people didn't move at all; they seemed busy picking out food or watching their kids. About 40% moved away from me, but no one looked disgusted. They were mostly looking at other things, like their grocery list or the food on the shelves, and they hardly seemed to notice me. About 30% moved toward me. Juanita and I both agree on this.

What did I learn?
Maybe people aren't taking special notice of me after all, and maybe I don't look really weird or disgusting. Maybe people in the grocery store are more interested in their shopping than in me.

How will I reward myself?
Bought myself a Mounds Bar.

FIGURE 10.1. *(cont.)*

FORM 10.1

Exposure Worksheet

FILL OUT THIS PART *BEFORE* THE EXPOSURE

My Exposure Situation (Be specific)

What aspect of the situation causes me the most distress?

What subtle ways of avoiding do I need to watch out for?

Preparing My Thoughts

Negative thoughts/predictions

Alternative thoughts

Goals for the Exposure (How will I know I did well?)

(cont.)

Adapted with permission of the publisher from Wilhelm, S. (2006). *Feeling Good about the Way You Look: A Program for Overcoming Body Image Problems*. New York: Guilford Press.

Exposure Worksheet *(page 2 of 2)*

FILL OUT THIS PART *AFTER* THE EXPOSURE

Distress Rating: Beginning_____ Half-time_____ Ending_____

Evaluating My Efforts

Did I reach my goal?

Did my negative thoughts/predictions come true?

What did I learn?

How will I reward myself?

FORM 10.2

Distressing Situations Worksheet

Situation	Degree of distress (0–100)	Degree of avoidance (0–100)
1.		
2.		
3.		
4.		
5.		
6.		
7.		
8.		
9.		
10.		
11.		
12.		
13.		
14.		
15.		

Adapted with permission of the publisher from Wilhelm, S. (2006). *Feeling Good about the Way You Look: A Program for Overcoming Body Image Problems*. New York: Guilford Press.

HANDOUT 10.1

Sample Completed Distressing Situations Worksheet

Situation	Degree of distress (0–100)	Degree of avoidance (0–100)
1. Walking toward a stranger after dark without looking away	40	30
2. Passing a stranger in the lobby at work without looking away	45	35
3. Saying hello to a coworker in the lobby	55	40
4. Walking toward a stranger during the daytime	60	50
5. Standing under the lights near the water cooler and talking to a coworker	62	70
6. Standing under the lights near the water cooler and talking to several coworkers	65	75
7. Sitting across from a stranger in the train without avoiding eye contact	66	75
8. Going to church, sitting in the back	66	80
9. Going to church, sitting in the middle	70	82
10. Letting my partner touch my face	70	85
11. Letting my child touch my face	80	100
12. Sitting across from my sister and brother in a restaurant	90	100
13.		
14.		
15.		

HANDOUT 10.2

Henry's Sample Completed Exposure Worksheet

FILL OUT THIS PART *BEFORE* THE EXPOSURE

My Exposure Situation (Be specific)

Talking to the tall receptionist.

What aspect of the situation causes me the most distress?

Wearing flat shoes and standing right next to tall women.

What subtle ways of avoiding do I need to watch out for?

Not really looking her in the eyes.

Preparing My Thoughts

Negative thoughts/predictions

1. *She'll think she's better than me and will be really unfriendly and arrogant.*
2. *I look like such a freak!!!!*

Alternative thoughts

1. *I'm really mind reading and fortune telling. Chances are that she's not that interested in my height. Usually she is very friendly, and she likes to talk about health insurance and things like that.*
2. *I'm also labeling myself negatively and using all-or-nothing thinking. Just because I'm short and not perfect doesn't mean I'm a freak. Nobody has ever said anything bad about my height. My girlfriend says she finds me attractive.*

Goals for the Exposure (How will I know I did well?)

1. *Stand 2–3 feet from the receptionist.*
2. *Maintain eye contact.*
3. *Ask at least one question.*
4. *Stay for at least 3 minutes.*
5. *Attend to conversation, not myself-defeating thoughts.*

(cont.)

FILL OUT THIS PART *AFTER* THE EXPOSURE

Distress Rating: Beginning 45 Half-time 40 Ending 20

Evaluating My Efforts

Did I reach my goal?

Yes, and I even talked to her for much longer than I had planned and I was able to focus on the conversation.

Did my negative thoughts/predictions come true?

No, they didn't. I really don't think she was particularly interested in my height.

What did I learn?

My height is probably not as important to others as I think.

How will I reward myself?

Watch my favorite TV show tonight.

CHAPTER 11

SESSIONS 7–9

Adding Ritual Prevention

SESSION SUMMARY

- ☐ Check mood and BDD symptoms.
- ☐ Briefly review the previous session.
- ☐ Set the agenda jointly with the patient.
- ☐ Review homework.
- ☐ Work on the agenda.
  - ☐ Identify your patient's rituals.
  - ☐ Provide education about rituals and how they reinforce BDD symptoms.
  - ☐ Monitor rituals and identify triggers.
  - ☐ Develop a hierarchy and choose situations for ritual prevention.
  - ☐ Select ritual prevention methods.
  - ☐ Identify short-term goals.
  - ☐ Help the patient manage discomfort during ritual prevention.
  - ☐ Help the patient counteract comparison rituals: Shifting attention and taking in the big picture
  - ☐ Encourage the patient to practice ritual prevention and plan rewards.
- ☐ Assign homework.
- ☐ Ask for summary of/feedback on the session.

SESSION FORMS AND HANDOUTS

BDI-II (or other depression inventory)

Personal Session Form (Form 2.1)

Therapist Session Form (Form 6.1)

Colleen's Sample Completed Ritual-Monitoring Form (Handout 11.1)

Ritual-Monitoring Form (plus several extra copies for homework) (Form 11.1)

Sample Completed Ritual Hierarchy Lists (Handouts 11.2 and 11.3)

Ritual Hierarchy List (Form 11.2)

Approaches to Controlling Rituals (Handout 11.4)

Exposure and Response Prevention Worksheet (plus several extra copies for homework) (Form 11.3)

Examples of Things I Can Notice When Interacting with Other People (Handout 11.5)

The Big Picture Worksheet (Form 11.4)

INTRODUCTION TO THIS SESSION

The goal of this treatment segment is to help your patients learn how to stop engaging in repetitive behaviors or rituals. These behaviors reinforce their BDD fears and ultimately contribute to the persistence of their anxiety. Patients will learn to identify their rituals, monitor the frequency of these, decrease the amount of time they spend performing them, and replace them with healthier behaviors. We also describe how to combine ritual prevention with cognitive restructuring and with reducing avoidance behaviors. It is important for your patients to practice response prevention (stopping rituals) as part of their ongoing exposure exercises. We describe the first session in detail, but this section is likely to require two, three, or possibly even more sessions before treatment can move on to the next skill (perceptual retraining). You and each patient will need to incorporate ritual prevention into ongoing treatment until the therapy ends.

In Chapter 10, you have learned how to apply exposure to help patients become more comfortable in situations they have avoided or endured with great distress. For nearly all patients, however, exposure addresses only half of the BDD problem, because the patients also have excessive appearance rituals focused on checking, hiding, or trying to fix their perceived defects. Thus it is important to introduce ritual prevention as soon as a patient has a basic understanding of exposure. Your treatment will be most powerful when you flexibly combine these two treatment strategies. Repetitive compulsive behaviors can include checking one's body in the mirror, checking the body area by looking at it directly, comparing one's appearance to others', excessive grooming and applying makeup, reassurance seeking, excessive exercising, frequently touching the body areas, compulsive tanning, excessive clothes changing, shopping for appearance-related products, and compulsively seeking information about cosmetic products or procedures online or in books. Skin picking and hair pulling are additional compulsive behaviors that can be due to BDD; we address these problems in more detail in a separate treatment module, because we use a somewhat different approach to treat them (see Chapter 15).

Most patients have more than one ritual. Most feel a very strong urge to engage in these appearance-related actions and find them hard to resist or control. The rituals typically consume 1 hour or more per day and can become so time-consuming that they take the place of other activities, such as working, hobbies, or spending time with family or friends. Focusing treatment on reducing the rituals enables patients to gain control over them.

Start ritual prevention soon after you have conducted 1 or 2 relatively easy exposures that can be completed without also having to limit rituals. Then start to incorporate ritual prevention into the exposure exercises. This is important, because a patient who is still ritualizing is less likely to learn from the exposures. For the very small group of patients with BDD who have no rituals, you can use exposure and the cognitive strategies described in previous and subsequent chapters.

Check Mood and BDD Symptoms

Review the BDI-II (or other depression inventory) that the patient has completed in the waiting room. Pay attention to the scale's total score and the suicidality item, and ask further questions about suicidality if clinically indicated (see Chapter 2). Also briefly inquire about BDD symptoms over the course of the week.

Hand out the *Personal Session Form* (Form 2.1), and remind the patient to record information she finds significant during the session.

Briefly Review the Previous Session

Briefly check in with the patient on her perception and understanding of the previous session.

Set the Agenda Jointly with the Patient

Convey the topics you'd like to cover during the session. Explain to your patient that she will learn a new skill called "ritual prevention," which she will use together with exposure. Ask your patient whether there are any issues she would like to cover in this session, and try to combine these with the work on ritual prevention.

Review Homework

Discuss your patient's homework from the previous session, which focused on exposure exercises and completion of relevant forms.

Work on the Agenda

Identify Your Patient's Rituals

You will use several strategies for identifying rituals: reviewing information from questionnaires and early assessment sessions; questioning the patient directly to identify the rituals that follow BDD thoughts; and patient self-monitoring.

Review Assessment Information

We suggest that you review the items about rituals in the BDD-SS (Form 4.3) and the *BDD Information-Gathering Form* (Form 4.4), to get an idea of which rituals your patient engages in and how frequent and distressing they are. You also will have identified some rituals during your initial assessment session and while developing the model of the patient's BDD symptoms. Some patients will be able to give you very accurate estimates of how much time they spend ritualizing in any given situation, whereas others won't be sure or may deliberately minimize their reporting, usually out of embarrassment and shame.

Ask about Common Rituals

Among the most common BDD rituals are comparing oneself to others in terms of appearance, checking one's appearance in the mirror, and excessive grooming behaviors. We describe these very briefly below, so that you can inquire about the details of these rituals with your patients (see Chapter 1 for a more comprehensive list).

Most people with appearance concerns tend to scrutinize others closely and to compare themselves to these others in terms of the body part(s) of concern. Unfortunately, patients with BDD tend to make upward comparisons, focusing on people they believe look better than themselves. They may also focus on individuals who look abnormal or disfigured with respect to the body part of concern. For example, a patient who is concerned about scarring may focus on burn victims. One patient of ours who was concerned about her height and body proportions compared herself to someone with dyschondrosteosis, a rare disorder characterized by unusually long arms, short legs, and short stature. Patients who make these downward comparisons are frightened that they look like the deformed persons and scrutinize them to convince themselves that they do not look as deformed. Generally, whoever the comparison targets may be, patients with BDD often end up feeling badly about how they look. Comparison rituals are usually associated with selective attention to the body part of concern; patients typically do not notice much else about themselves and the other person. In Chapter 12, on perceptual retraining, we describe how to decrease selective attention to the patient's own body.

Mirror checking is another very common ritual. This is usually done to determine how bad the body part of concern (hair, skin, nose, etc.) looks. This commonly occurs before a patient goes out to work or to other events where people are present, but it can occur at any time of the day or night. Often it occupies many hours a day. Mirror checking may be accompanied by excessive grooming rituals—putting on makeup, trimming hair, tweezing eyebrows, picking skin, or other actions designed to improve appearance. These and any other repetitive behaviors intended to reduce discomfort about appearance should be targeted for the ritual prevention techniques described below.

Although the rituals described above are especially common, be sure to ask your patient whether she performs any other repetitive behaviors in order to check, hide, or try to improve her appearance (see Chapter 1). These behaviors are limited only by a patient's ingenuity. For example, we've seen patients who repeatedly tied up their calves tightly with rope to make them smaller, drank gallons of water a day to widen their faces, and frequently touched doorknobs in the hope of improving their skin. You will want to identify all repetitive appearance-related behaviors so you can address them in treatment.

Provide Education about Rituals and How They Reinforce BDD Symptoms

Refer to your patient's BDD model to discuss briefly how rituals reinforce and feed her BDD symptoms. This happens in several ways:

1. The rituals (e.g., checking the mirror for long periods of time) keep her focused on her appearance rather than on other thoughts or activities (e.g., going for a bike ride).
2. Rituals may temporarily diminish anxiety, and thereby reinforce the ritualistic behavior. Most patients find that their rituals relieve their anxiety only temporarily.
3. Engaging in the rituals prevents the patient from ever seeing what would happen if she were to do without them.

Although you have already provided a rationale for stopping the rituals in Session 3, remind your patient of this rationale now. You might say:

> "Now that we've discussed some rituals you do, it seems that they aren't really very helpful. They keep you very focused on your appearance and upset about it. They also take up a lot of time and keep you from doing other things you'd enjoy a lot more. Today we are going to start 'response prevention,' which is simply preventing the rituals (ritual prevention). Learning this skill will help you get better control over your rituals, so you spend less time doing them and feel more comfortable without them. You've said that you wish you could leave the house in the morning without spending so much time trying to fix your hair and getting stuck in front of the mirror for an hour. Learning to cut back on this behavior will eventually enable you to feel more comfortable going out after spending much less time on your grooming. I'll explain some ways you can get better control over these excessive behaviors."

Because you've already done some work on exposure, you can tell your patient that her reactions to response prevention will probably be similar to how she reacted to exposure.

> "When you begin to resist a ritual, most likely you'll feel distressed at first and have some doubts about giving it up. This is because it *seems* to help you ward off your feared consequences. You might feel that the main reason a date went well was because you really prepared for it by spending several hours in front of the mirror plucking out unwanted facial hair and fixing your makeup. But in fact, it's these very rituals that maintain your body image concerns, because they prevent you from learning that your fears of being laughed at wouldn't have come true even if you hadn't spent hours doing and redoing your makeup and hair. Your distress would have decreased over time on its own.
>
> "Our goal is to enable you to get used to handling fearful situations without ritualizing, so your fears decrease and you discover that the rituals weren't necessary in the first place. Stopping the rituals also helps stop your mental association between your rituals and temporarily feeling better. With time, your urges to ritualize will subside. I know this is hard to believe at this point, but we'll work on this together so you can see for yourself."

Occasional patients don't avoid situations or aren't really uncomfortable in any situations unless they suppress their appearance rituals. The treatment of these patients would focus on having them expose themselves to situations that normally trigger rituals, and ultimately on encouraging them to eliminate those rituals. These patients can start by monitoring the rituals that are related to their most important goal (e.g., becoming comfortable in social situations without lengthy mirror checking beforehand).

Monitor Rituals and Identify Triggers

The first step is for the patient to monitor her rituals and identify what triggers them. Begin by educating your patient about the purposes served by monitoring rituals in situations that typically trigger them. It enables you and your patient to determine how frequently and for how long they occur. It also enables the two of you to identify triggers for rituals. For example, getting ready for work in the morning may trigger excessive mirror checking and makeup application. Other triggers might include seeing an attractive person or even feeling bored. Some patients find that the monitoring helps them realize how much time they waste on these behaviors, which motivates them to do response prevention. The process of monitoring rituals may also provide a temporary decrease in their frequency, especially if your patient writes down each ritual as soon it occurs. Patients who have difficulty estimating how long their rituals last will benefit from monitoring the rituals for several days to get an accurate estimate of the base rate of the behaviors. This will help them set realistic goals before starting response prevention.

Your patient will use the *Ritual-Monitoring Form* (Form 11.1) to monitor her rituals and identify triggers. Before explaining the monitoring assignment, review your patient's long-term goals. These are the same goals you reviewed together before starting the exposure strategies described in Chapter 10. It's important to keep the goals in mind, to encourage your patient to complete the work of self-monitoring and eventually reducing rituals.

Now select a situation that provokes rituals. Ask your patient to fill out Form 11.1 to indicate when the most recent ritual began, what triggered it, the type of ritual, what thoughts occurred, the feelings triggered by the thoughts, and the amount of time spent on the ritual. It's important for the patient to do the monitoring in detail—for example, specifying the day, the time of day, and the exact trigger situation. If the form is filled out more broadly and vaguely (e.g., the patient just writes in "mirror checking" once to reflect checking throughout the day), this information will be much less helpful when the patient is doing response prevention.

Showing the patient Colleen's completed form (see *Colleen's Sample Completed Ritual-Monitoring Form*, Handout 11.1) may help you explain how to complete Form 11.1 (You can give Handout 11.1 to the patient to use as a guide for completing this form.) Colleen, a 27-year-old nurse, believed that she had excessive facial hair. Although people told her she looked very attractive, she thought she looked like a "hairy monster." On days when she thought she looked particularly bad, she would call in sick. Her first exposure practice focused on going to work every day, no matter how hairy she thought she looked. Colleen decided to work on reducing the rituals related to going to work, because she had already decided that going to work regularly was an important exposure goal. As you can see in Handout 11.1, Colleen tracked her rituals related to going to work for 1 day. Note that for patients whose rituals fluctuate, ritual monitoring should occur over several days.

Now give your patient several blank copies of the *Ritual-Monitoring Form* (Form 11.1) and ask her to fill in the columns for rituals that occur during the coming week. For example, if she engages in rituals before going to work or out to the store, ask her to complete the form for several days for daily rituals and for selected days for rituals that occur less often.

Develop a Hierarchy and Choose Situations for Ritual Prevention

Next, show your patient the two *Sample Completed Ritual Hierarchy Lists* (Handouts 11.2 and 11.3), and then help her develop a hierarchy for response prevention by using the blank *Ritual Hierarchy List* (Form 11.2). Take trigger situations from the patient's completed version of Form 11.1 and transfer them to the *Ritual Hierarchy List* (Form 11.2). Also have the patient rate (on the usual scale from 0 to 100) how much distress she would feel if the ritual were interrupted, as well as the frequency of her rituals or the time she spends ritualizing.

For example, Colleen used the information from her *Ritual-Monitoring Form* (Handout 11.1) to rate how distressed she would feel on the 0–100 scale if her rituals were interrupted, and how frequently they occurred or how much time they took. As you can see in Handout 11.2, Colleen recorded her rituals in enough detail to help her set specific goals for later ritual prevention.

Next, ask your patient what situation she would like to choose to begin ritual prevention. Usually this will be an exposure situation the patient is already working on. However, if this exposure situation is not associated with any rituals, it may be best to pick an easier situation from the hierarchy. We suggest you select an exposure situation that will cause your patient moderate distress, but not severe distress, if the rituals are interrupted (e.g., one she rates from 40 to 60 on Form 11.2).

If your patient is very avoidant because of her BDD symptoms (e.g., she doesn't work or is largely housebound), and she is engaging in many rituals at home, we suggest targeting the rituals she does do at home. Let's use Tom as an example. He mostly stays in his house. His BDD is too severe for him to work or see any friends or family members. Tom goes out of his house for an hour each day to do an exposure and response prevention assignment, but he spends the rest of his day alone at home. Tom also needs to address the rituals he's doing at home, which take up about 10 hours a day. He will need to do these exercises at home *in addition to* the exposure and response exercises he does outside of his home. *Tom's Sample Completed Ritual Hierarchy List* (Handout 11.3) is another handout to provide your patient with an example.

If any of your patients are engaging in risky behaviors—such as drinking excessively to quell their anxiety in social situations, or spending so much money on makeup or clothes that they cannot pay their other bills—you'll need to prioritize response prevention that is focused on these behaviors. Be sure that behaviors such as these are included in your patients' hierarchies so you don't forget about them. Also, depending on their severity and the risk they pose to your patients' well-being, you may need to start focusing on such behaviors early in the treatment, even if they are high on the hierarchies and if starting to cut back on them would cause the patients a lot of anxiety.

Select Ritual Prevention Methods

It would be great if a patient could just stop all her rituals at once, but for most patients that's impossible. Therefore, you need to help your patient find ways to reduce the rituals as fast as possible. We recommend that you choose one or more of several strategies described below. The rituals you choose to work on will be based on each patient's *Ritual Hierarchy List* (Form 11.2) and relevant exposures the patient is currently doing. Or, as noted above, certain patients may benefit from also using response prevention for rituals that are not linked to exposures. In such cases, you'll want to start by targeting rituals that have lower distress ratings on the patients' hierarchies, as these will initially be easier to control than those with higher ratings.

Note that some response prevention strategies will work better for certain situations than for others, so you are likely to find that methods not used initially may be helpful later in the treatment for different rituals. If one technique doesn't work, try adding or following it with another.

Now briefly introduce the ritual prevention methods we discuss below to your patient:

> "Now I'm going to tell you about the different methods you can use to get better control over your rituals. After I describe them to you, together we can select which ones you want to try for the rituals you'll start working on first. Eventually you'll want to try out most of these techniques, to see which ones work especially well for you. Let me give you this handout to refer to while I go through the response prevention methods. We can refer to this handout throughout the treatment to select the techniques you'd like to try." [Give the patient *Approaches to Controlling Rituals*, Handout 11.4.]

Stimulus Control

Stimulus control requires patients to *manipulate their environment to avoid cues* that trigger or increase rituals. You can ask your patients to deliberately modify certain situations, activities, or objects that trigger the appearance rituals. For example, if your patients use tools like scissors (to cut their hair), rulers (to measure body parts), or hand mirrors for their appearance rituals, ask them to discard them or give the tools to someone else to keep for them temporarily. For Colleen, seeing her tweezers almost always resulted in hair plucking. Her solution was to give them to her husband and ask him to return them to her for only 5 minutes each week. Tom stopped carrying a pocket mirror with her and threw out a mirror she had on her desk at home. Sometimes patients ask whether they should cover all the mirrors in their house. This is a form of stimulus control, and this strategy might be helpful for a short period of time. However, in the long run, your patient will need to learn to deal with mirrors in a healthier way. (The current chapter provides many strategies for doing so, and Chapter 12, which focuses on perceptual retraining for mirror checking, does as well.) For a patient who shops excessively for beauty products or clothes, you might want to recommend that she stop carrying credit cards or going to her favorite stores.

In addition, you can ask your patient to leave the trigger situation (e.g., walk away from the bathroom mirror) once a ritual starts and engage in an alternative behavior that you and the patient select in advance. Examples of alternatives might be to call a friend, draw a picture, or go for a bike ride.

Some patients find it helpful to put notes to themselves on doors, walls, or mirrors with messages that help them leave (or never even enter) triggering situations. One of our patients put a note on her bathroom door that said, "Are you *really* sure you want to go in there?" This helped her to turn around and not go in. Another patient simply wrote "STOP." It can also be helpful to write down a list of alternative activities that a patient can keep readily available when she gets the urge to ritualize. She may feel so anxious at those times that it may be hard to think of something else to do. Reading the list can help her focus her thinking and choose another activity to do instead.

Selective Ritual Prevention

Selective ritual prevention means initially allowing rituals *only in certain situations*, but not in others. At first, have the patient prevent the rituals directly related to the exposures she is doing, usually beginning with briefer rituals accompanied by a weaker urge. For example, consider recommending that the patient discard a mirror kept in a desk drawer at work, so that checking at the desk while working can be eliminated. Or if a patient is spending several hours a day at work and home researching cosmetic surgery on the Internet, have her stop doing this at work first prior to addressing the rituals at home.

Decreases in the Time Spent Ritualizing

For very time-consuming rituals accompanied by intense urges and high anxiety, your patient can *gradually reduce the amount of time spent and/or the number of rituals*. Be sure to have the patient first establish how much time she is spending on ritualizing, using the *Ritual-Monitoring Form* (Form 11.1). Then you and the patient can agree on immediate goals for the maximum time to be allowed for each ritual on a given day. Encourage your patient to challenge herself, but also to be realistic. For example, because Colleen spent about 40 minutes every morning before she went to work checking the mirror and tweezing, her therapist asked her to reduce this by 10 minutes every day. In Colleen's case, it was a good idea to work on the mirror checking and tweezing together, because the tweezing only occurred during mirror checking. A timer can be very useful for this strategy. The first day Colleen set the timer to 40 minutes, the next day to 30 minutes, then to 20 minutes, and so forth, until eventually she ritualized for only a few minutes and then not at all. Encourage your patient to decrease the rituals as fast as possible. Once the alarm goes off, no matter whether your patient feels the ritual is complete or not, she will have to stop.

A similar strategy is to *reduce the number of repetitions* of a given ritual. For example, if your patient applies and re-applies facial powder 10 times per day, have her decrease the powder applications gradually until eventually she stops completely.

This response prevention strategy also includes gradually decreasing the use of camouflage. For example, you could have a patient gradually wear less and less makeup, and then do some exposures without wearing any at all. You could also have a patient gradually move her hat farther and farther back from her forehead, then stop wearing it in certain situations, and then stop wearing it altogether.

Ritual Delay

Your patient can also decrease rituals by *postponing them for as long as possible.* If your patient has multiple rituals pertaining to the long-term goal she is working on, start with the ritual that's easiest to postpone first. For example, an urge to check a certain body part by looking at it or touching it could be delayed for 30 minutes, after which your patient should attempt to postpone it again, perhaps for another 30 minutes. Encourage your patient to postpone the ritual for as long as possible.

Postponement of rituals can also decrease their frequency, giving your patient time to utilize the cognitive strategies described in Chapter 9, which in turn tend to weaken the desire to ritualize as your patient's perspective changes. Often, a patient is more amenable to postponing a ritual than to trying the other strategies described above. However, eventually your patient has to give up the ritual altogether. If this does not occur naturally after the patient has been delaying rituals, you'll need to use one of the other strategies described here.

Competing Responses

Competing responses are *healthy behaviors that the patient engages in to replace appearance rituals.* These should be activities that are physically incompatible with the appearance rituals. In social situations, they must also be unobtrusive. Competing responses should focus on the same muscle groups used in the appearance compulsions, such as making a fist whenever your patient experiences the urge or initial action of picking up tweezers to pluck and even out her eyebrows. A patient who has an urge to touch or count his supposedly thinning hair while reading could hold his book tightly with both hands or grip the arms of his chair. Other physical competing responses include knitting, squeezing a soft ball, or manipulating marbles whenever the urge to ritualize strikes.

Ask your patient to maintain a competing response for at least 2 minutes, preferably until the urge subsides. If the first competing response doesn't work, design another. As you are designing competing responses, keep the following principles in mind: The response should be physically incompatible with the appearance ritual; it should be socially unremarkable; and your patient should be able to maintain it for long enough that the urge to ritualize dissipates. In Chapter 15, we say much more about using competing responses to decrease BDD-related skin picking and hair pulling.

Increases in Healthy Behaviors

No matter which ritual reduction strategies you choose with your patient, remember to encourage her to increase healthy behaviors over the course of the treatment. This is especially important if your patient is ritualizing for many hours per day. Removing rituals without filling the void leaves her open to rapid return of the rituals. Encourage your patient to get a volunteer or paid job, read books, play an instrument, meet friends, or engage in other activities that are inconsistent with the rituals and consistent with her values and goals.

Identify Short-Term Goals

Before beginning actual exposures with response prevention, you should take a look at Colleen's sample completed *Exposure and Response Prevention Worksheet* (Figure 11.1), in which she set goals for overcoming her rituals. As you can see, this form is similar to the *Exposure Worksheet* (Form 10.1) presented and described in Chapter 10. However, an important difference is that approaches to ritual prevention are listed as goals, and you and your patient need to agree on the initial short-term response prevention goals to work on. List these in the "Goals . . . " section on a blank copy of the *Exposure and Response Prevention Worksheet* (Form 11.3). To find a balance between challenging your patient and pushing her so hard that she gets frustrated, it's helpful to start with situations that cause only moderate distress at the outset. Colleen's example (in Figure 11.1) provides a good model for setting response prevention goals. In her "Goals . . . " section, she focused on rituals she performed during her exposures that caused her only moderate distress. She and her therapist decided to completely stop her least distressing rituals (taken from her completed *Ritual Hierarchy List*, Handout 11.2), while she also increased healthier behaviors.

Now you can help your patient fill in the first sections of the *Exposure and Response Prevention Worksheet* (Form 11.3), and can assign exposure while stopping rituals in this situation for homework. Generally, you will probably need to do this during the next session, after your patient has monitored her rituals and completed the *Ritual Hierarchy List* (Form 11.2) for homework.

Decide on specific, achievable, and objective goals for the exposure and response prevention, and ask your patient to write them down on Form 11.3. From this point forward, the goals should include stopping rituals altogether or changing some rituals. It's also critical for your patient's goals to be realistic. Goals focusing on reducing time, frequency, or repetitions of rituals enable the patient to measure whether she has achieved them.

For response prevention that is not linked to an exposure, have the patient select one or two of the response prevention techniques above and start applying them to one or two of the rituals that are lower on her hierarchy during the upcoming week. The patient can fill out the relevant

FILL OUT THIS PART *BEFORE* THE EXPOSURE/RESPONSE PREVENTION

My Exposure and/or Response Prevention Situation (Be specific)
Going back to work on Monday morning, try to reduce comparing and mirror checking.

What aspect of the situation causes me the most distress?
When I see attractive women (either patients or colleagues).

What subtle ways of avoiding, or rituals, do I need to watch out for?
Checking my appearance in the bathroom mirror, getting stuck there.

Preparing My Thoughts

Negative thoughts/predictions
Everyone will notice my facial hair. They'll think I'm disgusting.

Alternative thoughts
Their world does not revolve around my facial hair. They probably could not care less.

Goals for the Exposure/Response Prevention (How will I know I did well?)

1. *Do not compare myself to others or scrutinize their faces for facial hair. Notice other things about them, like what they are talking about, the sound of their voice, what kind of mood they seem to be in, what their concerns are, etc.*
2. *Do not check the mirror for more than 2 seconds when at work. While in the bathroom washing my hands, just look at my hands, not in the mirror.*

FILL OUT THIS PART *AFTER* THE EXPOSURE/RESPONSE PREVENTION

Distress Rating: Beginning *80* **Half-time** *50* **Ending** *20*

Evaluating My Efforts

Did I reach my goals?
For the most part I occasionally compared myself (maybe 5 times), but was always able to redirect my attention to other things quickly. I only checked the mirror once, and only for a couple of seconds.

Did my negative thoughts/predictions come true?
No.

What did I learn?
That I enjoy work more when I am less focused on my facial hair.

How will I reward myself?
I am excited that I did well with regard to my Exposure and Response Prevention work. The success is my reward.

Adapted with permission of the publisher from Wilhelm, S. (2006). *Feeling Good about the Way You Look: A Program for Overcoming Body Image Problems*. New York: Guilford Press.

FIGURE 11.1. Colleen's sample completed *Exposure and Response Prevention Worksheet*.

Ritual	Response prevention technique
Looking for hair products on the Internet	Don't turn on my computer until 10 A.M. each day. If I catch myself searching for hair products, I'll get up and walk away from the computer.
Calling my mom to ask if my hair looks OK	When I get the urge to call, delay calling for at least 30 minutes and read my book instead.

FIGURE 11.2. Tom's response prevention techniques.

sections of Form 11.3 to assist with this. Figure 11.2 gives you another example of how rituals might be linked to ritual prevention strategies.

Help the Patient Manage Discomfort during Ritual Prevention

After you and your patient have decided on the method and goals for preventing rituals, remind the patient that she will initially feel more anxious, but this will diminish over time. Changing BDD rituals can cause significant discomfort, as can exposure. When your patient first begins a response prevention exercise, her distress rating could even go up to 80 or 90, but will gradually drop down to a 60 or 70 and, with repetition, to much lower ratings of 20, 10, or even 0. Thus it is critical for the patients not to give into the urge to ritualize when her discomfort increases, because then she robs herself of the opportunity to experience the decrease in distress she will only feel if she continues the exercise. Most patients who have sought treatment accept the fact that they need to face their fears. The following dialogue shows how to approach a patient's concern:

THERAPIST: When you first resist your rituals, you'll probably feel distressed initially. I can understand that you might not want to give up your rituals, because you may feel like the rituals have helped prevent bad things from happening. For example, you might feel that the main reason a date went well is because you really prepared for it by spending several hours in front of the mirror plucking out unwanted hair. But as we've discussed, the rituals have lots of downsides. They take up so much time, and they feed the BDD by keeping you focused on how you look. Also, they prevent you from learning that your fears—for example, being laughed at—might not have come true even if you hadn't ritualized. If you never go out until you've done your rituals, how will you get to see how things would have gone if you hadn't done your rituals?

PATIENT: Well, my parents did force me to go out to a family party this week without doing my hair and makeup first, and it was terrifying. I just ended up leaving the party and hiding in the bathroom.

THERAPIST: Trying to stop your rituals all of a sudden is really hard, and it's understandable that you felt anxious. We'll approach this very systematically, and we'll plan the response prevention together, to make it more doable for you. At first, learning this skill will make you a little anxious. It's important that you don't give into the ritual when your discomfort increases, because then you'll rob yourself of the opportunity to experience the decrease in distress that you'll only feel if you work on the exercises over the long term. You might need all your willpower to do this. But with practice, you'll find that it gets easier and easier to control your rituals. The urge to do your rituals will weaken. How does this sound to you?

For the most part, patients get out of CBT-BDD whatever they put in to it. It's normal to experience some distress as part of this program. So if your patients are willing to make this investment, it's pretty likely that they'll improve. Some patients have asked whether they should do relaxation exercises when they get anxious. In our experience, these don't work well in combination with exposure or ritual prevention. However, we occasionally use relaxation in the treatment of skin picking, which we describe in Chapter 15.

Often cognitive strategies can help prepare patients for the exposure and response prevention exercises, and help them understand that many of their fears are not rational and that their worst predictions usually don't come true. But even with this preparation, patients will become uncomfortable at various points. Help them prepare for this by reminding them that tolerating the discomfort helps them get much better in the long run. The cost of the short-term suffering is small in comparison to what they've been through before they came for treatment.

Help the Patient Counteract Comparison Rituals

Because patients with BDD selectively attend to their flaws, they often compare the body parts that they perceive as flawed to the same body parts of others. For example, if a patient dislikes her own nose, she is likely to compare it with other people's noses. Comparison rituals are very common; virtually all patients engage in this behavior. These rituals are also usually very distressing to patients, because they usually just reinforce their negative views of their appearance and can even make them feel worse. In addition, comparing can be very time-consuming and is particularly difficult to prevent.

Some of the ritual prevention strategies described above may be helpful for comparison rituals. For example, your patient may be able to cut down on the time she spends comparing during the day, or in a particular situation. These approaches may be particularly helpful if your patient compares herself with models on TV or in magazines. For instance, you can have her use stimulus prevention methods such as stopping a subscription to a fashion magazine that triggers comparing. She can also cut down the time she spends reading such magazines or limit the number of people she compares herself to while reading a magazine.

In our experience, however, it can be very helpful to supplement these more standard strategies with the following approach, especially when patients interact with other people. We call this approach "taking in the big picture." This exercise consists of broadening the patient's focus from specific body parts or appearance in general to other aspects of life and conceptually fits with the attention shifting exercise we introduced in the exposure chapter (Chapter 10). Patients need to turn on their senses and try to notice what is really happening in a particular situation—in other words, to try to see the big picture. Usually, when comparing herself with other people, all a patient with BDD really notices is the other person's eyes, or skin tone—or whatever body part the patient dislikes about herself. She focuses on these body areas, thinking things such as "Her eyes are so much prettier than mine; I can't stand it!" Or "She has such gorgeous hair; I have a rat's nest on my head." Or "Why can't I have clear skin like everyone else at this meeting? I feel so ugly!" Such thoughts make your patient feel miserable. Another problem is that when the patient is caught up in this compulsive comparing, she is missing out on everything else that's going on—for example, what the other person is saying, what kind of mood the person seems to be in, whether the person seems to be upset, what else is going on in the room, whether there's a funny smell coming from the kitchen, and so forth. In other words, your patient misses out on just about everything that's going on.

A powerful way to counteract comparison rituals is to try to have your patient tune into these other things. Ask her to shift from a BDD focus (i.e., her appearance concern) to another focus. Encourage the patient to "turn on her senses" and to pay attention to the task at hand. So, for example, if she is in a meeting at work, she can focus on the discussion with her colleagues. She can listen to the different contributions of her coworkers and can take a look at relevant written materials. If she is at a gym, she can try to focus on what a particular exercise feels like in all the different parts of her body. If she is looking at others, she should really try to see the big picture and notice *all* the features of other people, not just the body part she is comparing to her own feature of concern. We've provided a handout for your patient that lists some of the things she can notice; ask her to try to notice and focus on these things while interacting with other people. This handout is called *Examples of Things I Can Notice When Interacting with Other People* (Handout 11.5). Then have her fill in *The Big Picture Worksheet* (Form 11.4) after she interacts with another person or a group of people, and encourage her to notice as much as possible about the situation in question.

When your patient is noticing things about people other than their appearance, it's important for her not to stay in the "comparison mode." For example, it isn't helpful for the patient to write, "She has a nice voice, and I don't," or "Her personality is so much better than mine." Making comparisons like these, even if not focused on appearance, keeps the patient feeling bad and focused on her inadequacies. Instead, her descriptions of other people and the environment should be relatively neutral. Comparison rituals are extremely common, and this is why we are describing the strategies of "shifting attention" and "seeing the big picture" here. However, you will find that you can apply these strategies more broadly. In fact, you might be able to apply them any time your patient is caught up in BDD-related thinking and not focusing on the situation at hand.

Encourage the Patient to Practice Ritual Prevention and Plan Rewards

If time permits in your first session (or, more likely, in your second session) on ritual prevention, see whether you can identify an appropriate situation in or near the clinic where you and your patient can actually practice exposure and response prevention during the session. Whether ritual prevention practice is done during the session or at home, addressing your patient's thoughts before the assignment by having her fill out the top half of the *Exposure and Response Prevention Worksheet* (Form 11.3) will make her practice easier. It can be helpful to ask the patient to imagine every aspect of the exercise ahead of time, to identify negative predictions that can be tested during the practice. Using the techniques from Chapter 9, you and the patient can address the negative thoughts she has listed in the section entitled "Preparing My Thoughts" on the worksheet.

Also, ask your patient to rate her distress before, during, and after an exercise. After your patient has completed the exercise, help her review whether she reached her goals, and record this in the appropriate space on Form 11.3. Like exposure, ritual prevention is an opportunity for your patient to learn whether her scary predictions and anxiety-provoking thoughts come true if she does not ritualize. Discuss and write down what your patient has learned from the ritual prevention practice.

Finally, encourage your patient to plan rewards for successful completion of exposure and response prevention exercises.

ASSIGN HOMEWORK

- Assign monitoring of rituals for homework on a daily basis for the next several weeks or until the patient's ritualistic behaviors are much reduced. Have the patient fill out the form right after she has done a ritual. Give the patient *Colleen's Sample Completed Ritual-Monitoring Form* (Handout 11.1) as a guide.
- Have your patient complete or revise her response prevention hierarchy (if necessary after additional ritual monitoring). Give the patient *Colleen's Sample Completed Ritual Hierarchy List* (Handout 11.2) as a guide. You can also give her *Tom's Sample Completed Ritual Hierarchy List* (Handout 11.3) as a guide if you decide to try additional response prevention.
- Do exposure exercises that incorporate ritual prevention into the goals. Ask your patient to complete copies of the *Exposure and Response Prevention Worksheet* (Form 11.3) regularly during the program.
- If your patient engages in comparing rituals, have her complete *The Big Picture Worksheet* (Form 11.4). Have her fill out several copies of this worksheet each week for the rest of the treatment.

ASK FOR SUMMARY OF/FEEDBACK ON THE SESSION

Ask the patient to briefly summarize the major points covered during the session. Also ask whether she had any concerns about the session or your behavior, and respond appropriately.

KEEP WORKING ON RITUAL PREVENTION THROUGHOUT THE TREATMENT

As is the case for exposure (see Chapter 10), it is very important to keep working on response prevention throughout this entire treatment. Be sure that it's part of the patient's homework every week. This will enable the patient to continue to make progress by getting the rituals she initially works on under better and better control, and moving on to more difficult rituals. An ideal way to accomplish this is to assign the *Exposure and Response Prevention Worksheet* (Form 11.3) for homework at every session. Ideally, the patient will complete at least one of these exercises every day throughout the treatment. This worksheet incorporates the core CBT-BDD skills of cognitive restructuring, exposure, and response prevention, so the patient can keep working on all of these skills. Keep having the patient gradually try increasingly challenging assignments by moving up her exposure and response prevention hierarchies over the course of the next couple of sessions. This will help ensure that she continues to make progress throughout the treatment. Before you move on to introduce your next core treatment component, you want to be sure to provide a couple of sessions for the patient to practice and combine the skills she has learned so far, while also progressing up her hierarchies. Below is an outline of what those sessions might look like.

SESSION SUMMARY FOR SESSIONS 8 AND 9

- ☐ Check mood and BDD symptoms.
- ☐ Briefly review the previous session.
- ☐ Set the agenda jointly with the patient.
- ☐ Review homework (which included work on cognitive skills, exposure, and response prevention).
- ☐ Work on the agenda.
    - ☐ Have the patient continue to practice cognitive skills, and work her way up to increasingly challenging exposure and ritual prevention exercises. (Remember to leave the office to work on exposure and response prevention exercises.)
- ☐ Assign homework (refining cognitive skills, exposure, and response prevention).
- ☐ Ask for summary of/feedback on the session.

FORM 11.1

Ritual-Monitoring Form

Time started	Trigger situation	Thoughts	Feelings	Ritual	Time spent ritualizing

Fill out this form right after you do a ritual. Fill out at least one form each day.

Adapted with permission of the publisher from Wilhelm, S. (2006). *Feeling Good about the Way You Look: A Program for Overcoming Body Image Problems*. New York: Guilford Press.

FORM 11.2

Ritual Hierarchy List

Trigger situation and ritual	Distress if ritual was interrupted (0–100)	Frequency of rituals or time spent ritualizing

FORM 11.3

Exposure and Response Prevention Worksheet

FILL OUT THIS PART *BEFORE* THE EXPOSURE/RESPONSE PREVENTION

My Exposure and/or Response Prevention Situation (Be specific)

What aspect of the situation causes me the most distress?

What subtle ways of avoiding, or rituals, do I need to watch out for?

Preparing My Thoughts

Negative thoughts/predictions

Alternative thoughts

Goals for the Exposure/Response Prevention (How will I know I did well?)

FILL OUT THIS PART *AFTER* THE EXPOSURE/RESPONSE PREVENTION

Distress Rating: Beginning _____ Half-time _____ Ending _____

Evaluating My Efforts

Did I reach my goal?

Did my negative thoughts/predictions come true?

What did I learn?

How will I reward myself?

Adapted with permission of the publisher from Wilhelm, S. (2006). *Feeling Good about the Way You Look: A Program for Overcoming Body Image Problems*. New York: Guilford Press.

FORM 11.4

The Big Picture Worksheet

Rather than just focusing on your appearance concerns, try to attend to the situation you are in. Often this will mean that you will shift attention from how you think and feel about your appearance concerns to what is going on around you.

Date and Situation

What I Noticed

What percentage of your attention was focused on your appearance concerns? _____

HANDOUT 11.1

Colleen's Sample Completed Ritual-Monitoring Form

Time started	Trigger situation	Thoughts	Feelings	Ritual	Time spent ritualizing
7:15 A.M.	Before leaving house and going to work	I look like a hairy monster. Everyone will laugh and tease me!	Terrified	Mirror checking and tweezing	40 minutes
8:10 A.M.	Seeing patient who doesn't seem to have facial hair	I'll never look like that. She looks perfect. I'm so ugly. I'll never be happy looking like this.	Ashamed	Comparing myself to patient	10 minutes
8:25 A.M.	Same as above (seeing female patient who doesn't have facial hair)	The patient might have noticed my facial hair. She was repulsed.	Anxious	Mirror checking	15 minutes
10:05 A.M.	Saw myself in the restroom mirror when washing hands	I wish I didn't have to go out and face everyone. They'll notice all these hairs. I just want to go home.	Anxious, depressed	Mirror checking when washing hands in restroom	7 minutes
11:55 A.M.	Saw myself in the restroom mirror when washing hands	Let's see what I look like before I go on the street.	Slightly anxious	Mirror checking (before going home)	3–4 minutes

HANDOUT 11.2

Colleen's Sample Completed Ritual Hierarchy List

Trigger situation and ritual	Distress if ritual was interrupted (0–100)	Frequency of rituals or time spent ritualizing
1. Before leaving house: Mirror checking and tweezing	60	40 minutes
2. At work: Comparing my appearance to others' appearance	45	2 times
3. At work: Mirror checking	40	4–7 minutes, 2 times

HANDOUT 11.3

Tom's Sample Completed Ritual Hierarchy List

Trigger situation and ritual	Distress if ritual was interrupted (0–100)	Frequency of rituals or time spent ritualizing each day
1. Mirror checking	60	5 hours
2. Comparing my appearance to people on TV	50	3 hours
3. Combing my hair	50	1 hour
4. Calling my mother and asking her if I look OK	45	30 minutes
5. Looking for hair products on the Internet	40	2 hours

HANDOUT 11.4

Approaches to Controlling Rituals

Stimulus Control: You manipulate your environment to avoid cues that trigger or increase rituals.

BDD examples:
- Stop carrying a pocket mirror.
- Take your mirror off your desk at work.
- Give tweezers used for hair plucking to partner to keep; get them from partner to use for only 5 minutes a week.
- Get rid of credit card for clothing store.
- Leave the bathroom as soon as you start checking the mirror, and call a friend, draw a picture, or go for a bike ride instead.

Selective Ritual Prevention: You initially allow rituals only in certain situations, but not in others.

BDD examples:
- Don't check mirrors at school or work.
- Stop researching cosmetic surgery on the Internet while at work.
- Don't comb your hair in the car.

Decreases in the Time Spent Ritualizing: Gradually reduce the amount of time spent and/or the number of rituals. You can also reduce number of repetitions of a given ritual.

BDD examples:
- Cut down eyebrow tweezing by 10 minutes each day.
- Cut down mirror checking by 15 minutes each day; set a timer and leave the mirror as soon as it goes off, whether you want to leave or not.
- Cut down asking a loved one whether you look big enough by two questions a day.
- Cut down tanning by 20 minutes each week.

(cont.)

Ritual Delay: Postpone rituals for as long as possible.

BDD examples:

- Postpone looking at the cellulite on your legs for 30 minutes.
- Postpone checking your makeup for 20 minutes.
- Postpone measuring your thighs for 30 minutes.

Competing Responses: These are healthy behaviors done to replace appearance rituals. These should be activities that are physically incompatible with the appearance rituals. In social situations, they must also be unobtrusive. Competing responses should focus on the same muscle groups used in the appearance compulsions, such as making a fist whenever you experience the urge or initial action of picking up tweezers to pluck and even out your eyebrows.

BDD examples:

- Squeezing a soft ball when getting the urge to pick your skin.
- Making a fist when getting the urge to feel the bump on your nose.
- Picking up knitting needles and starting to knit when getting the urge to feel for facial hairs.

Increases in Healthy Behaviors: Removing your BDD rituals without filling your time with other activities might leave you vulnerable to return to your rituals. Develop hobbies and activities to fill your time in a meaningful way.

BDD examples:

- Get a volunteer job.
- Meet friends.
- Take a class.

HANDOUT 11.5

Examples of Things I Can Notice When Interacting with Other People

- The sound of their voices
- The tone of their voices
- The smell of their perfume
- Their sense of humor
- What the conversation is focusing on
- Details of the conversation (what they said and what I said)
- What kind of mood they are in
- Whether they seem upset about something
- Whether they seem alert or fatigued
- Whether they seem happy
- What they are wearing
- What else is going on in the room: Are other people there? If so, what are they doing?
- Is the situation quiet or noisy? If it's noisy, what are the noises?
- Are there any smells in the room? If so, what are they?
- Can I hear other people talking? If so, what do they seem to be talking about?
- Can I feel anything (e.g., the taste of food in my mouth, whether the chair I'm sitting on is padded or hard)?

CHAPTER 12

SESSION 10

Perceptual Retraining for Mirror Checking

SESSION SUMMARY

- ☐ Check mood and BDD symptoms.
- ☐ Briefly review the previous session.
- ☐ Set the agenda jointly with the patient.
- ☐ Review homework.
- ☐ Work on the agenda.
  - ☐ Explain the rationale and goals for mirror retraining.
  - ☐ Assess your patient's relationship with mirrors.
  - ☐ Develop a hierarchy for mirror exposures.
  - ☐ Provide perceptual retraining during mirror exposures: seeing the big picture.
  - ☐ Remind the patient to engage in response prevention during mirror exposures.
  - ☐ Encourage the patient to practice and move up the hierarchy.
  - ☐ Coach the patient in using metaphors.
- ☐ Assign homework.
- ☐ Ask for summary of/feedback on the session.

SESSION FORMS AND HANDOUTS

BDI-II (or other depression inventory)

Personal Session Form (Form 2.1)

Therapist Session Form (Form 6.1)

Distressing Mirror Situations Hierarchy (Form 12.1)

Sample Completed Distressing Mirror Situations Hierarchy (Handout 12.1)

Mirror Retraining Worksheet (plus several extra copies for homework) (Form 12.2)

Exposure and Response Prevention Worksheet (plus several extra copies for homework) (Form 11.3)

Thought Record (plus several extra copies for homework) (Form 9.1)

BDD Information-Gathering Form (from initial assessment) (Form 4.4)

INTRODUCTION TO THIS SESSION

Most people with BDD have problems with mirrors and other reflective surfaces: they check them excessively, avoid them, or both. Some patients spend many hours a day checking their appearance in the mirror or in other reflective surfaces. We have treated several patients who had car accidents because they were checking their appearance in the rearview mirror while driving. Patients may be late for work or for social events because they get stuck checking their appearance in a mirror before leaving the house. Some have problems with work or school because they so frequently go to the bathroom to check their appearance in the mirror.

Patients with BDD may also avoid mirrors, or may use only small and cloudy mirrors for fear of becoming distressed when they see their reflections. Some patients avoid looking in mirrors only when they're undressed; others can look at certain body areas but avoid looking at other areas. Some people alternate between mirror checking and mirror avoidance, both of which maintain their negative thoughts and feelings about their looks.

When patients with BDD look at their reflection, they usually focus selectively on the body parts of concern ("hot spots"), while ignoring other body parts. They also often get very close to the mirror, which causes their "defects" to look more prominent and distorted. Imagine how a small scar will look after a patient stares at it from 2 inches away for 3 hours a day! It becomes all that the patient sees. Some patients use magnifying mirrors or especially bright lights to scrutinize the perceived defects even more closely, which further fuels their distorted view of how they look.

Many patients compulsively check not only mirrors, but other reflective surfaces—anything that is shiny will do. These can include store or car windows, car bumpers, reflecting glass on pictures, or metal toasters. Some patients even check themselves in tweezers or spoons. Such images are especially distorted and can fuel intense distress and despair.

While they look at their reflections, some patients simply scrutinize themselves, whereas others examine their faces or bodies from different angles. During mirror checking, many patients try to fix the problems they perceive; for example, they may also pluck hairs, shave, comb their hair, apply makeup, or pick their skin. Others manipulate their faces (e.g., pull on their lips) to try to improve their looks.

While checking themselves in reflective surfaces, most patients engage in negative, judgmental, and emotionally charged self-talk, such as "Look at those huge, disgusting scars!" This negative self-talk, combined with selective attention to flaws and disregard for attractive or acceptable body parts, results in very poor body image.

It is common for patients with BDD to have "good mirrors" (mirrors that they think make them look a little bit better than, or not as bad as, they fear) and "bad mirrors" (mirrors that they think make them look especially bad). Some patients tend to focus their excessive checking on good mirrors and their avoidance on bad mirrors. Like most BDD rituals, mirror checking often makes people feel worse but sometimes makes them feel a little better (which has the unfortunate consequence of fueling more checking). The outcome can depend on whether they look in a "good mirror" or a "bad mirror," on environmental factors (e.g., the lighting in the room), or on other factors (e.g., whether they just got a "bad" haircut or have a pimple at the time they check).

Nearly all patients with BDD have problems with mirror avoidance or checking, as well as with selective attention to flaws while they are looking at themselves; thus they are likely to benefit from the techniques described in this chapter. You can start working with mirrors after your patient has a basic understanding of both exposure and response prevention. Usually this will occur about two sessions after you have introduced response prevention (see Chapter 11). One to two sessions that focus on mirror exposures and perceptual retraining will usually suffice. However, material from this session should be assigned as homework every week. In addition, you can include it on the agenda of future sessions as needed.

You will need a small mirror (although this should be larger than a pocket mirror or a compact mirror) and a full-length mirror to use during these sessions.

Check Mood and BDD Symptoms

Ask your patient for the BDI-II (or other depression inventory) he has completed in the waiting room. Pay attention to the scale's total score and the suicidality item, and ask further questions about suicidality if clinically indicated (see Chapter 2). Also briefly inquire about BDD symptoms over the course of the week.

Hand out the *Personal Session Form* (Form 2.1), and remind the patient to record information he finds significant during the session.

Briefly Review the Previous Session

Briefly check in with the patient on his perception and understanding of the previous session.

Set the Agenda Jointly with the Patient

Convey the topics you would like to cover during the session (perceptual retraining for mirror checking). Ask the patient whether there are any issues he'd like to cover in this session; if so, try to weave them into the perceptual retraining session.

Review Homework

Discuss your patient's homework from the previous session. At this point in treatment, the patient should be practicing all of the core skills (cognitive strategies as well as exposure and ritual prevention at home).

Work on the Agenda

Explain the Rationale and Goals for Mirror Retraining

Earlier in the treatment, you will have established that the patient has difficulties with mirrors. As noted above, this is true for virtually all patients with BDD. You can go back to the patient's BDD model and discuss how he has already learned one approach to dealing with mirrors, which is response prevention. The goal of response prevention is for him to get better control over his excessive mirror checking.

Next, you can explain that the patient is going to learn an additional skill to feel more comfortable when he looks in mirrors. This is called "mirror retraining." The goals of mirror retraining are (1) to help the patient change how he looks in the mirror to a *mindful, nonjudgmental* way; and (2) help the patient come to see himself *more holistically*, resulting in improved self-perception. The following specific goals are typical for most patients:

- "Gain a more holistic view of myself, instead of focusing on and checking 'hot spots.'"
- "Observe and describe my entire body objectively, without judging or evaluating it."
- "Observe and describe my entire body while I am a normal distance from the mirror, rather than a few inches away."
- "Stop using tools that distort appearance and interfere with a holistic view, such as magnifying mirrors."
- "Decrease subtle and overt avoidance behaviors (such as covering my hair with a hat) and rituals (such as applying makeup or picking my skin) when I am viewing myself in a mirror."
- "Tolerate and accept my appearance and emotions."
- "Decrease the frequency of maladaptive mirror-checking episodes."

At this point, the patient may ask, "Why do mirror retraining? Isn't it better to stop looking in mirrors altogether?" We suggest telling your patient that you *do* recommend response prevention with mirrors—that is, cutting back on and eventually stopping excessive mirror checking. This may involve getting rid of unnecessary mirrors. Some of our patients have had as many as 30 mirrors—on every wall in their homes, in all of their pocketbooks, in their cars, on their desks at work, and so on. We encourage our patients to get rid of most of these mirrors as part of stimulus control when they are doing response prevention (see Chapter 11). We also encourage our patients to cut down on the frequency of mirror checking and the time they spend in the mirror.

However, you can explain to your patient that most people need to have at least a few mirrors in their lives. Most people use a mirror each day for normal grooming. In addition, the world is full of reflecting surfaces (mirrors in hotel lobbies or stores, reflecting windows, etc.). Although we encourage our patients *not* to check themselves in surfaces such as these, or to seek out mirrors to do checking, they may nonetheless catch unanticipated glimpses of themselves in these surfaces or need to look in the mirror each morning when grooming. When this happens, we want them to be prepared for this, by being able to see themselves in a more holistic and nonjudgmental way. In other words, we want them to see the "big picture." This is why we have them learn mirror retraining.

Assess Your Patient's Relationship with Mirrors

As a first step, obtain a basic overview of how your patient generally deals with mirrors and how much distress mirrors provoke. Begin by asking the patient to write down 10–15 mirror-related situations he avoids or can only manage by using certain rituals in front of the mirror (e.g., letting the light hit his skin in a certain way). Help the patient generate this list by reminding him of the dimensions that make looking in a mirror more or less difficult. Here are several examples:

- Type and size of mirror
- Distance from the mirror
- Duration of mirror observation
- Lighting
- Use of camouflage (e.g., makeup, hat, certain clothing)
- Use of tools such as magnifying mirrors
- Angle of view
- Time of day

Ask about any other idiosyncratic aspects of mirror use. For example, one patient avoided touching his face while looking in the mirror. If your patient has any difficulty identifying the features associated with mirror discomfort and avoidance, you can begin by assigning homework to observe all experiences in which a mirror is present, regardless of whether he actually looked in the mirror. Your patient should note his discomfort level and all aspects of the situation that seemed to influence the discomfort.

Develop a Hierarchy for Mirror Exposures

Your next task is to transform the mirror situations into a list of specific exposure tasks. Vary the list according to the features that increase discomfort, to form a hierarchy from least to most disturbing mirror experiences. Include only those situations that are actually feasible for mirror practice (e.g., it may not be feasible for the patient to do a mirror exposure while nude in a dressing room at a department store), and make those situations as specific as possible. You and the patient can use the *Distressing Mirror Situations Hierarchy* (Form 12.1) to create this list. You can give *Sample Completed Distressing Mirror Situations Hierarchy* (Handout 12.1) to your patient to use as a guide for filling out his own worksheet.

To determine the order of situations on the list, ask your patient how distressing each situation is on the scale from 0 (not at all) to 100 (highest ever experienced), as you have done for exposures in previous sessions. Next, ask your patient to rate how much he avoids each mirror-related situation (0 = never avoids, 50 = avoids 50% of the time, and 100 = always avoids). Encourage your patient to use the full range of the scale for both distress and avoidance. Handout 12.1 gives an idea of the level of distress provoked by various mirror exposures for one patient.

You can begin mirror practices in situations that provoke distress and avoidance ratings near 40, since this degree of anxiety is tolerable for most patients. Ask your patient to complete a copy of the *Exposure and Response Prevention Worksheet* (Form 11.3) before doing the exposure.

Provide Perceptual Retraining during Mirror Exposures: Seeing the Big Picture

We now describe an important part of mirror exposures. Rosen (1998) first described a strategy that combines mirror exposure with mindful emotional processing. Mirror exposure involves systematic exposure to the mirror reflection while asking patients to take a *different perspective* than they typically do. Instead of focusing on their "hot spots," patients are asked to look at the big picture, to see themselves more holistically.

Mindful emotional processing involves changing what your patient attends to and thinks during the mirror exposure. Discourage any negative judgments and emotionally charged self-descriptions (e.g., "I look like Pinocchio—my nose is huge and disgusting!"). Instead, ask the patient to describe his appearance in an *objective, nonjudgmental* way (e.g., "My nose is 2 inches long," "My eyes are almond-shaped and a deep brown color"). During this process, the patient learns to use neutral language without all-or-nothing negative adjectives like "huge" or "gross." He also learns to avoid "should" statements ("I should get my hair cut right away—it looks really ratty"). He will gradually learn to tolerate and accept minor appearance flaws as he moderates his language and refocuses his attention. We have used Rosen's method successfully for our patients with BDD over the years.

Mirror exposure does not involve staring at the perceived defects in the mirror. It also does not involve exaggerating the perceived flaws (e.g., we typically do not recommend asking a patient to apply rouge all over his face if he thinks his skin is too red). In our experience, this is not helpful. In fact, it may just reinforce maladaptive beliefs, and a "nonholistic" view of oneself. In fact, we are suggesting something quite different. The patient learns to look at and describe the "defective" areas, but to use entirely neutral language, such as references to size and shape. He should spend no more time describing the defective areas than he spends describing any other areas of his body.

Below is some guidance on how to introduce mirror exposure to your patient.

THERAPIST: You've told me that you often spend several hours a day looking at the mole on your chin in the mirror. This fits right in with the discussions on selective attention to things you dislike about yourself that we had a few weeks ago [when the therapist and patient discussed self-defeating thoughts and cognitive restructuring].

PATIENT: Yeah, I know. I just focus on negative things and tend to blow them out of proportion.

THERAPIST: Yes, and we also discussed that at the same time, you discount your positive qualities.

PATIENT: Maybe.

THERAPIST: Anyway, today I want to talk a little bit more about your problem with selective attention to flaws. I'd like to address it in the context of working with mirrors. Can you see my little mole right here? (*Patient assents.*) What do you think would happen if I kept staring at it and ignored the rest of my face?

PATIENT: Hmm, I don't know. Would the mole look different?

THERAPIST: Yes, probably so. If I kept staring just at my own mole, and at nothing else, after a while, it would look huge and seem like that was all there was to my face. And it would overshadow other aspects of my face that I feel neutral about such as my nose, or that I actually like—such as my eyes. Now that I've pointed it out, do you think my mole is the most important thing about my face?

PATIENT: No. Certainly not.

THERAPIST: OK, now what if we both stare at it for a while? I'll use a mirror, and you can just stare at my mole. Remember to focus only on the mole.

PATIENT: This is a little weird, but OK.

THERAPIST: Keep staring for a little bit (*Therapist times this for 60 seconds*). Now tell me, does it seem like it's a more important part of my face? Does it seem bigger or darker?

PATIENT: Yes, it really does. I think I see what you're getting at.

THERAPIST: Right. A minute ago, you hardly noticed the mole, but now after focusing on it exclusively, it's gained a lot of importance in our minds. And that happened after only 1 minute! Imagine what would happen if we did it for much longer. That's what focusing on a small thing does. Have you ever had the experience of looking at a word for a long time, and it seems like it is spelled wrong or looks weird? That's the same phenomenon.

PATIENT: So are you saying that I perceive my mole differently from how it really is, because I keep looking at it for so long every day?

THERAPIST: Yes, because you keep staring at it, after a while your mole appears more prominent. So, starting today, we want to help you perceive yourself more accurately when you look in the mirror. We call this exercise a "perceptual retraining exercise." We'll practice by having you describe your entire body, from top to bottom, as objectively as you can. I'd like you to start by describing your hair and then work your way down to your toes. Usually it's a good idea to use inches or millimeters as you describe the width or size of different body parts, because using these units of measurement helps you stay objective. As you repeat this exercise, you'll eventually realize that your mole is not as prominent as you have been thinking. I'm asking you to look at *all* of yourself, and not just zero in on the parts you don't like. Can you see how this way of looking in the mirror is very different from what you normally do?

PATIENT: Yes, normally I'd just zero in on my mole and look at it from different angles, but you want me to take a broader perspective and try to be objective even about my mole. But what if I get stuck staring at the mole and think something awful?

THERAPIST: Just gently remind yourself that you are supposed to be completely objective about your appearance. It would be like trying to describe someone you saw on the street to an artist who would draw the person. So you could say to yourself, "My mole is brown and about 3 millimeters in diameter," and then move on to the next part of your body. It's very important that you learn to replace your negative self-descriptions with more objective, neutral statements. You may eventually find that there are parts of your body you like but haven't been paying attention to.

PATIENT: Well, maybe!

THERAPIST: Yes, maybe! Also, it's important to describe *all* of your body, from head to toe. After all, there's much more to how you look than just your mole. When other people see you they see all of you. We're trying to help you see yourself this way because it's a more accurate view of how you look. And another important thing is to look at yourself from a normal distance. What do you think this would be? What's the distance most people see you from?

PATIENT: Well, I guess usually from the distance where you are now, maybe a few feet away.

THERAPIST: Yes, that's a pretty typical distance.

PATIENT: So you're saying I shouldn't get up really close to the mirror, like an inch away?

THERAPIST: Exactly. As we just saw, that gives you a very distorted view of how you look. Also, you need to see all of you in the mirror so you can describe yourself, and that will be hard if you're just an inch away. If you're using a full-length mirror, you'll want to see yourself from head to toe. If you're using a smaller face mirror, you'll want to see from the top of your head down to your neck and the top of your shoulders.

PATIENT: OK.

THERAPIST: Remember not to do any kinds of rituals while you do this exercise. Don't touch your mole or fix your appearance in any way. Don't zero in on the mole or stare at it. Just describe what each body part looks like, and then move on to the next one.

PATIENT: What should I do if I get so disgusted by my mole or some other body part that I don't want to look at it at all?

THERAPIST: Try to make yourself look at it and describe it in a neutral way. Remember that even subtle avoidance behaviors are likely to interfere with your success in this exposure practice. Just do the best you can to keep going. And look at your other body parts, too—parts you think look OK, and parts you actually kind of like.

PATIENT: I'm not sure I can keep going. It's sort of scary.

THERAPIST: You're right; at first this exercise can be anxiety-provoking. But remember, this is just like the other exposure exercises you've already done. It will get easier with practice. Try to be patient. If you do get anxious, try to take it as a reminder that you need to practice more. Also remember that we won't start with the most challenging item on your hierarchy—we'll try to keep your anxiety at a manageable level by taking a gradual approach. We'll start with one that you rated about a 40. So today we'll keep the light a little dim in my office. As you get more comfortable, we can do the mirror retraining under brighter lights.

Because this exercise can make the patient very anxious, he may refuse to do it. If so, ask him whether you can make it easier for him in some way. For example, he could select the angle at which he looks at the mirror, how close he is to the mirror, or whether he keeps his hat on or not.

We recommend modeling this exercise for your patient. It's helpful to start at the very top of the body and systematically work down to the feet. This helps ensure that all major aspects of the body are looked at. This also involves ending with the feet in a full mirror exercise, or with the neck in a face mirror exercise. This can be advantageous because the feet and neck are rarely disliked body areas. It can help to end with a body area that the patient likes or feels neutrally about, rather than one he dislikes.

Here is an example of how a therapist might model the mirror exercise:

"Let me just show you what your mirror exercise might look like, and we can adjust it to fit your appearance. [Looks in a mirror from a normal distance while describing herself.] My hair is reddish-brown, straight, and about shoulder-length. I have thin bangs that go down to the top of my eyebrows. My skin is light. My face has two wrinkles going horizontally across; they're both about a millimeter wide and a couple of inches long. I also have a couple of vertical lines between my eyebrows. My eyebrows are light brown, shaped like an arch, and about 2½ inches long. My eye color is hazel, and my eyelashes are black, and my eyes are almond-shaped. They're about 1½ inches wide and almost an inch high. My nose is about 2–3 inches long and straight. My cheeks are a little reddish on the cheekbones. My ears are about 3 inches long and 2 inches wide. I'm wearing silver earrings. My lips are dark pink, of medium fullness. My mouth is about 3 inches wide. My teeth are fairly white, and a couple of them are a little crooked. My chin protrudes a little, maybe a few millimeters. My jawline is kind of square. My face is oval, my neck is . . . "

Complete this exercise for your face only or for your entire body, depending on how you instruct your patient during the first mirror exposure. Some patients will find it easier to start by looking only at their heads in the mirror, whereas others may prefer to begin with a large mirror to see their full bodies. Even if you start with a small mirror, we strongly recommend that you ultimately use a larger mirror to provide patients with a more holistic view of themselves. As for other exposure exercises, position the mirror at a distance that provokes moderate but not extreme discomfort—but also be sure that it is not too close, as this will not encourage a holistic perspective. Encourage your patient to start the first exercise in the office, speaking aloud about what he sees. Whenever the patient gets stuck on a body part, remind him gently to move on to the next one. If he uses a negative label for a specific body part (e.g., "disfigured," "too dark," "grotesque"), remind him to be objective and nonjudgmental and to describe the body part again. The same is true if the patient uses "shoulds" (e.g., "I should get new pants—these make me look really fat"). The entire exercise should take about 10 minutes.

If you feel comfortable using humor, you might, if the patient misses a body area, say something like "Do you have any ears?" You can also say something like "Pretend I'm blind and can't see you. Can you give a little more detail about your shoulders [or other body area that was too briefly described]?"

Congratulate the patient after he completes this exercise. It can be very hard for patients to do. It's hard for them to look at themselves in the mirror and describe themselves, especially in front of another person.

It's important to rate anxiety on the 0–100 scale both before and after the mirror retraining. We provide a form for this, the *Mirror Retraining Worksheet* (Form 12.2). If the patient's anxiety increases to a very high level (e.g., 90 or above), and does not improve over the course of the exposure, you will need to try to figure out what happened. Was he too close to the mirror? Did he zero in too much on the disliked areas? Did he end the exposure with checking the disliked areas? Or did he engage in negative self-talk during the exercise? However, keep in mind that it is normal for patients to feel very anxious during this exercise. Some patients might even feel nauseous. Do not interrupt the exercise if this happens. These symptoms will likely improve if you repeat mirror retraining a few times.

Remind the Patient to Engage in Response Prevention during Mirror Exposures

It is very important that the patient *not* engage in any rituals during the mirror retraining, such as excessively zeroing in on and checking the disliked areas, fixing his hair, or picking his skin. A common pitfall is that many patients compulsively check their disliked body areas during this exercise. Watch their eyes as they describe the disliked body areas. If they seem to be looking more intently at these areas, or for a longer time than they have looked at other areas, remind them to avoid checking and looking too much at the areas they don't like and to move on to the next area.

Also, your patient may successfully complete the exercise—for example, ending with describing his foot size and his shoes—but then compulsively zero back in on the "defective" areas before turning away from the mirror. This undermines the positive effects of the exercise, because the patient has ended with checking behavior, has "undone" his holistic perspective to some extent, and now feels awful. Help the patient understand that this isn't helpful, and that the last thing he looks at should be his feet, or his neck if he is starting with a smaller mirror. If the patient happens to dislike these parts of his body, he could try ending with a less disliked, nearby body area.

In addition to practicing daily systematic and planned mirror retraining exercises, your patients will also need to gradually cut down mirror checking that occurs spontaneously over the course of the day. This approach is the same as that discussed in Chapter 11.

Encourage the Patient to Practice and Move Up the Hierarchy

Your patient may need to repeat the first mirror retraining exercise several times until he becomes more comfortable. It can also be helpful to reverse roles, with the patient giving you feedback on how you are doing with the exercise. Once the distress rating has decreased to 10 or 20, encourage your patient to move on to the next mirror-related item on his *Distressing Mirror Situations Hierarchy* (Form 12.1). Ask the patient to complete another *Mirror Retraining Worksheet* (Form 12.2) for the next situation.

Coach the Patient in Using Metaphors

Various metaphors can help your patient tolerate negative thoughts about his body parts. For example, you might suggest that your patient view intrusive thoughts and images of his disliked mole as leaves on a river that he will just allow to float by without interfering with them. The leaves require no special attention or diversion of energy and can just be left alone.

Similarly, you can tell the patient:

> "It's often best just to let appearance preoccupations go by. It's OK to mentally note that they are there, but then note that they are 'just thoughts' and just let them go. It's probably best not to fight them actively, as this just focuses more attention on them and probably won't be successful. If you try not to think of a pink elephant, what do you think of? A pink elephant [see also Wegner, 1989]. Similarly, trying *not* to think about how you look can just keep you focused on how you look. In addition to letting the thoughts just float by, it can be helpful to just try to *gently refocus* on something else that is going on around you—for example, what someone is saying to you, the movie you're watching, the temperature in the room, the feel of the chair against your body. Again, it's key to *gently* let the appearance thoughts go by without interfering and *gently refocus* on other things. A 'letting go and gentle refocusing' approach is likely to work better than trying to battle the thoughts and forcing yourself to focus on something else."

The following extended metaphor is adapted with permission of the publisher from Marsha Linehan's *Skills Training Manual for Treating Borderline Personality Disorder* (Linehan, 1993, p. 94). Linehan notes that her version is adapted in turn "from one I was told by a Zen teacher, who read it in a book by another spiritual teacher, Anthony de Mello, S. J."

> A man bought a new house and wanted a beautiful lawn. He worked on it every week, doing all that the gardening books recommended. But the lawn always seemed to have dandelions growing in it. First he pulled them out, but they grew back. Then he bought weed killer, which worked for

> a while, but the dandelions grew back again after the summer rains. He worked harder and pulled them out until none were left. Next summer, he thought he would have no dandelions, but alas, they came up again. He thought the problem was the type of grass he had, so he spent a fortune for new sod. This worked for some time and he was very happy, but just as he started to relax, a dandelion came up. A friend suggested this was because his neighbors' yards had dandelions, so he tried to get all his neighbors to kill their dandelions. By the third year, he was exasperated, and there were still dandelions. After consulting all the local experts and gardening books, he wrote to the U.S. Department of Agriculture for advice. Finally he got a reply and was very excited, but the note said: "Dear Sir: We have considered your problem and have consulted experts. After careful consideration, our advice is that you learn to love those dandelions."

As the metaphor suggests, some patients—especially those who have tried hard to change their appearance but remain frustrated with the outcome—will need to learn to accept their body parts just as they are.

Assign Homework

Encourage your patient to practice mirror retraining and fill out the *Mirror Retraining Worksheet* (Form 12.2) every day until the next session. For mirror homework assignments, you and your patient will have to agree on specific retraining exercises based on the *Distressing Mirror Situations Hierarchy* (Form 12.1). In addition, ask your patient to continue completing copies of the *Thought Record* (Form 9.1) and to engage in other, non-mirror-related exposure and response prevention exercises (with the help of the *Exposure and Response Prevention Worksheet*, Form 11.3).

From now until the next session, your patient should invest about 10–20 minutes per day in mirror retraining and about 1 hour per day in CBT-BDD exercises from previous sessions.

Ask for Summary of/Feedback on the Session

Ask the patient to briefly summarize the major points covered during the session. Also ask whether the patient had any concerns about the session or your behavior, and respond appropriately.

Continue Mirror Retraining Throughout Treatment

Just as with the previous skills the patient has learned—cognitive restructuring, exposure, and response prevention—it is important that the patient continue to do mirror retraining throughout the rest of the treatment. *Ideally, mirror retraining is done twice a day for 5–10 minutes each time.* Having the patient record an anxiety rating before and after retraining on the *Mirror Retraining Worksheet* (Form 12.2) can help both you and the patient see whether he is doing the retraining correctly (if so, his anxiety should diminish over time when he is doing the same retraining). A variation of this exercise is to videotape the patient while he is conducting the mirror retraining, or even in the context of another exposure and response prevention exercise.

You might also consider taking photographs of your patient. Reviewing the videos or still images with the patient is another way to help the patient gain a more "objective" perspective on what he looks like.

Occasional patients find the mirror retraining too anxiety-provoking at this point in the treatment. If they are very frightened, see if there's a way to make it easier—for example, doing it in dimmer light or using a mirror they think makes them look less terrible. You can also remind them that they are currently experiencing this anxiety many times a day anyway (when they are checking mirrors), and that the purpose of the mirror retraining is to help them gradually feel less anxious when they do look into mirrors. If the retraining still seems too hard, you can try coming back to it later in the treatment.

FORM 12.1

Distressing Mirror Situations Hierarchy

Situation	Degree of distress (0–100)	Degree of avoidance (0–100)
1.		
2.		
3.		
4.		
5.		
6.		
7.		
8.		
9.		
10.		
11.		
12.		
13.		
14.		
15.		

FORM 12.2

Mirror Retraining Worksheet

Rate your anxiety on a scale from 0 (no anxiety) to 100 (worst anxiety ever), both before and after the mirror retraining.

Date and time	Mirror situation	Anxiety before	Anxiety after

HANDOUT 12.1

Sample Completed Distressing Mirror Situations Hierarchy

Situation	Degree of distress (0–100)	Degree of avoidance (0–100)
1. Looking at little compact mirror that is hard to see in dim light	35	40
2. Looking in window of storefront next to workplace, on cloudy day	40	40
3. Using round face mirror (not magnified), with overhead bathroom light on	50	50
4. Using round mirror (not magnified) to comb hair, with bath cabinet lights on	60	55
5. Using round magnifying mirror, with all bathroom lights on	70	80
6. Seeing face and upper body in mirror in work bathroom, with no one else present	75	70
7. Seeing face and upper body in mirror at work bathroom, with two coworkers present	80	70
8. Trying on hats in department store, using counter mirror, with others present	85	80
9. Full-length bedroom mirror, when dressed for work, in daylight	90	90
10. Trying on clothes in dressing room at department store, using large mirror	90	95
11. Full-length mirror in bedroom, when wearing underwear only, with only hall light on	95	100
12. Full-length mirror in bedroom, when naked, with bedroom light on	100	100
13.		
14.		
15.		

CHAPTER 13

SESSIONS 11–20

Advanced Cognitive Strategies and Moving Forward

SESSION SUMMARY

- ☐ Check mood and BDD symptoms.
- ☐ Briefly review the previous session.
- ☐ Set the agenda jointly with the patient.
- ☐ Review homework.
- ☐ Work on the agenda.
  - ☐ Explain core beliefs and the rationale for working on them.
  - ☐ Identify deeper-level beliefs and refine the patient's BDD model.
  - ☐ Educate the patient about deeper-level beliefs.
  - ☐ Use cognitive strategies to evaluate and modify deeper-level beliefs.
  - ☐ Help the patient identify healthier core beliefs.
- ☐ Assign homework.
- ☐ Ask for summary of/feedback on the session.

SESSION FORMS AND HANDOUTS

BDI-II (or other depression inventory)

Personal Session Form (Form 2.1)

Therapist Session Form (Form 6.1)

Completed *Your Personal BDD Model* (Form 7.1)

Core Belief Record (plus extra copies) (Form 13.1)

My Positive Traits (Form 13.2)

Advanced Cognitive Strategies (Handout 13.1)

Thought Records (plus extra copies) (Form 9.1)

INTRODUCTION TO THIS SESSION

After you have introduced perceptual retraining, you will often find it helpful to have the patient practice all of the previously learned core treatment components (cognitive restructuring, exposure, ritual prevention, and perceptual retraining) for a couple of sessions before moving on to the advanced cognitive strategies. Earlier in treatment, you have encouraged your patient to focus on automatic thoughts (e.g., "This guy just stared at my pimple"). However, as treatment progresses, you will learn more about the deeper-level beliefs your patient holds. These beliefs may include assumptions and rules such as the following:

"If I have wrinkles, others won't respect me."
"I must be attractive to be happy."

These intermediate beliefs are usually based on even deeper negative core beliefs, which are global, overgeneralized, and negative beliefs about the self or the world. They can usually be expressed in very simple sentences, such as those shown in Figure 13.1.

To ensure long-term maintenance of treatment gains, you will need to address these deeper-level beliefs. This chapter will teach you how to identify and modify such beliefs. We recommend doing this work with all patients. The effect can be quite powerful.

A patient may mention deeper-level beliefs in conversations earlier in the treatment. Once you have identified such a belief, you need to decide whether to work on it right away or later in therapy. We often do not address deeper-level beliefs until Session 13 or 14, but you need to be flexible. Base your decision about when to address them on your patient's progress so far in treatment. If your patient is working well with the basic cognitive and behavioral strategies described in earlier chapters and has a good understanding of the CBT model of BDD, working on deeper-level beliefs is usually a good next step. But if your patient is struggling to understand the model or to counteract negative automatic thoughts, complete basic exposures, or block rituals, it probably makes more sense to work on these skills first.

The cognitive strategies we have presented in Chapter 9 are useful for working on deeper beliefs. We encourage you to have the patient complete copies of the *Thought Record* (Form 9.1), both in session and as homework, that focus on deeper-level beliefs. In this chapter, we present some additional, more advanced cognitive strategies to help you identify and modify your patient's deeper-level beliefs. We suggest that you try all of the strategies in this chapter. (The survey method, however, is optional, because the patient needs to have people in her life whom it would be reasonable to survey and from whom answers would help her learn something new. Not all patients have such people in their lives.)

• I am bad.	• I am unlovable.
• I am inadequate.	• Others will reject me.
• I am defective.	• I am undesirable.
• I am not good enough.	• I am weak.
• I am a loser.	• I am worthless.
• I am a failure.	• I am unworthy.

FIGURE 13.1. Typical negative core beliefs.

There is no need to finish all of the material in this chapter in one session. You can complete it in the next session, and you can weave aspects of it into future sessions as needed. Some of the techniques can be assigned as homework.

Check Mood and BDD Symptoms

Check the BDI-II (or other depression inventory) the patient has completed in the waiting room, and check the score on the suicidality item as in previous sessions, responding as appropriate. Briefly explore the patient's general mood and discuss BDD symptoms since the last session. Hand out the *Personal Session Form* (Form 2.1), so that the patient can record information she finds significant during the session.

Briefly Review the Previous Session

Briefly check in with the patient regarding her perception and understanding of the previous session.

Set the Agenda Jointly with the Patient

Convey the topics you'd like to cover during the session, and try to incorporate any issues the patient would like to discuss into today's session.

Review Homework

Discuss your patient's homework from the previous session.

Work on the Agenda

Explain Core Beliefs and the Rationale for Working on Them

Explain to the patient that so far the two of you have worked on her thoughts about appearance—examining them to see whether they are accurate and helpful, identifying cognitive errors, and developing more accurate and helpful thoughts. Now you're going to work on her deeper-level beliefs, also known as "assumptions," "rules," or "core beliefs." Explain what these beliefs are and how they can have a powerful effect on our view of ourselves, our mood, and our lives. It may be helpful to use the metaphor of peeling an onion. So far, the thoughts you've been working on together are like the outer onion skin—more "surface-level" beliefs. Now you're going to peel the onion and get to the deeper layers, which are the core underlying beliefs that the patient has about herself. Then explain that in today's session, you're going to do some exercises together that will focus on these deeper beliefs. This will help the patient identify them, think about them, and examine them, rather than simply accepting them as fact.

Identify Deeper-Level Beliefs and Refine the Patient's BDD Model

Previously your patient has learned how to notice thinking errors and to develop rational responses by evaluating and disputing these maladaptive thoughts. You have taught your patient to complete copies of the *Thought Record* (Form 9.1) to facilitate this learning. These cognitive techniques are an important part of CBT-BDD, and you should encourage your patient to practice them daily. So far, the cognitive strategies have focused on thoughts that are easily accessible in your patient's mind and are prompted by everyday situations. These have been primarily beliefs about appearance. Now you need to connect those thoughts to her deeper underlying beliefs). If your patient doesn't learn to identify and modify these core beliefs, she may be more likely to relapse.

From the outset of therapy, you have been conceptualizing your patient's BDD symptoms. When you first helped the patient complete *Your Personal BDD Model* (Form 7.1), you considered how her thoughts, feelings, and compensatory behaviors (appearance rituals, avoidance) interacted. Over the course of treatment, you have learned more about the typical situations and thoughts that upset her. Usually such thoughts are connected to deeper-level assumptions, rules, or core beliefs—global, overgeneralized beliefs about the self or the world. Now that you've learned more about your patient, it is time for the two of you to refine your conceptualization of her BDD model. It's usually advantageous to keep track of new information by revising your patient's individualized model on her completed copy of Form 7.1 and writing new information in the appropriate boxes. To determine the sources of your patient's symptoms, ask her questions such as these:

> "What did you learn or conclude about yourself and about the importance of appearance while growing up?"
>
> "What kinds of experiences might have contributed to the development of deeper-level beliefs about yourself and those around you?"

Sources of core beliefs may include parental teachings about appearance; parents' behavior toward the patient; modeling by other important people (family members, etc.) who focused on appearance; and experiences that conveyed strong negative messages about self-worth, usually related to appearance. You can directly ask your patient about the following:

- Parents' or other adults' attitudes and behaviors related to appearance (e.g., children were not allowed to leave the house until they were perfectly groomed).
- Parents' or other adults' own plastic surgery that conveyed messages about the importance of facial or body attractiveness.
- Emotional, physical, or sexual abuse.
- Racial discrimination (e.g., an Asian child was considered too short, according to Western values) or other cultural experiences or values.
- Actual appearance flaws and circumstances around these (e.g., severe acne in adolescence, scars from an accident, birthmarks).
- Significant teasing during childhood.

Ask Questions

Sometimes your patient directly expresses her personal rules (e.g., "I have to look perfect at all times"). These rules often involve "should," "must," or "have to." In this case, you can easily elicit related assumptions and underlying core beliefs by just asking what would happen if your patient were to violate a rule or stop doing an appearance ritual:

THERAPIST: If you didn't try to look perfect, what would happen?

PATIENT: Then I'd be defective and others would reject me.

At times your patient may directly express a core belief (e.g., "I am bad," "I am unlovable") during a therapy session or on a *Thought Record*, and you can refer back to this and note the core belief on the BDD model. You should also look for any recurring theme in sessions that indicates a core negative belief. Comment on the theme you have noticed, and inquire whether your patient is aware of this and whether it happens commonly in many situations.

THERAPIST: I've noticed that you've referred several times to feeling inadequate about meeting other people's expectations. [Therapist provides specific details from this or previous sessions.] Do you think you often feel inadequate in relation to other people?

PATIENT: I suppose that's true. I hadn't thought about it like that, but I always feel like I'm trying to catch up, or I'm not making the grade.

THERAPIST: So it sounds to me that you might be holding a basic belief about yourself like "I'm inadequate." If that sounds right to you, we might want to look at where that comes from. It seems a little curious, given your apparent competence in your work and in some other areas you've told me about.

Use the Downward Arrow Technique

One of the best ways to elicit deeper-level beliefs is called the "downward arrow" technique (Burns, 1999). Begin by selecting one of your patient's thoughts that seems related to a deeper-level belief. Then repeatedly ask for the meaning of this thought. To do this, you can repeat the same basic question about the meaning of the thought over and over ("What would that mean?" . . . "If that were true, what would that mean?"). Or you can vary how you ask the question a little, as in the following sequence:

"What would that mean?"
"If that were true, why would that be so bad?"
"What's the worst part about that?"
"And if that were true, what would that mean about you?"

Consider the example of Frank, who was excessively concerned that his sideburns were uneven. His compensatory strategies include shaving rituals and not leaving the house when he thought his sideburns were imperfect. The exchange below illustrates the use of the downward arrow method to identify core beliefs.

THERAPIST: You told me that it's very difficult for you to leave the house when your sideburns are uneven. Suppose you were to leave the house with imperfect sideburns. What would be so bad about that?

PATIENT: Then I'd look like I let my appearance go.

THERAPIST: Let's assume this was true and you let your appearance go. What would that mean about you?

PATIENT: That I'm worthless scum.

THERAPIST: Is there anything else?

PATIENT: No, I'd just be scum. Who would even want to talk to me?

THERAPIST: What would it mean if no one wanted to talk to you?

PATIENT: I'm a horrible person; no one could love me.

The therapist stopped the questioning at this point, because Frank showed a major change in affect and directly stated a core negative belief about himself ("I'm unlovable"). As noted above, core beliefs usually start with the phrase "I am . . . , " and for patients with BDD, they are usually statements about self-worth and/or lovability.

Once you and your patient have identified some negative core beliefs via direct questioning or the downward arrow technique, write it on the *Core Belief Record* (Form 13.1). Discuss how much your patient believes each "old" core belief. Then, *after* you use some of the strategies described below to evaluate the core beliefs, help the patient develop one or more alternative beliefs and list these on Form 13.1.

Note that an alternative belief shouldn't just be the opposite of a negative core belief, because these are usually implausible. Therefore, avoid using the word "not" when you and the patient are developing an alternative belief. For example, if the old belief was "I am hideous," a reasonable alternative belief might be "I look good enough," rather than "I am not hideous" or "I look good," which may be too strong for the patient to believe. Useful new core beliefs contain some positive traits that the patient will identify when doing the self-esteem pie and other exercises that are described below.

Next, ask your patient for evidence that supports the old core belief. Sometimes the patient will report a childhood memory of someone teasing him in support of the old core belief. Discuss this evidence and whether it was true then and is true now. Use any of the several methods described below to evaluate the patient's interpretation. Next, collect evidence that contradicts the old belief and supports a new, alternative belief.

Educate the Patient about Deeper-Level Beliefs

If you suspect that your patient has a certain rule, assumption, or core belief, present it to the patient. Also educate your patient about how the particular belief operates. The exchange below shows how Frank's therapist helped Frank understand the effect of another of his core beliefs: "I am worthless."

THERAPIST: Tell me how the belief "I am worthless" affects your thinking on a daily basis.

PATIENT: It makes me absolutely miserable, but it's how I see everything that's happening to me.

THERAPIST: So, for example, if someone looks at you, how does the belief affect what you might think in this situation?

PATIENT: Well, I'd automatically assume that the person was criticizing me and thought I looked like a creep.

THERAPIST: Would you actually know what the person was thinking?

PATIENT: It wouldn't matter; I'd just assume it. I wouldn't even stop to consider anything else.

THERAPIST: OK, so this is a very automatic response. Now, what if something good happens? Let's say someone gives you a compliment.

PATIENT: Oh, I can't accept it! I just assume people are complimenting me because they feel sorry for me.

THERAPIST: So, no matter what happens, you interpret it to match your belief. And if something doesn't fit your belief—like a compliment about your appearance, for example—you just change the meaning of the compliment, so your interpretation of the compliment fits with your belief.

PATIENT: Yes, that's true.

THERAPIST: It looks to me like your strategy just reinforces your belief that you are worthless. It's hard for you to consider any other alternatives, so you reinterpret the compliment to fit what you believe. What do you think?

Use Cognitive Strategies to Evaluate and Modify Deeper-Level Beliefs

After you have identified a problematic assumption or belief and educated your patient about it, you can start helping your patient evaluate and modify it. Below we present a number of cognitive strategies for working on maladaptive deeper-level beliefs.

Cognitive Restructuring (Modifying Self-Defeating Thoughts)

Standard cognitive restructuring skills, as discussed in Chapter 9, can be applied to core beliefs. Each core belief can be written down on a standard *Thought Record* (Form 9.1). The patient can then identify the cognitive errors in the belief and develop a more rational and helpful belief. We have found that doing the self-esteem pie and the other exercises described below will facilitate cognitive restructuring of core beliefs, as these exercises help open the patient's mind to less negative views of herself that can be integrated into her new alternative thought. Don't feel pressured to use all of the strategies below in one session. Instead just choose the ones that seem especially relevant for your patient, and save the other ones for later (or don't use them at all).

Self-Esteem Pie

Many patients with BDD are unaware of the large impact their body image has on their self-worth. Often they see themselves almost entirely in terms of the things they hate about how they look. They're usually unaware of, overlook, or minimize many of their positive traits. Such patients tend to "discount the positive" about themselves and to focus excessively on the negative. It can be very helpful for them to develop a more balanced perspective of their positive and negative traits, and to learn not to discount or overlook the positive ones. This is another example of seeing the "big picture."

First, you want to find out what your patient values about herself. First, ask her to list all the components of her self-esteem, *both positive and negative*—such as intelligence, accomplishments, abilities, work habits, relationships, personality, social status, and appearance. It's important at this point in the exercise *not* to help the patient recognize her positive traits; that comes later. At this point, simply have the patient list her positive and negative traits, without eliciting additional traits.

Then ask the patient to draw a large circle to represent a pie, and to divide this pie into different-size pieces that represent the amount contributed by each part of herself to her overall self-esteem. Pay attention to how much of the patient's self-worth is based on looks. How much of the appearance piece of the pie is positive, and how much is negative? What do the other slices consist of?

As an example, consider Cora. She told her therapist:

> "You probably think I am really superficial, but I think this all has to do with my face. It's just so red. It looks horrible . . . I look like a freak. For a while I thought I had rosacea, but the doctors tell me that I don't have it. They act as if I have nothing, and it's not a big deal. But for me it is. On bad days I'm so ashamed about the way I look, that I don't even want to leave the house. I feel really worthless."

Cora's initial self-esteem pie is presented in Figure 13.2. Most of her self-image was based on her appearance, and most of her appearance evaluations were negative. Cora's self-image was also based on her intelligence and personality, about which she felt pretty good, but she had mixed feelings about her accomplishments. Overall, her self-image was more negative than positive, because she placed so much value on the color of her skin. After she completed the chart, her therapist spoke about the large negative appearance piece. It was pretty obvious that changing the importance Cora placed on her looks would dramatically improve her self-image.

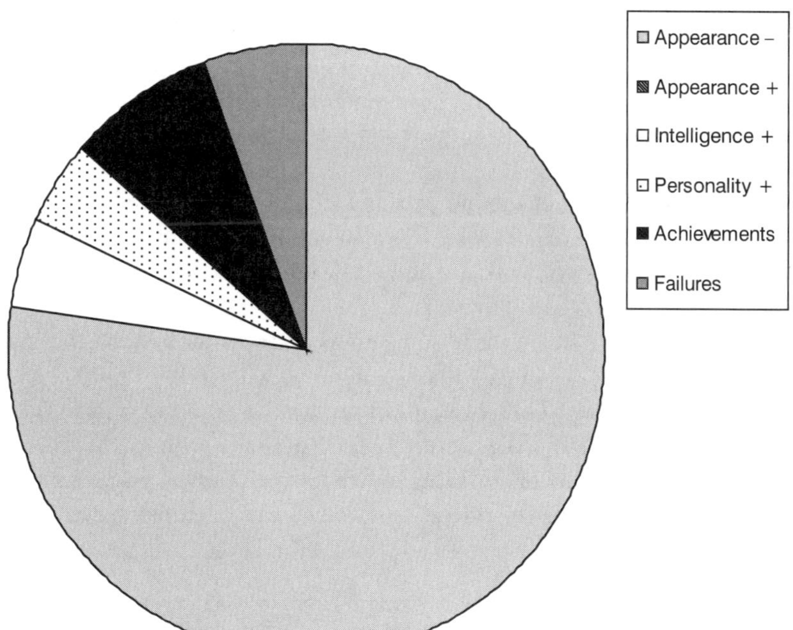

FIGURE 13.2. Cora's original self-esteem pie.

Cora was very hard on herself (as most patients are) when completing this pie. For example, in the area of achievements, the main reason she put herself down was that she compared herself to her best friend, who had a doctoral degree. In doing so, she didn't consider what she had accomplished, such as raising children who had "turned out well," being able to sell some of her paintings in a local art gallery, and her current work on her bachelor's degree (now that her children were grown). Thus, instead of considering the things she could be proud of, she based her self-evaluation on a limited number of areas in which she felt she wasn't as accomplished as some other people she knew. In addition, Cora underestimated her positive personality qualities, taking it for granted that she had many friends and got along with almost everyone she met.

After the therapist encouraged Cora to list some of her achievements (we describe how to do this with your patient below), she began seeing herself differently. She was able to recognize some of her talents, strengths, and successes. Because the therapist was concerned about Cora's negative view of her looks, the therapist asked:

THERAPIST: What about your eyes? Your smile? Your legs? The way you dress? Your height? Your weight?

PATIENT: I'm a stylish dresser, which I feel good about. I also like being tall. I don't care for my smile, because my teeth aren't straight, but I like my eyes and eyebrows.

Based on these new insights, Cora decided to revise her self-image pie a little. First she decreased the negative appearance slice; this made room for larger and newly recognized and acknowledged positive achievement, personality, and accomplishment pieces. Her new self-esteem pie is presented in Figure 13.3. Because she was now able to see the whole picture rather than just focusing on her complexion, her self-worth improved, and she felt better. To ensure that Cora could easily remember what she learned from this exercise, her therapist helped her develop a "rational self-esteem statement" (this statement is discussed further below) and write it down:

> Although my skin doesn't look exactly as I'd like it to, that doesn't mean I am inadequate. I have many good qualities: I am a great friend. I am a good mom and have successfully raised three kids. I have pretty eyes, and I dress well. I am smart and I am artistic.

Cora carried the revised drawing of the pie with her in her purse, so she could look at it whenever she felt inadequate because of her looks. It is also noteworthy that as Cora's mood improved during the pie exercise, the "horrible skin" she had described in her original thought changed to "skin that doesn't look exactly as I'd like it."

Like Cora, most of us have strengths in some areas and weaknesses in others, and are average in many domains. Patients who focus mainly on areas where they "don't measure up" will have largely negative self-esteem. Therefore, it's important for your patients to put their imperfections in perspective and see the big picture. Many patients with BDD base most of their self-worth on the single dimension of appearance. Not surprisingly, a minor scar or pimple can cause their self-worth to plummet. To address this, encourage each patient to identify as many strengths as possible.

Listing the Patient's Positive Traits

As the next step in this exercise, have your patient fill out the *My Positive Traits* form (Form 13.2). Ask her to think more about her positive traits and whether there are any additional ones

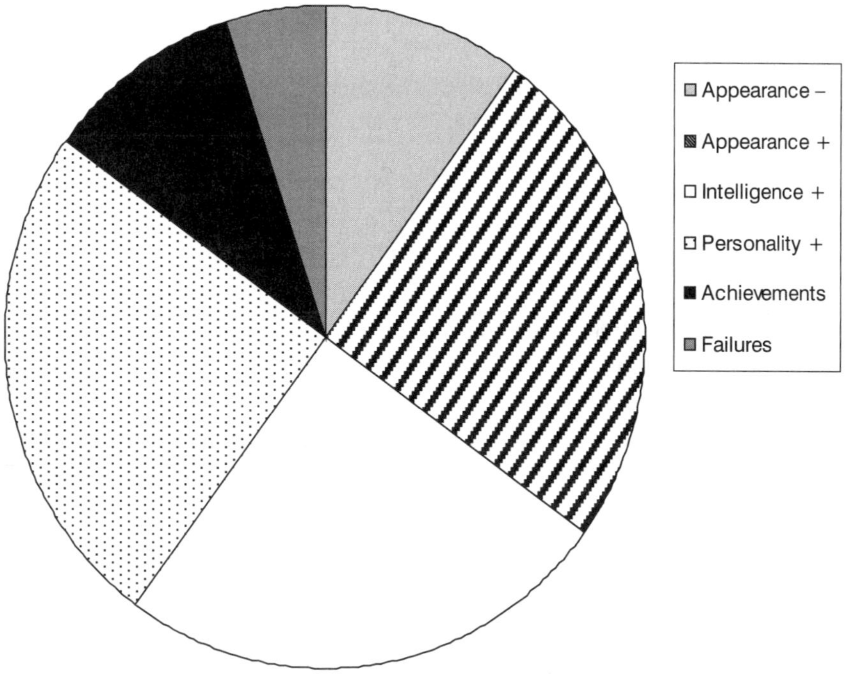

FIGURE 13.3. Cora's more balanced self-esteem pie.

she didn't write down when she drew her first pie. Now you can ask the patient questions to help her identify those positive features:

- *Intelligence.* Can you understand things? Can you solve problems? Do you know trivia? Do you have a good vocabulary? Have you ever helped anyone with something? Can you concentrate? Do you remember things?
- *Accomplishments/competence.* What do you/did you do well? Do you have skills at doing things around the house (cooking, gardening, entertaining, solving problems, etc.)?
- *Creative and artistic abilities.* Do you write poetry, play an instrument, paint, or the like?
- *Athletic abilities and health.* Do you play a sport? Are you fit, strong? Do you keep yourself physically healthy?
- *Work habits.* Do you work hard? Are you prepared? Do you arrive on time, meet deadlines, and try your best? Are you responsible? Do you care about doing a good job?
- *Relationships.* Do you have any assets that make others happy to be with you? Are there people who consider you a friend? Do you have any good relationships (with friends, parents, children, siblings, colleagues, classmates, etc.)? In difficult relationships, are there aspects that are good? What do you contribute to these relationships?
- *Personality.* What qualities do others like about you? Are you caring, friendly, outgoing, generous, empathetic, polite, respectful, reliable, responsible? Do you have a sense of humor? What makes you a good spouse, mother, parent, and so on? Are you persistent, strong?

- *Social status.* Do you have a nice house or apartment, a car, a good job, and so forth?
- *Appearance.* Do you like other aspects of your appearance (your clothing style, shoes, height, weight, hair color, complexion, face, lips, eyes, mouth, chin, cheekbones, ears, nose, eyebrows, posture, shape of your face, shape of your hands, arms, legs, etc.)?

It's important to include as many positive traits as possible on the patient's list. On the other hand, you don't want to be overly positive by listing traits that are not really characteristic of the patient. Otherwise, the traits will not be believable, and the exercise will lose credibility. You can also note your observations of positive traits you think the patient has (if the patient does not list these traits herself) and ask whether your observations are accurate. For example, you might ask, "During our conversations, I've gotten the sense that you're a hard worker and take your job responsibilities very seriously. Do you think that's true of you? What would your coworkers say?" If the patient agrees, you can encourage her to add this to the list.

If the patient has trouble identifying positive traits, you could ask her to name a person she knows and admires. Ask her to describe what she admires and likes about this person. Then ask whether any of this person's traits are characteristic of herself (e.g., kindness, caring about people, being a hard worker). You could also ask how a friend (if she has one) would describe the patient. What positive traits would a friend mention?

We've found that regardless of how little patients think they have in their lives, or how few accomplishments or talents they believe they have, they can usually come up with quite a few positive traits. You can provide additional guidance to help lengthen a patient's list, if necessary. For example, a young housebound patient who was on disability because of BDD and could not name any friends was able to come up with a long list of positive traits that she felt good about. These included such things as being a nice person, treating her little nephew well, paying her bills on time, obeying the law, keeping her apartment clean, not giving people any trouble, being honest, not overspending her disability check, and so on.

This self-esteem exercise involves getting the patients to think hard about what she values: What does she value in other people, what do other people value in her, and what does the patient value in herself? You can also address values by asking the patient to think about what she wants to have people say about her at her funeral. Or, when she is on her deathbed and is thinking back over her life, what does she want her life to have been like? Does she want to be remembered for her kindness, for her accomplishments, or for being a good friend or parent—or for having perfectly even eyebrows? (The funeral/deathbed portion of the exercise may not be appropriate for a suicidal patient, so you will need to use your clinical judgment here.)

Translating the List of Positive Traits into a New Self-Esteem Pie

After asking these questions and having the patient make this list of positive traits, encourage your patient to draw her self-esteem pie again. Have her fill in all the strengths first, and leave the weaknesses and appearance items for last. Ask your patient to try to come up with as many pie pieces as she can.

After the patient draws the new pie, ask her what she thinks of it. Try to help her see that it's a more accurate picture of herself. If the patient discounts the new pie, ask whether maybe she is discounting the positive about herself. In other words, is there a cognitive error in her thinking?

Next, have the patient write down a "rational self-esteem statement" in the space allotted for this at the bottom of *My Positive Traits* (Form 13.2). This is basically a rational response, which, as we have noted in Chapter 9, is a brief summary of the highlights of your patient's ideas. The statement is most helpful if it's relatively short, so the patient can remember it easily when negative thoughts pop up. After your patient has written this response down on Form 13.2, encourage her to refer to it between sessions. An example of a rational self-esteem statement has been presented above for Cora. Another example of such a statement is this:

> I'm basically a good person. I'm nice to people, honest, and hard-working. People come to me when they're having a hard time. Also, I'm a good guitar player and a good cook, and I exercise and keep myself healthy.

You can then say something like the following to your patient (tailor this to her individual beliefs as appropriate):

> "Having more than one area that matters in your self-image is also a way to stabilize your self-esteem, because you're less vulnerable. Let me give you an example. If you value your clear skin above anything else in yourself, a pimple is a major disaster. It can shake your entire self-perception, because you have nothing to balance it with. However, if you just see beautiful skin as just one of many positive characteristics, even a multiple-zit attack can't send you into a depression, because you still have lots of other things going for you."

At the end of this exercise, your patient should walk away with a more balanced self-esteem pie and a long list of qualities that form the basis of her positive self-esteem.

What Would You Teach Your (Imagined) Children?

Patients with BDD often have rules and assumptions for themselves they would never impose on anyone else. An effective strategy for challenging these beliefs is to encourage a patient to take another perspective by asking how he would advise his own child (preferably of the same gender) and why. The goal here is to help the patient identify and state aloud his own alternative, more rational beliefs to strengthen them. The exchange below illustrates how Frank's therapist used Frank's imagined son as a reference point.

THERAPIST: So, Frank, you've told me that you believe that if your sideburns are uneven, you shouldn't leave the house.

PATIENT: Yeah, that's true. I either have to fix them or stay home.

THERAPIST: How much time per year would you say you spend fixing your sideburns?

PATIENT: Well, I spend almost an hour a day, I think.

THERAPIST: If we add that up, how much time per year?

PATIENT: OK, about 6–7 hours per week. Multiply that by 50 or so, and that's about 350 hours a year.

THERAPIST: OK. Let's assume you had an 18-year-old son. Would you tell him that he can't go out until his sideburns are perfect? Even if it would mean that he misses school or parties? Would you suggest that he set aside at least 350 hours every year to fix his sideburns?

PATIENT: No, of course not. I'd never do that.

THERAPIST: Why wouldn't you recommend this?

PATIENT: Because it's a complete waste of time, and I know that this could ruin his life.

THERAPIST: So what would you teach him about sideburns and the importance of his appearance?

PATIENT: It's not that important. He should look OK, but it's much more important to just be himself with his friends, even if he doesn't look perfect.

THERAPIST: Why is that more important than how he looks? Wouldn't his friends reject him if his sideburns weren't perfectly even?

PATIENT: I see what you're saying. That makes no sense. Of course his looks don't matter that much.

THERAPIST: What would you tell him does matter?

PATIENT: Well, things like being a good friend, being honest, going out with his friends, playing sports, and stuff like that.

THERAPIST: That's good advice. So now how would you feel about recommending what you just taught your son for yourself? What's the next step here?

In the line of questioning above, note how the therapist imbedded the cost of the appearance rituals in terms of time and interference with other activities versus the benefits of looking perfect. Also note the direct questions and "devil's advocate"–style restatement of Frank's belief, to encourage him to state an alternative belief about the importance of appearance to others that would contradict his own assumptions and behavior. Finally, the therapist pressed the point about Frank's taking his own advice and what actions that would entail.

If your patient says something to his imagined child that is inconsistent with developing healthier beliefs (e.g., "Well, you shouldn't go to the party if you look bad"), you will need to step in. Using a Socratic style, ask the patient, "Would you really say this to your child? Or do you think you were talking to yourself?"

In this exercise, as well as the "reversing roles" exercise below, it may take a little practice for the patient to take a genuinely different perspective. Try to help him with this. We have found that doing the self-esteem pie first can help these exercises go better, as the patient has already given some thought to traits other than appearance that are important.

Reversing Therapist and Patient Roles

Another strategy that may enable the patient to take a different perspective is to role-play a role reversal: Have your patient play the part of the therapist, and you play the part of your patient. The patient may be reluctant to do this, but encourage him to give it a try. Most patients will find it helpful.

THERAPIST: Frank, you've told me you feel like you'd be "worthless scum" if you were to pay less attention to your appearance and let your sideburns grow a little uneven. Now let's reverse roles. If I was your patient, and you were my therapist, suppose I told you this? How would you deal with that?

PATIENT: Well, if I was your therapist, I'd point out to you that sideburns are just a small part of how you look overall. Also, appearance isn't everything, and there are so many things that determine a person's worth.

THERAPIST: Like what?

PATIENT: Like if you're someone who contributes something positive to your environment. Like being a good friend, hard worker, stuff like that . . .

THERAPIST: And are you a good friend? Do you work hard?

PATIENT: I'm very supportive of the people I care about, so I guess I'm a good friend. I know I'm a good worker, and I do work hard.

THERAPIST: So how does that fit with your initial idea that you're worthless?

PATIENT: It doesn't, really.

Like the previous exercise, the role reversal requires the patient to articulate aloud alternative beliefs that contradict the negative ones, gradually whittling away at them. Note that a single application of reversing roles or advising one's child is likely only to weaken core beliefs, not to remove them completely. Thus these strategies must be repeated in varying forms when negative core beliefs occur.

Picturing the Extreme

Another strategy Frank's therapist used to modify Frank's beliefs about himself was to have Frank picture a "worthless scumbag," which was a term Frank had used to describe himself.

THERAPIST: Suppose I told you, "I recently met this guy who totally let himself go. Boy, he was such a worthless scumbag!" What kind of person would you picture?

PATIENT: I would picture someone who is really despicable and contemptible.

THERAPIST: What would this person do?

PATIENT: Well, he would be a real lowlife. He wouldn't be working and would be really lazy. You know—dirty, sleazy, and filthy. Like that.

THERAPIST: Hmm. Interesting. It doesn't really describe you, does it?

PATIENT: No, I'm not that bad!

THERAPIST: So how accurate is the label "worthless scumbag" for you?

PATIENT: I guess it doesn't really describe me.

THERAPIST: OK. If it doesn't really describe you, what do you think you need to do?

Again, the therapist pressed for the next step: how to translate the discrepant belief into action.

Turning the Tables

Still another strategy for helping patients take another perspective on their fears and beliefs is "turning the tables," illustrated as follows. As long as she could remember, Melanie had been concerned about her looks. She was quite successful at work, but since her mid-30s she had been very worried about thinning hair, her increasing wrinkles, and her sagging facial features. She was afraid that others would consider them a sign of reduced ability. She told her therapist:

> "Many of the people who work with me are younger. If I continue to age like this, my colleagues won't respect me any more."

Embedded in Melanie's' statement was a deeper-level belief about not being respected by others. The therapist decided to address this assumption by turning the tables. The therapist began with questions about Melanie's own view of her colleagues' appearance.

THERAPIST: If one of your colleagues was losing her hair or getting wrinkles, I'm curious whether you'd respect her less? Would you think to yourself, "She's really ineffective now"?

PATIENT: Well, I don't know . . . probably not. Aging is part of being human. It's normal. And it takes a really long time before a person actually starts to be less capable. If I'd drop or disrespect everyone because they're getting older, pretty soon I'd be all by myself.

THERAPIST: So it sounds like you don't actually judge your coworkers' value by their looks. What is it that you value in them?

PATIENT: A good work ethic, being dependable, prepared, intelligent, competent, of course, and friendly, I guess.

THERAPIST: Uh-huh. To what degree do you think you have those traits?

PATIENT: Hmm . . . I'm pretty sure I have a good work ethic, because I usually come in early and I don't take long breaks. I also know that I'm reliable, because I do what I commit to, meet deadlines, and so forth. It's hard to say how smart and competent I am. Others sometimes come to me for advice, so I guess I have some valuable skills. In general, my projects turn out pretty well.

THERAPIST: Anything else?

PATIENT: Well, now that I think of it, I was a major player in turning the company around a couple of years ago when we had a lot of financial difficulties. I suppose I've gotten quite a bit of praise and recognition for that. . . . And I think people consider me friendly. I try to help others, respond to their questions. I'm pretty patient with their mistakes.

The next step for Melanie was to come up with a rational response that succinctly summarized what she had learned while evaluating her thoughts. As we have noted in Chapter 9, and have reiterated in this chapter in describing the rational self-esteem statement on Form 13.2, a rational response is a brief summary of the highlights of all your patient's ideas. Again, such a response is most helpful if it's relatively short, so the patient can remember it easily when negative thoughts occur. And, again, encourage your patient to write this rational response down so she can refer to it between sessions. Here is the rational response Melanie developed:

> Even if others notice I'm getting older, they'll still respect me. Their respect is based on my work ethic, dependability, intelligence, and nice personality.

Survey Method

Although turning the tables eased some of Melanie's anxiety about others' not respecting her, she was still not entirely convinced. When the therapist asked her how much she believed her new rational response, she said, "Only about 70%. And I still believe it a little—maybe 40%—that they don't respect me because of my wrinkles." To strengthen Melanie's conviction, her therapist suggested that she conduct a survey. This suggestion reflects an important principle of cognitive therapy: to keep addressing a problem from different angles until more rational beliefs are solidified. When one strategy is only partly successful, another should be added.

Melanie and her therapist decided that Melanie would conduct a survey of relevant people to determine whether her assumption about their opinions was correct. Melanie agreed to ask three trusted colleagues what they thought of her and her performance in the last year. Together, she and the therapist decided how she would ask the question so that the colleagues would give clear answers. After Melanie conducted the survey, she told her therapist that the answers were all positive and included comments like "You are a helpful and supportive colleague, hard-working, competent," "You are a real asset to the social atmosphere of our firm," and "You're smart, and you get promoted often." No one mentioned decreasing abilities or commented on her appearance. Melanie felt pretty good about these answers, which gave her further evidence to support her rational response. She now rated her belief at 95% for the response. In turn, this change in attitude made her more comfortable and more self-confident at work.

The survey method can be very helpful in providing your patient with a different perspective. There is a caveat, however: Be careful that this strategy doesn't turn into a reassurance ritual, especially if your patient has a frequent problem with asking others for reassurance. Also, the patient needs to have people in her life to ask such questions of, as it may not be appropriate to ask these questions of strangers. If family members are the only people in the patient's life, and they've given such feedback previously without a positive effect, it probably will not be helpful for the patient to ask them again. Thus the survey method may not be ideal for certain patients.

Help the Patient Identify Healthier Core Beliefs

Now you and your patient can go back to the *Core Belief Record* (Form 13.1) and add new core beliefs based on what the patient has learned from the exercises described above. As a reminder, a new core belief shouldn't just be the opposite of a negative core belief, because these are usually implausible. Therefore, avoid using the word "not" when you and the patient are developing an alternative belief. For example, if the old belief was "I am a freak," a reasonable alternative belief might be "I look OK," rather than "I look great" or "I look good," which may be too strong for the patient to believe. Again, useful new core beliefs contain some positive characteristics that the patient has identified in the process of doing the self-esteem pie and other exercises in this session.

Assign Homework

The homework should incorporate cognitive strategies with exposure and response prevention as well as perceptual retraining. Possible homework assignments for modifying negative beliefs include the exercises listed below, many of which are based on or extend the strategies described above. Give your patient *Advanced Cognitive Strategies* (Handout 13.1) to help her with the homework.

- Review and revise your original BDD model.
- Use the downward arrow method when negative emotions (e.g., depressed mood, crying) occur, to identify the core belief(s) behind the emotions.

- Write down what you might tell your (imagined) children about appearance-related thoughts and behaviors.
- Write down what you might tell yourself if you were a therapist.
- Form a mental picture of what a negative label would actually represent in real life whenever you use a negative label aloud or in your mind. Check if the label really fits.
- Conduct a survey of friends, colleagues, or others, based on our discussion about this during the session.
- Draw in the pieces of a self-esteem pie after determining the relative weights of the various components of the pie.
- Complete the *Core Belief Record* (Form 13.1) for each negative belief that comes up this week.

Ask for Summary of/Feedback on the Session

Ask the patient to briefly summarize the major points covered during the session. Also ask whether the patient had any concerns about the session or your behavior, and respond appropriately.

Moving Forward (Sessions 12–20)

During Session 11, you may not finish all of the core belief exercises recommended in this chapter. That's not a problem: Just integrate the exercises you didn't get to into the next few sessions, and refer back to the exercises your patient finds beneficial for the remainder of the treatment.

Once you have introduced the advanced cognitive strategies, continue combining all core treatment components in subsequent sessions. Follow the session structure we have outlined earlier for all of these sessions, and combine the skills in a way that makes sense for your patient.

If none of the optional treatment modules (see Chapters 15–18) are relevant to your patient, she will continue to practice all of the core treatment components—both in session and in homework—until the relapse prevention sessions at the end of treatment. However, if any of the optional modules are relevant to your patient, you can move on to those, starting in the next session. Feel free to combine the strategies outlined in the core components with the modular interventions. Alternatively, you could spend another session or more practicing the core treatment components before moving on to the optional modules.

The bottom line is that the pace of treatment, and the exact points at which different skills are introduced, will vary somewhat for each individual patient and should be tailored to the patient, based on her progress to date and her treatment needs. Once a new skill set is learned—whether it is a core treatment component or a module component—it should continue to be practiced and incorporated into future sessions and homework assignments until the treatment ends.

FORM 13.1

Core Belief Record

Old core belief #1: ______________________________

How much do you believe this right now? (0–100) _____

Evidence that supports old core belief (try to counter it):

Alternative belief #1: ______________________________

How much do you believe this right now? (0–100) _____

Evidence that supports old core belief (try to counter it):

Old core belief #2: ______________________________

How much do you believe this right now? (0–100) _____

Evidence that supports old core belief (try to counter it):

Alternative belief #2: ______________________________

How much do you believe this right now? (0–100) _____

Evidence that supports old core belief (try to counter it):

Adapted with permission of the publisher from Beck, J. S. (2011). *Cognitive Behavior Therapy: Basics and Beyond* (2nd ed.). New York: Guilford Press.

FORM 13.2

My Positive Traits

Think about and write down your positive traits. Consider different areas that matter to you. For example, can you understand things? What do you/did you do well? Do you have skills at doing things around the house (cooking, gardening, entertaining, solving problems, etc.)? Do you write poetry, play an instrument, paint, or the like? Do you play a sport? Do you work hard? Are you responsible? Are there people who consider you a friend? Do you have any good relationships (e.g., friends, parents, children, siblings, colleagues)? Do you have a nice house or apartment, a car, a good job, and so forth? Do you like other aspects of your appearance (your clothing style, shoes, height, weight, hair color, complexion, face, lips, eyes, mouth, chin, cheekbones, ears, nose, eyebrows, posture, shape of your face, shape of your hands, arms, legs, etc.)?

Rational Self-Esteem Statement

HANDOUT 13.1

Advanced Cognitive Strategies

The strategies described below will help you look at and evaluate your core beliefs. Core beliefs are deeper-level beliefs. They are global, overgeneralized, and negative beliefs about yourself or the world. They can usually be expressed in very simple sentences, such as "I am worthless," "I am inadequate," or "I am unlovable."

1. **Cognitive restructuring, using a copy of the *Thought Record*.** In the "Thoughts" section, write down underlying rules (e.g., "I should always look perfect") or negative core beliefs (e.g., "I am worthless") instead of appearance beliefs. Identify cognitive errors, and develop more rational and helpful alternative beliefs.

2. **Self-esteem pie and self-esteem list (the *My Positive Traits* form).** Review and remind yourself of positive traits. Add items to the self-esteem list if you think of new ones.

3. **What to tell your (imagined) children.** If you find yourself getting bogged down in negative thoughts or negative beliefs about yourself (negative core beliefs), take a different perspective by offering advice to your own child or your imagined child (preferably of your own gender). Have your child express your thoughts, and offer him or her more accurate and helpful advice.

4. **Reversing therapist and patient roles.** This is another strategy for taking a different perspective. If you find yourself getting bogged down in negative thoughts or negative beliefs about yourself (negative core beliefs), take a different perspective by playing the role of your therapist. Ask questions or make comments to yourself that a therapist would make. Try to make these questions and comments as accurate and helpful as possible.

5. **Picturing the extreme.** If you're starting to focus on negative core beliefs (such as "I'm totally worthless"), try picturing the extreme. Ask yourself, "What would a totally worthless person be like?" Answer this in some detail. Then ask yourself, "Does this really describe me? If not, why not?"

6. **Turning the tables.** Pretend that another person is expressing your negative thoughts or core beliefs (e.g., "If I have any wrinkles, I'm really unlikeable"). What would you say to other people if they said this to you? Would you not like them if they had a wrinkle? Is there a more accurate and helpful view? If so, what is it?

(cont.)

7. **Survey method.** Actually ask some people what they think about you and your beliefs. For example, you could ask what they think of you or your performance at work. Do they mention the parts of your appearance you don't like, or say that they don't like you because of them? What is a more accurate and helpful view?

8. **Identify healthier core beliefs.** After using the methods above, try to develop some new, healthier, more accurate, and helpful core beliefs. This is a very important step.

CHAPTER 14

TERMINATION SESSIONS, RELAPSE PREVENTION, AND BOOSTER SESSIONS

SESSION 21

SESSION SUMMARY

- ☐ Check mood and BDD symptoms.
- ☐ Briefly review the previous session.
- ☐ Set the agenda jointly with the patient.
- ☐ Review homework.
- ☐ Work on the agenda.
  - ☐ Discuss your patient's feelings about stopping treatment.
  - ☐ Review the *BDD Treatment Methods List* (Handout 14.1).
  - ☐ Attribute progress to your patient.
  - ☐ Plan for the future.
  - ☐ Prepare the patient to cope with stressors.
  - ☐ Help the patient plan what to do with extra time.
  - ☐ Schedule self-treatment sessions.
  - ☐ Review current medications.
  - ☐ Discuss cosmetic treatment.
- ☐ Assign homework.
- ☐ Ask for summary of/feedback on the session.

SESSION FORMS AND HANDOUTS

BDI-II (or other depression inventory)

Personal Session Form (Form 2.1)

Therapist Session Form (Form 6.1)

BDD Treatment Methods List (Handout 14.1)

Graph of Progress in Therapy (Handout 8.2)

Self-Therapy Session Form (Form 14.1)

Introduction to This Session

The goal of the relapse prevention sessions is to prepare patients for the ending of therapy. These sessions will explore patients' feelings about the ending of treatment, help reinforce their learning, prepare them for possible setbacks after therapy has ended, and maximize their long-term gains. The material covered in this chapter should be applied during the last two treatment sessions.

Approximately 2 months before treatment is scheduled to end, remind your patient that the last two treatment sessions will occur every 2 weeks rather than weekly. This gives him an opportunity to prepare for the ending of the treatment not only through experiencing a decrease in session frequency, but also through practicing self-therapy sessions before the treatment ends. Your patient may become anxious or frustrated about the ending of therapy, despite the initial agreement regarding the number of sessions. If this happens, use Socratic questioning to help him identify his thoughts about the spacing of sessions and eventual termination. Some patients are afraid of functioning without your support, fearing that they will not be able to handle problems on their own. Other patients may feel prepared but are sorry about ending their relationship with you. This chapter provides suggestions for dealing with various feelings about stopping therapy and for helping patients maximize their long-term gains.

Check Mood and BDD Symptoms

Check the BDI-II (or other depression inventory) the patient has completed in the waiting room, and check the score on the suicidality item as usual, responding as appropriate. Briefly explore the patient's general mood, and discuss BDD symptoms since the last session. Hand out the *Personal Session Form* (Form 2.1), so that the patient can record information he finds significant during the session.

Briefly Review the Previous Session

Briefly check in with the patient regarding his perception and understanding of the previous session.

Set the Agenda Jointly with the Patient

Set today's agenda by indicating that you plan to review homework, to begin to discuss the patient's feelings about ending treatment, and then to review what the patient has learned during therapy. Suggest that it is now time to review what you and the patient have done in therapy up to this point, in order to identify the cognitive and behavioral strategies that have worked best so far and decide how to plan for the coming weeks and months. Ask the patient whether there are any issues he'd like to include in the session, and work these into the agenda.

Review Homework

Review the previous homework assignment, and reinforce or correct the patient's efforts. If you spot mistakes, use Socratic questioning to help your patient consider possible solutions. At this final stage in treatment, encourage him to use what he has learned during the therapy to draw conclusions and make decisions.

Work on the Agenda

Discuss Your Patient's Feelings about Stopping Treatment

Remind your patient that next week's session will occur 2 weeks later and will be the final session of treatment. You can use standard Socratic questioning to help your patient identify and evaluate any problematic thoughts, as well as positive ones. Invite your patient to express his feelings and thoughts about ending the treatment (e.g., "Tell me how you're feeling about our stopping therapy."). Avoid interrupting, and continue to invite more comments until you're sure your patient has had sufficient opportunity to express what's on his mind. However, do not devote the entire session to this, as you might in a supportive or psychodynamic treatment.

Briefly indicate how you yourself feel about ending treatment. Comment on your experience in working with the patient, especially the positive features and strengths the patient has brought to the therapy. There will be more time to comment on this in the final session. Help your patient adjust to the ending of treatment by asking about the potential advantages and disadvantages of stopping sessions. For example, advantages might include learning to rely more on oneself and having more time for other activities. One disadvantage might be the lack of someone to speak to regularly, but this might be offset by gaining self-reliance and identifying other sources of support.

Review the *BDD Treatment Method List* (Handout 14.1)

Review what has been accomplished during treatment, with the aim of reminding your patient of all the therapy methods that have proved useful to him. You can ask him to get out his binder, to make it easy to review all the forms used during treatment and the therapy techniques they represent. You can use the metaphor of a toolbox, describing each technique as a tool. The list of strategies provided in the *BDD Treatment Methods List* (Handout 14.1) will help the patients identify the methods he has found most useful. Review this list carefully and discuss each technique; remind your patient how you used the technique during the therapy, and ask whether he will want to keep using it in the future when BDD symptoms reoccur. This process will take some time, so allow half or more of the first relapse prevention session for this purpose.

Attribute Progress to Your Patient

Throughout treatment, reinforce your patient for his hard work and progress. It's important for the patient to understand that he has accomplished the changes in BDD symptoms and mood himself, rather then crediting the improvement to the therapist. Helping him clarify how he accomplished these gains at the end of the process may also prevent relapse, as this strengthens the patient's self-efficacy beliefs. Engage in a discussion of the specific actions and strategies the patient used that seemed to produce the most gains.

Plan for the Future

Discuss what course your patient's BDD symptoms are likely to follow in the future:

"You've probably guessed that your BDD symptoms may return again at some point. Many people tend to revert to their past self-defeating habits when they experience stressful situations, or when their mood is low or they are very tired. During our treatment, you've worked hard. You now have the tools to help yourself during the next months and years. I expect that you'll generally be able to maintain your treatment gains, and you may even improve more in the coming months. But you do need to be prepared for lapses, when you'll have to struggle to keep your progress."

Ask your patient what he expects to happen during the coming year with regard to his appearance concerns. Be sure to discuss any unrealistic expectations. You can say something like this:

"Don't expect that your progress over the next few months will be a straight course. Remember what treatment has been like. It wasn't always easy for you, so expect ups and downs, but try to avoid day-to-day comparisons. Instead, keep the big picture in mind. Also, if you keep practicing your CBT-BDD skills, you may find that you gradually get even better."

Your goal here is to help your patient avoid overreacting when a minor setback occurs. You can refer back to the *Graph of Progress in Therapy* (Handout 8.2) to illustrate that it's normal to have low points, but that setbacks usually get shorter and less severe as time passes.

In addition, discuss the difference between a lapse and a relapse:

"Let's talk a little bit about a 'lapse.' A lapse is a temporary period during which some of your BDD symptoms come back. A lapse doesn't mean that you'll 'relapse'—that is, go back to where you were before you started this treatment. Just because you become afraid you look bad and start checking the mirror again on one day doesn't mean you'll return to your old fears and habits. When you have a surge in your symptoms, this may be a signal that you're under more stress than usual and will need to use your problem-solving skills to cope with the stressors."

Prepare the Patient to Cope with Stressors

Encourage your patient to identify stressful situations that might happen within the next few months and might be likely to exacerbate BDD symptoms. Some examples might be unexpected social expectations or responsibilities (such as speaking to a group or doing something in a public setting); meeting someone who's unusually attractive; hearing family or friends comment on movie stars or acquaintances' physical features; new media information about appearance-related products or cosmetic surgeries; or a serious loss (e.g., job loss, illness or death of a family member or friend).

Now ask your patient to choose one of these possible stressful events, to anticipate potential problems, and to practice coping strategies through visualization. Have your patient describe how he expects to react in this visualization, and help your patient identify any cognitive errors or problematic beliefs. Ask about other ways of interpreting the situation. Next, focus on what exposure methods are likely to be needed to reduce the discomfort, along with how to prevent avoidance and rituals that might make the problem worse. Encourage the patient to use the

BDD Treatment Methods List (Handout 14.1) to identify specific educational, cognitive, exposure, response prevention, or other strategies he thinks will work best.

Help the Patient Plan What to Do with Extra Time

If your patient used to have very time-consuming BDD symptoms, help him plan what he can do with the extra time he now has in his life. To identify potential problems, you can ask the patient, "How is your life different now from how it used to be? How are you spending most of your time?"

During this treatment, you have encouraged your patient to find healthy alternatives to replace BDD symptoms. If this hasn't happened, prompt your patient to resume some activities he used to pursue before he developed BDD, or to come up with new, realistic, and healthy activities. These new activities might include joining a book group or other regular social event, finding a job, doing volunteer work, taking a class for fun, or joining a support group. An activity should be social rather than solitary, to give the patient regular opportunities to meet people he enjoys and to practice exposures without avoidance and rituals. If the patient has accomplished some of these things during the treatment, encourage him to continue these activities. Activities such as these will make life more enjoyable and rewarding. In addition, many patients say that the busier they are, the less time there is for BDD in their lives.

Schedule Self-Treatment Sessions

You and your patient should also discuss a self-therapy plan. During self-therapy sessions, your patient will cover the same material he used to work on with you during the session. The only difference is that he is now his own therapist, as you will not be present. Begin self-sessions during the first relapse prevention session, so that your patient can apply this method during weeks when sessions aren't scheduled, and so that you can both see how this goes before the therapy ends. We recommend starting with self-therapy sessions on the same day and same time of usual office visits; for example, if your patient used to meet you on Mondays at 4:00 P.M., this time should now be used for self-therapy sessions. This plan will probably increase the likelihood that your patient will remember to follow through with these sessions. Encourage your patient to schedule self-sessions well ahead and mark them on the calendar. Suggest starting with weekly self-sessions, and then tapering to twice a month, then once per month, once per season, and finally once per year. Remind the patient that if he seems to be experiencing a BDD lapse—which may or may not occur—this would be a good time to schedule an additional session or more frequent sessions as needed. Provide your patient with several copies of the *Self-Therapy Session Form* (Form 14.1) to serve as a useful guide in planning these sessions.

Review Current Medications

If your patient is taking psychotropic medications, ask about his general thoughts regarding changes in medications, if any. For example, if your patient is doing well and considering reducing his current medications, warn him that cutting back on medications too quickly can precipitate anxiety and/or depression, depending on the medication, and that this in turn can lead to more BDD problems. Thus it will be important for the patient to discuss a plan for tapering off medications with the prescribing physician.

Discuss Cosmetic Treatment

If your patient had previously planned to obtain dermatological treatment, cosmetic surgery, or other cosmetic treatment, but has put this on hold during CBT-BDD, discuss your patient's intentions about this now that therapy is ending. Use Socratic questioning to help your patient evaluate the advantages and disadvantages of surgery or other cosmetic treatment, in light of what he has learned during the therapy and of his past experiences with such treatments. If your patient is still considering cosmetic treatment but is ambivalent about it, suggest that he delay the decision until after his new plans for social or other activities, and/or self-therapy sessions, are in place. This will afford him more time to judge whether such treatment is truly needed and will support a positive body image. The MI strategies described in Chapter 5 can be especially helpful when your patient is ambivalent about this issue. Remember to use these techniques to help the patient consider all sides of the question.

Assign Homework

Ask your patient to review all copies of the *Personal Sessions Form* (Form 2.1) he has completed during treatment, to identify the important points. Ask him to make two lists. One will include all the important learning points and can be titled "What I Have Learned." The second is a list of the methods that worked best for him to resolve the BDD symptoms and related problems (e.g., depressed mood). This can be titled "Treatment Strategies." These lists will serve as ready summaries of information learned and treatment methods likely to be useful in the future. You and your patient can compare the list of treatment methods to the *BDD Treatment Methods List* (Handout 14.1) to help him select the most useful strategies.

Ask for Summary of/Feedback on the Session

Ask your patient to summarize the major points covered during the session. Ask for any comments and questions about what he has learned during the session. Finally, ask the patient for feedback about the session, including anything that bothered him. Respond to any concerns in an understanding manner, and decide how to address them.

SESSION 22 (FINAL SESSION)

SESSION SUMMARY

- ☐ Check mood and BDD symptoms.
- ☐ Briefly review the previous session.
- ☐ Set the agenda jointly with the patient.
- ☐ Review homework.
- ☐ Work on the agenda.
  - ☐ Review weeks since the last session and self-treatment sessions.
  - ☐ Schedule booster appointments and tell the patient how to prepare for them.
  - ☐ Congratulate the patient on "graduation."

☐ Assign homework.
☐ Ask for summary of/feedback on the session.

BDI-II (OR OTHER DEPRESSION INVENTORY)

Personal Session Form (Form 2.1)
Therapist Session Form (Form 6.1)

Introduction to This Session

The goal of this last session is to continue to prepare your patient for the ending of therapy. Cover any remaining issues, particularly as they pertain to symptoms and relapse prevention.

Check Mood and BDD Symptoms

Check the BDI-II (or other depression inventory) the patient has completed in the waiting room, and check the score on the suicidality item as usual, responding as appropriate. Briefly explore the patient's general mood, and discuss BDD symptoms since the last session. Hand out the *Personal Session Form* (Form 2.1) so that the patient can record information he finds significant during the session.

Briefly Review the Previous Session

Briefly check in with the patient regarding his perception and understanding of the previous session.

Set the Agenda Jointly with the Patient

Remind your patient that this is the last session. Set today's agenda by indicating that you plan to review homework and to discuss any remaining symptoms. In addition, let your patient know that you are going to ask him about the self-therapy sessions and educate him about how to prepare for the booster sessions. And, as always, ask the patient whether there are any issues he'd like to include in the session.

Review Homework

Review the previous homework assignment, and reinforce or correct the patient's efforts. If you spot mistakes, use Socratic questioning to help your patient consider possible solutions. At this final session of treatment, encourage the patient to use what he has learned during the therapy to draw conclusions and make decisions.

Work on the Agenda

Review Weeks since the Last Session and Self-Treatment Sessions

Discuss with your patient whether any kinds of problems have occurred since the last session and, if so, how he has handled them. Praise your patient for using CBT-BDD skills, and ask him how well they worked. If your patient's use of the strategies did not work well, discuss how he can handle similar problems next time. If he did not use CBT-BDD skills, ask why not, and discuss how he can remember to use these skills next time and fully integrate them into his day-to-day life.

Also review your patient's experience with the self-therapy sessions, and remind him to conduct weekly self-therapy sessions until the first booster session. Discuss any problems he may have encountered with self-treatment, and discuss ways to conduct these sessions successfully in the future. Remind your patient that it's important to schedule these regularly. Come up with a schedule for self-therapy sessions during this session.

Schedule Booster Appointments and Tell the Patient How to Prepare for Them

Booster sessions are typically provided 1 month and 3 months after the end of treatment, so be sure to schedule these sessions now. Advise your patient that he should come to the booster sessions even if he is feeling good, as the goal of these sessions is to *prevent* symptom recurrence. Let your patient know that the booster sessions are an opportunity to review what is going well and how he can improve further.

Tell the patient that if he is not doing well, it is equally (or even more) important for him to come to the booster sessions, so that he can sharpen his skills. These sessions are an opportunity to check on any reemergence of maladaptive strategies. Thus your patient should be prepared to discuss what kind of problems have arisen since the end of treatment and how he has coped with them.

Congratulate the Patient on "Graduation"

In the final session, ask your patient to reflect on the entire course of the therapy. Have him describe what he has learned about himself in general, and how this will help as he looks forward to the immediate future. Help your patient be as specific as possible about this future view.

Comment honestly about the progress you have observed, and about your patient's special skills and abilities that facilitated this progress. Reinforce hard work and the learning that has occurred during treatment with positive statements (e.g., "I was especially impressed by how you stuck to the task of looking for alternative ways of viewing your thoughts"). Ask for feedback about the treatment in general and your style as a therapist. Finally, express honest feedback to the patient, if advisable: "It was great working with you," "I'll miss working with you," "I'm so glad our work together helped," "I have a lot of confidence in you." Congratulate your patient for completing or "graduating" from the program.

Assign Homework

Ask your patient to continue with regularly scheduled self-sessions, and to prepare for booster sessions as described above.

Ask for Summary of/Feedback on the Session

Ask your patient to summarize the major points covered during this last session. Ask for any comments and questions about what he learned during the session. Finally, ask the patient for feedback about the session and the treatment, including anything that bothered him. Respond to any concerns in an understanding manner, and decide how to address these.

BOOSTER SESSIONS

Patients who have made gains in treatment are good candidates for booster sessions to prevent relapse. The frequency of booster sessions can be gradually reduced, and you can offer as many as seem helpful for a particular patient. We typically recommend at least two booster sessions. As described above, the first booster session is usually scheduled for 1 month after the end of treatment, and the second one for 3 months after the end of treatment. Sometimes therapists offer additional booster sessions (e.g., once per season and then once per year).

SESSION SUMMARY

- ☐ Check mood and BDD symptoms.
- ☐ Briefly review the previous session.
- ☐ Set the agenda jointly with the patient.
- ☐ Review homework.
- ☐ Work on the agenda.
  - ☐ Review weeks since the last session and self-treatment sessions.
  - ☐ Schedule future booster appointment.
- ☐ Assign homework.
- ☐ Ask for summary of/feedback on the session.

SESSION FORMS AND HANDOUTS

BDI-II (or other depression inventory)

Personal Session Form (Form 2.1)

Therapist Session Form (Form 6.1)

Self-Therapy Session Form (Form 14.1)

Introduction to This Session

The goal of each booster session is to prevent symptom recurrence.

Check Mood and BDD Symptoms

Check the BDI-II (or other depression inventory) that the patient has completed in the waiting room, and check the score on the suicidality item as you did during regular treatment sessions, responding as appropriate. Briefly explore the patient's general mood, and discuss BDD symptoms since the last session. Hand out the *Personal Session Form* (Form 2.1) so that the patient can record information he finds significant during the session.

Briefly Review the Previous Session

Briefly check in with the patient regarding his perception and understanding of the previous session.

Set the Agenda Jointly with the Patient

Remind your patient that this is a booster session. Set today's agenda by indicating that you plan to review homework, and to discuss any symptoms or problems your patient has encountered. Let your patient know that you are also going to ask about his self-therapy sessions. Ask the patient whether there are any issues he'd like to include in the session.

Review Homework

Review the previous homework assignment, and reinforce or correct the patient's efforts. If you spot mistakes, use Socratic questioning to help your patient consider possible solutions.

Work on the Agenda

Review Weeks since the Last Session and Self-Treatment Sessions

Discuss with your patient how he has done since the last session. Have any kinds of problems occurred since the last session, and if so, how has he handled them? Praise your patient for using CBT-BDD skills, and ask him how well they worked. If your patient's use of the strategies did not work well, discuss how your patient can handle similar problems next time. If he did not use CBT-BDD skills, ask why not, and discuss how he can remember to use these skills next time.

Also review your patient's experience with the self-therapy sessions. Did he conduct these sessions, and if so, how often? Was the patient able to schedule the sessions on a regular basis, or was it hard to do this? What did he do during the sessions? If the patient did not do self-therapy sessions, was he able to integrate CBT-BDD strategies in his life in other ways? Were any CBT-BDD techniques especially helpful? If so, reinforce use of these techniques. If certain techniques were not used in self-therapy or were not helpful, discuss with the patient why this was the case, and help the patient think through whether and how such approaches might be useful in future sessions. Collaboratively discuss approaches to resolving any other challenges or problems that might have arisen since your last session.

Remind the patient to continue to conduct weekly self-therapy sessions and the use of CBT-BDD skills in general. Plan future self-therapy sessions, and ask whether the patient needs additional copies of the *Self-Therapy Session Form* (Form 14.1). If the patient is not willing to do self-therapy sessions, encourage the use of CBT skills more broadly.

Schedule Future Booster Appointment (at First Booster Session Only)

If this is the first booster session, schedule a second booster session for 3 months after the end of treatment.

Assign Homework

Ask your patient to continue with self-therapy sessions, to complete self-session forms, and to prepare for the second booster sessions (if this is the first one).

Ask for Summary of/Feedback on the Sessions

At the end of each booster session, ask your patient to summarize the major points covered during the session. Ask for any comments and questions about what he learned during the session. Finally, ask the patient for feedback about the session, including anything that bothered him. Respond to any concerns in an understanding manner, and decide how to address these.

FORM 14.1

Self-Therapy Session Form

Date of session: ____________________

Mood check:

Important changes in symptoms:

Homework check: How did I do on homework I set for myself last week? What got in my way? How can I learn from this experience for next time?

What skills have I been practicing well?

(cont.)

Adapted with permission of the publisher from Wilhelm, S., & Steketee, G. (2006). *Cognitive Therapy for Obsessive-Compulsive Disorder.* Oakland, CA: New Harbinger publications.

Self-Therapy Session Form *(page 2 of 2)*

Where am I still having troubles, and what should I do about this?

What are my treatment goals for the coming week?

What homework assignment will help me meet these goals?

Date for next session:

HANDOUT 14.1

BDD Treatment Methods List

Reeducate yourself.

1. Refresh your memory about BDD problems by rereading any of the following handouts that are relevant:
   a. *What Is Body Dysmorphic Disorder?*
   b. *Information about Body Shape and Weight Concerns*
   c. *Information about Muscle Dysmorphia*
   d. *Information about Steroid Use*
   e. *Information about Other Body-Shaping Substances*
   f. *Information about Cosmetic Treatment for BDD*
2. Review the *Standard BDD Model* handout, your completed *Your Personal BDD Model* Form, and the *BDD Model with Treatment Techniques* handout.

Use cognitive strategies.

1. Review the various types of thinking errors by rereading any of the following handouts that are relevant:
   a. *Types of Maladaptive Thinking*
   b. *Examples of Cognitive Errors Associated with Weight, Shape, and Muscularity Concerns*
   c. *Examples of Cognitive Errors Involving Cosmetic Treatment*
   d. *Examples of Cognitive Errors in Depressive Thoughts*
2. Record automatic negative thoughts in situations that trigger BDD fears, using the *Keeping Track of Your Thoughts* or *Thought Record* form. Identify the pattern of these thoughts.
3. Review the *Questions to Evaluate Negative Thoughts* handout, and select the questions that are most relevant to your negative thinking in specific situations.
4. Generate plausible alternative rational ideas, and decide how much you believe the automatic thoughts or the alternative ones and which ones are more likely to be true. Respond to negative predictions about the immediate and long-term future with alternative predictions. Decide which predictions are more likely to be true.
5. Evaluate the pros and cons of your thoughts. (For thoughts about skin picking, hair plucking/pulling, or getting cosmetic treatment, you can use the relevant *Pros and Cons Worksheet*.)
6. Take another perspective by considering how you might advise a friend or relative with your same concerns, or remembering how others you trust have advised you.

(cont.)

Use advanced cognitive strategies that focus on core beliefs.

Use the *Advanced Cognitive Strategies* handout.

1. Do cognitive restructuring with core beliefs.
2. Review your self-esteem pie.
3. Do the exercise "What to tell your (imagined) children."
4. Do the exercise "Reversing therapist and patient roles."
5. Do the exercise "Picturing the extreme."
6. Do the exercise "Turning the tables."
7. Do the exercise "Survey method."
8. Identify healthier core beliefs.

Use exposure strategies.

1. Review the situations on your *Distressing Situations Worksheet*, and add any new ones that have cropped up.
2. Use copies of the *Exposure Worksheet* to work on facing fears and handling anxiety in new situations.
   a. Identify the trigger for distress.
   b. Identify negative thoughts and predictions.
   c. Identify cognitive errors.
   d. Think of alternative rational thoughts and predictions.
   e. Shift attention toward the task at hand.
   f. Set clear goals for exposures.
   g. Rate your distress periodically during the exposure.
   h. Decide whether you reached the goal.
   i. Notice whether the negative thoughts or the alternative thoughts actually came true.
   j. Determine what you learned from the experience.
   k. Reward yourself if your goals were met.
3. When you are doing new exposures, select specific, measurable, and achievable goals.
4. Plan your daily life to include regular exposures to social situations, and use your cognitive skills to modify anxious thoughts and manage discomfort in these situations.

Block rituals and avoidance behaviors.

1. Use the *Ritual-Monitoring Form* to record rituals and avoidance.

(cont.)

2. It is best to prevent or stop the ritual altogether right from the start. However, when rituals are hard to resist, use one or more of the following methods to reduce or eliminate them:
   a. Use stimulus control to remove triggers for rituals from your environment.
   b. Allow rituals only in certain situations, but not others.
   c. Decrease the time you spend ritualizing.
   d. Delay the rituals.
   e. Use competing responses, which are activities that focus on the same muscle groups used during appearance compulsions, but are physically incompatible with the rituals.
3. Substitute healthy behaviors for rituals or avoidance. For example, spend time talking with friends rather than fixing your makeup in the mirror.
4. If your exercising becomes excessive, find a moderate level, and practice this consistently.
5. If you begin to weigh yourself too often and are anxious about it, weigh yourself weekly, not daily (or if necessary, do it monthly, not weekly).
6. Wear clothes that fit—not too loose, not too baggy.
7. Eat a healthy diet—not a rigid one.
8. Stop comparing yourself with others; shift your attention—take in the big picture.
9. Stop using steroids or any other substances you take for some aspect of your appearance.
10. Use ritual prevention for behaviors related to cosmetic treatment.
11. Incorporate response (ritual) prevention into your exposures, and use copies of the *Exposure and Response Prevention Worksheet* to record your results.

Use mirror retraining.

1. Describe yourself in a neutral and objective way, without negative self-talk.
2. Describe yourself from head to toe. Describe *all* body areas. Don't spend more time on the body areas you dislike than on other body areas.
3. Stand at a normal distance from the mirror, not really close.
4. Don't do any mirror checking. In other words, don't zero in and focus on what you don't like, especially at the end of the mirror session.
5. Take in the big picture!
6. Use the *Mirror Retraining Worksheet* to record your results.

PART IV

OPTIONAL MODULES FOR PATIENTS WITH RELEVANT SYMPTOMS

The core interventions described in Part III (Chapters 9–14) are relevant for all patients. However, they may not sufficiently reduce specific symptoms (e.g., BDD-related skin picking) that certain patients with BDD have. So, in addition to the core skills described earlier, you can select the specialized treatment modules described in Chapters 15–18 to address individual patients' needs. These modules increase the flexibility of CBT-BDD, enabling you to personalize the treatment for each patient. Some patients may not require any of these modules, whereas others will potentially benefit from several or even all of the modules in addition to the core interventions.

Typically, you will select specialized modules after patients are familiar with the core CBT-BDD skills. However, as noted above, in some cases (e.g., severe depressed mood, strong urge to seek surgical treatment, damaging skin picking, central focus on weight or body build), you may need to use a module earlier in the treatment. Your decision as to whether your patient needs one or more of these specialized modules should based on your patient's feedback, your own clinical judgment, and elevated scores on aspects of BDD measures.

CHAPTER 15

Skin Picking and Hair Pulling

Does Your Patient Need This Module?

This optional module is intended for patients who engage in repetitive skin picking or hair pulling to try to improve their appearance. About one-third of patients with BDD repeatedly pick their skin to remove perceived imperfections, such as pimples. They may use their fingers or tools, including tweezers, pins, needles, nail cutters, or knives. This behavior can consume hours a day and can cause visible disfigurement and tissue damage, with consequent sores, scars, or infections. Thus, ironically, although the patients' goal is to improve their appearance, the outcome can be seriously damaging to their skin and their looks. The most common site for picking is the face, followed by the back, neck, scalp, ears, chest, arms, and legs. Patients often describe feeling "mesmerized" while picking. Many patients use cosmetics and clothing to cover areas they have picked.

Some patients with BDD also pluck or pull their hair—for example, to make "unruly" eyebrows even or remove "excessive" neck, facial, or other body hair. Bald patches may result, which may lead to further pulling and plucking episodes, usually with the goal to undo the damage caused by previous hair plucking. To differentiate BDD-related hair pulling or plucking from trichotillomania, ask patients why they do this. If their goal is to improve a perceived defect in appearance, the hair pulling/plucking can be considered a BDD symptom.

We suggest applying the following criteria to determine whether a patient could benefit from the strategies in this module: (1) an elevated score on the BDD-SS (Form 4.3) (≥5 for the questions about skin picking/hair pulling); (2) the patient's input regarding the behaviors described above and related symptoms she considers problematic; and (3) your clinical judgment that the module is relevant. If any of these criteria are met, this should prompt discussion of whether this module should be used with the patient.

Session Structure

The standard agenda outlined in earlier chapters for all CBT-BDD sessions should be followed.

SESSION SUMMARY

- ☐ Check mood and BDD symptoms.
- ☐ Briefly review the previous session.
- ☐ Set the agenda jointly with the patient.
- ☐ Review homework.
- ☐ Work on the agenda.
  - ☐ Identify and monitor skin-picking and/or hair-plucking/pulling rituals.
  - ☐ Identify triggers for skin picking and/or hair pulling/plucking.
  - ☐ Determine behavioral chains.
  - ☐ Identify thoughts and emotions related to picking or plucking/pulling.
  - ☐ Identify consequences of picking and/or plucking/pulling.
  - ☐ Show the patient how to apply cognitive strategies for picking and/or plucking/pulling.
  - ☐ Help the patient start ritual prevention strategies.
  - ☐ Encourage the patient to find healthier ways to regulate emotions.
- ☐ Assign homework.
- ☐ Ask for summary of/feedback on the session.

SESSION FORMS AND HANDOUTS

BDI-II (or other depression inventory)

Personal Session Form (Form 2.1)

Therapist Session Form (Form 6.1)

Completed BDD-SS (Form 4.3)

Ritual-Monitoring Form (plus several extra copies for homework) (Form 11.1)

Pros and Cons Worksheet for Skin Picking (Form 15.1)

Pros and Cons Worksheet for Hair Plucking or Hair Pulling (Form 15.2)

Thought Record (plus several extra copies for homework) (Form 9.1)

Types of Maladaptive Thinking (Handout 9.2)

Completed *Your Personal BDD Model* (Form 7.1)

BDD Model with Treatment Techniques (Handout 8.1)

INTRODUCTION TO THIS SESSION

The overall goal of this optional module is to reduce skin picking and/or hair pulling by doing these things:

- Increasing your patient's awareness of these behaviors and their triggers.
- Increasing your patient's insight into the pros and cons of skin picking and hair pulling.
- Teaching your patient strategies to prevent or reduce these behaviors.

Generally one or two sessions should suffice to introduce the methods described below. Several of these strategies may already be familiar to your patient from work on ritual prevention and cognitive restructuring. However, if your patient has caused significant physical damage through skin picking and/or hair pulling, you might consider focusing on these behaviors before working on other BDD rituals. In this case, be sure to read Chapter 11 and to introduce ritual prevention to the patient before proceeding with the strategies described below.

In this module, you should strive to do the following:

- View patients' urges to pick their skin or pull their hair as compulsive behavior, much like checking mirrors and comparing themselves to others.
- Be nonjudgmental; these patients are usually very ashamed of their behavior.
- Take a balanced approach toward dermatological treatments. For example, mild acne might benefit from a topical treatment to reduce blemishes and thereby minimize the triggers for skin picking. (In our experience, however, such treatment is usually ineffective for overall BDD symptoms.) On the other hand, it is counterproductive for your patients to make emergency phone calls or visits to a dermatologist just because of a small blemish (see Chapter 17 on cosmetic treatment for more detailed information). Also, it is not advisable for patients with BDD whose acne is mild or nonexistent to receive treatments that are usually reserved for severe acne, such as isotretinoin (Accutane) or dermabrasion.

Many of the strategies we describe below have been adapted from "habit reversal training," a behavioral approach initially developed in the 1970s (see Azrin & Nunn, 1973). Habit reversal training is a multicomponent treatment, and its original version included many different strategies (e.g., awareness training, competing-response training, contingency management, and relaxation training), but awareness training and competing-response training appear to be the most critical components. In this CBT-BDD module, we enhance these two original habit reversal training techniques with other strategies we have found helpful in reducing skin picking and hair plucking/pulling as symptoms of BDD.

Check Mood and BDD Symptoms

Check the BDI-II (or other depression inventory) that the patient has completed in the waiting room, and check the score on the suicidality item as usual, responding as appropriate. Briefly explore the patient's general mood, and discuss BDD symptoms since the last session. Hand out the *Personal Session Form* (Form 2.1), so that the patient can record information she finds significant during the session.

Briefly Review the Previous Session

Briefly check in with the patient regarding her perception and understanding of the previous session.

Set the Agenda Jointly with the Patient

Convey the topics you'd like to cover during the session, and ask the patient whether there are any items she would like to include in the agenda.

Review Homework

Discuss your patient's homework from the previous session.

Work on the Agenda

Identify and Monitor Skin-Picking and/or Hair-Plucking/Pulling Rituals

To reduce skin-picking or hair-pulling behavior successfully, your patient needs to be aware when it occurs. So start by assessing the behavior in detail. As noted earlier, the severity ratings for skin picking and hair pulling on the BDD-SS (Form 4.3) will give you an initial idea of how frequent, distressing, or impairing a patient's rituals are. Some patients can provide you with very accurate estimates of their skin-picking and hair-plucking/pulling frequency. Even so, most patients will benefit from monitoring their rituals for several days with the *Ritual-Monitoring Form* (Form 11.1), to determine when they occur, their frequency, and their duration. *Continue this monitoring throughout treatment until the rituals are eliminated, so you can track progress over time.*

In a patient's first session on skin picking or hair plucking/pulling, ask your patient to give you an estimate of the amount of time she engages in those rituals per day, and also ask her to track the actual frequency of the rituals during the following (and later) weeks with Form 11.1.

Identify Triggers for Skin Picking and/or Hair Plucking/Pulling

The self-monitoring strategies described above will begin to increase your patient's awareness of picking and pulling behaviors. This is very important, as patients often describe being in a trance-like state while picking or pulling. After discussing the frequency of skin picking and hair pulling, ask the patient about situational triggers, associated thoughts, and feelings. Some picking or pulling rituals may be triggered by specific situations. For example, it is common for picking to occur after a patient has already seen or felt a skin imperfection. Most patients report being alone at home while picking their skin or plucking/pulling their hair. Also, certain emotions, especially tension and boredom, can trigger skin picking. It is very important for your patient to be aware of the situations that trigger pulling/plucking and picking.

After this discussion, remind your patient to fill in the relevant columns on the *Ritual-Monitoring Form* (Form 11.1) to track the specific triggers, thoughts, and feelings for occurrences of picking and plucking/pulling during the coming week.

Determine Behavioral Chains

Next, discuss specific physical movements involved in the patient's picking or plucking/pulling actions. Find out the sequence or chain of these behaviors, because each preceding behavior often serves as a cue for subsequent behaviors, and thus the early behaviors can be used as warning signals for the behaviors that lead to an actual picking or plucking/pulling episode. This will help the patient learn when to implement alternative behaviors to interrupt the chain.

You need to help the patient to increase her awareness of the behavior. Her goal is to detect the onset of picking or pulling behavior as early in the behavioral chain as possible. Ask questions like the ones in the following exchange:

THERAPIST: You've already told me that you usually pick your face in the bathroom in the basement of your house. What events lead up to the picking? Is there anything you do before the picking?

PATIENT: Yes, I turn on both sconces and the overhead light, so it's really bright. And then I lean over the sink.

THERAPIST: What happens next?

PATIENT: I run my hand over my skin to see if there are any bumps, and if I feel anything uneven, I start picking it.

The more details you can get the patient to provide for the behavioral chain, the better. For example, what hand does she use? What tools does she use? These details will help when you and the patient are devising response prevention exercises.

Identify Thoughts and Emotions Related to Picking or Plucking/Pulling

Ask your patient why she picks her skin or plucks or pulls her hair. Usually the patient will tell you she does this to improve her appearance, but she might also say that skin picking or hair pulling reduces tension or boredom. In addition to a discussion in the session, the self-monitoring at home will shed light on thoughts and feelings that trigger skin picking.

Identify Consequences of Picking or Plucking/Pulling

Next, ask your patient about the results of picking or pulling. Be sure to ask about physical consequences (e.g., bleeding, scarring, bald spots, lack of eyebrows); emotional consequences (e.g., guilt, shame); and behavioral consequences (e.g., avoidance behaviors like hiding bald spots or red marks with makeup or clothing). You'll want to refer to these in the next section of this module.

After collecting all of the information described, write down a general chain of events with your patient that represents as accurately as possible the behavior pattern your patient usually exhibits. Again, this will lay important groundwork for the interventions described below.

THERAPIST: Let me see if I have the general picture right. Picking is especially problematic when you need to go out. It usually begins with a thought that your skin might look bad, and then you touch your face with your right hand to see if you feel any bumps. You usually feel something, and then you go to the mirror to look at the bump, while telling yourself you won't pick. But telling yourself this doesn't seem to stop you, and it doesn't really matter how big the bump is, because even a tiny one will provoke picking. So then you scratch at it with your fingernail, and sometimes this hurts, but you keep doing this anyway—often till you draw blood. Your thoughts are focused on smoothing out the skin to make it look better, but it's hard to stop doing it, even when you realize that you're making it look red or bloody. Do I have this right so far?

PATIENT: Ugh, it sounds terrible, but I guess that's what I'm doing.

THERAPIST: OK. I want to make sure I am getting the sequence and all the details right, so we can work on the critical parts of the sequence. If I heard you correctly, when you're looking in the mirror, you also think to yourself that you'll just do a little more and then stop—but actually you almost never stop after telling yourself this, because the urge to pick is so strong. Look at the sequence as I put it on paper here, and tell me if you think this is everything and if I have it in the right order. We can check it by having you monitor the picking this week, to make sure we haven't left anything out.

Show the Patient How to Apply Cognitive Strategies for Picking and Plucking/Pulling

Discuss and Write Down Pros and Cons of the Behavior

The preceding discussion with the patient has set the stage for examining the pros and cons of her picking and plucking/pulling behavior. Patients often have the misconception that they are improving their skin/hair by picking or plucking it, or at least they tell themselves this to justify their actions. Ask your patient to think through and write down as many pros (advantages) and cons (disadvantages) of picking or hair pulling as possible. Consider the following example:

THERAPIST: If we looked at this objectively, what do you think are the advantages of plucking your facial hairs?

PATIENT: Well, I feel better right when I do it—you know, less frustrated or stressed out. I don't look as hairy. Sometimes I need to pluck the eyebrows so that they are really symmetrical, and this is hard to do . . . and if I don't get it right I have to keep plucking and plucking.

THERAPIST: OK, what else?

PATIENT: I guess there's not much else I can think of.

THERAPIST: What are the disadvantages?

PATIENT: Um, bald patches on the eyebrows, sometimes red marks, but I hide those pretty well with eyebrow pencil and makeup. It hurts after I pluck in the same area, sometimes for a while.

THERAPIST: Anything else?

PATIENT: Like what?

THERAPIST: You've said you have bald patches, red marks, and some pain. You've mentioned feelings of embarrassment, and you try to hide the bald patches and marks. Is that a pro or a con?

PATIENT: Oh, not good—that's a con. Yeah, it doesn't work that well, and I waste a lot of time, too. I think I'm getting that the hair plucking probably does me more harm than good. Still, it's such a strong urge.

THERAPIST: Yes, it is. We'll work on that. But it's important first to be clear on whether the plucking works mainly for you or against you.

Use a Socratic style to ask questions that express curiosity or wonder about what the patient thinks and believes, rather than asking leading questions (ones you know the answers to and want the patient to figure out). Make sure that the patient evaluates any pros and cons she may not have considered previously. Ideally, the list of cons will be longer than the list of pros—which usually reflects reality. Pros may include improving the patient's appearance or feeling briefly better. Disadvantages may be the amount of time consumed, skin damage, bald spots, shame or embarrassment, looking worse, not going out and doing things after bloodying or damaging the skin, and the risk of longer-term scarring or hair loss. Less obvious to many patients is that skin picking and hair plucking/pulling intensify the BDD problem by keeping the patients focused on their appearance, especially when the behaviors actually damage appearance. If there are clear disadvantages a patient hasn't thought of, you can ask directly about these, again using a Socratic questioning style:

THERAPIST: Is the time you spend on picking a pro or a con? Is it something you mainly enjoy doing?

PATIENT: No, I don't enjoy it. In fact, I really hate it, and it interferes with other things.

THERAPIST: OK, the time it takes is problematic. So should we add that to the list of cons, maybe with a comment about the things it keeps you from doing?

After the patient reviews the pros and cons of these behaviors, you can have her write down the percentage of picking/plucking/pulling episodes after which she feels better and the percentage after which she feels worse. She can write this at the bottom of the *Pros and Cons Worksheet for Skin Picking* (Form 15.1) or the *Pros and Cons Worksheet for Hair Plucking or Hair Pulling* (Form 15.2). In our experience, patients often say that they feel better only a small percentage of the time, but they usually haven't previously realized this. This realization can be an additional impetus for them to try the strategies below.

Address Maladaptive Thoughts Related to the Behavior

Have your patient use the *Thought Record* (Form 9.1) to address unhelpful, invalid, or self-defeating thoughts related to skin picking or hair plucking/pulling, such as unrealistic goals for the skin or hair (e.g., "My skin should be absolutely clear"). Help your patient to identify the cognitive errors (see *Types of Maladaptive Thinking*, Handout 9.2) in such statements (e.g., all-or-nothing thinking, "should" statements) and develop rational responses to them, such as the following:

> "Having perfectly clear skin is not a realistic goal; it's pretty normal to have a few imperfections. The problem starts when I can't accept them and start picking at them for several hours at a time. That's when I make it worse. I just have to accept that my skin is a little imperfect, and that's OK."

As described in Chapter 9, you can also use cognitive restructuring with a belief such as "It will definitely turn out better this time," or "I just need to take care of this one hair." Again, help your patient to identify the cognitive errors in such beliefs and to examine the evidence that supports or refutes the beliefs.

Help the Patient Start Ritual Prevention Strategies

Introduce the reason for ritual (response) prevention and why it's likely to be helpful. Refer back to the patient's completed copy of *Your Personal BDD Model* (Form 7.1) and to the *BDD Model with Treatment Techniques* handout (Handout 8.1) to illustrate the problematic nature of these behaviors and the intent of ritual prevention. The goal is for the patient to gradually cut down and eventually completely stop skin picking and/or hair pulling/plucking:

> "So it seems that you've decided the skin picking is really a liability without much advantage to you, and it ultimately keeps you focused on your appearance to the exclusion of other thoughts and activities. We've already been working on preventing your other rituals, like mirror checking. Today I'd like to go over how the various ritual prevention strategies we've already talked about might apply to your skin picking. Our aim is to help you get better control over this ritual, so you spend less time on it and feel more comfortable when you don't do it."

The general principles for ritual prevention are the same as those described in Chapter 11. However, keep in mind that picking or plucking/pulling often occurs outside a patient's awareness. Therefore, your patient will need to invest more time in monitoring and in identifying triggers, behavioral chains, and so forth than patients with other rituals may require. Be sure that your patient can detect picking or plucking/pulling behavior reasonably well before you move on to ritual prevention. Though you can try all of the strategies described in Chapter 11, in our clinical work we have had particularly good results with (1) *stimulus control strategies*, in which patients manipulate their environment to avoid cues that trigger or increase rituals; and (2) *competing responses*, which involve activities that are physically incompatible with the appearance rituals.

Stimulus Control Strategies

Earlier in this module, you have discussed with the patient the triggers for these rituals, as well as the behavioral chains. The triggers and early behaviors in the chain should be conceptualized as warning signs, and the patient should try to remove herself from a situation as soon as these occur. To implement stimulus control methods, for example, you can ask your patient to stay out of the bathroom, keep the lighting low so that visibility is poor, or get rid of unnecessary mirrors (e.g., compact mirrors or magnifying mirrors) used for picking or plucking/pulling. You could also suggest putting a sticky note on the bathroom mirror that reads "STOP!" to remind the patient to stop picking. The sticky note can also have a smiley face on it, to help the patient visualize how good she will feel if she does not give in to the urge to pick.

If the patient uses tools to pick or pluck (e.g., tweezers, knives), ask her to remove these from her environment if possible, or at least to make it much harder to use them when the urge to do this strikes. These tools can cause considerable skin damage, which is occasionally life-threatening (some patients have cut through large blood vessels by mistake). For example, the patient could discard her tweezers or ask someone else to keep them except for 5 minutes each week. She could put her sewing kit (with needles she uses for picking) away in the back of a closet where it is difficult to reach. Razor blades could be replaced by razors with built-in blades that can't be used for picking.

Engaging in stimulus control as soon as early warning signs occur is an important part of treatment. To help the patient use this method effectively, be sure to discuss different ways to remove the triggers ahead of time. The patient can make a list to refer to when she feels an urge to pick or pull. For example, if a patient routinely picks her skin when she is standing in front of the bathroom mirror, the list might include leaving the bathroom and calling a friend, going for a walk, running an errand, reading a magazine, or going for a bike ride. Usually behavioral chains are easier to interrupt in the early stages (e.g., when the patient has just entered the bathroom) than in later stages (e.g., when the patient has already touched the imperfection on the skin). Talking about this in advance will help motivate the patient to attend to the early warning signs and to control the stimulus early in the process. Even if the patient fails to detect the early signal, remind her that every second counts, and that it's never too late to engage in a response prevention strategy.

Competing Responses

Competing responses are very helpful in preventing skin picking and hair plucking/pulling. As described in Chapter 11, competing responses are healthy behaviors that are physically incompatible with the rituals to be prevented. Competing responses should focus on the same muscle groups used in the appearance compulsions. In social situations they must be unobtrusive, and the patient must be able to maintain a competing response for a minute, or until the urge to pick or pull decreases.

Together with your patient, generate a short list of activities that could be used as competing responses. One good strategy is to make a fist when the urge occurs or when your patient begins the initial action of picking up tweezers to pluck her eyebrows or feels the urge to scratch or pick her skin. This strategy tends to work very well for most patients. However, patients who prefer to keep their hands busy could use a soft ball or play with marbles when urges occur. Enjoyable hobbies that involve use of the hands (e.g., doing embroidery or knitting) can also be good competing responses. The disadvantage of involving tools in competing responses is your patient will have to have the tools she needs for these responses (e.g., the soft ball, marbles, or knitting needles) in the locations where the picking or pulling often occurs. Another option is to help the patient decide always to knit or do some other handiwork while watching TV in the evenings if TV watching is a common trigger for picking.

You can also encourage the patient to combine response prevention techniques. For example, in addition to trying to avoid going into the bathroom to pick, if the patient does go in she could cut back on the time spent picking by immediately making a fist and then going for a walk.

Encourage the Patient to Find Healthier Ways to Regulate Emotions

Patients often say that although they initially might have started picking or pulling to improve their appearance, over time these behaviors have assumed an emotion-regulating function. In other words, they are using skin picking and hair plucking/pulling to decrease unpleasant feelings, like tension or boredom. Discuss other possible ways to regulate emotions (going to the gym, listening to a meditation or relaxation tape, taking a hot bath, listening to music, etc.). Assign one or more of these as alternative behaviors whenever triggering emotions such as boredom or stress occur during the coming weeks.

Many of the techniques described in this chapter have originally been developed for patients with severe hair-pulling problems. If your patient is interested in reading more about this, you might want to recommend the book *Help for Hair Pullers* (Keuthen, Stein, & Christensen, 2001) or the workbook *Trichotillomania: An ACT-Enhanced Behavior Therapy Approach* (Woods & Twohig, 2008).

Assign Homework

- Assign ritual monitoring; ask the patient to complete the *Ritual-Monitoring Form* (Form 11.1) for several weeks or until the skin picking or hair plucking/pulling stops.
- Give the patient several blank copies of the *Thought Record* (Form 9.1), to enable her to observe and dispute the irrational thinking that justifies the rituals.
- Ask your patient to use stimulus control and competing responses for ritual prevention.
- Assign alternative positive behaviors in response to negative emotions that might trigger the picking or pulling.

Ask for Summary of/Feedback on the Session

Ask the patient to briefly summarize the major points covered during the session. Also ask whether the patient had any concerns about the session or your behavior, and respond appropriately.

FORM 15.1

Pros and Cons Worksheet for Skin Picking

Pros	Cons

Percentage of skin-picking episodes I feel better after: ______________________

Percentage of skin-picking episodes I feel worse after: ______________________

FORM 15.2

Pros and Cons Worksheet for Hair Plucking or Hair Pulling

Pros	Cons

Percentage of hair-plucking or hair-pulling episodes I feel better after: ______________

Percentage of hair-plucking or hair-pulling episodes I feel worse after: ______________

CHAPTER 16

WEIGHT, SHAPE, AND MUSCULARITY

DOES YOUR PATIENT NEED THIS MODULE?

Use this optional module if your patient reports (1) excessive concerns about body weight, and/or about body parts that the patient describes as too fat but that are actually normal-looking; or (2) excessive concern that his body is too thin, too small, or not muscular enough (i.e., muscle dysmorphia). Most patients in the latter group will be men.

You can use the following criteria to determine whether this section is needed: (1) an elevated score on the BDD-SS (≥5 for the weight/shape/muscularity questions); (2) the patient's input regarding weight/shape/muscularity concerns and related symptoms he considers problematic; and (3) your clinical judgment that the module is relevant. If any of these criteria are met, this should prompt discussion of whether this module should be used with the patient.

The *BDD Information Gathering Form* (Form 4.4), as well as the BDD-SS (Form 4.3), will help you determine whether a patient meets the criteria listed above. In addition, the following questions may be useful:

"Have you been upset about your weight or your body shape?"
"Have you felt ashamed or embarrassed about your weight, your shape, or your body build?"
"Do you think you look too big, overweight, or fat?"
"Have you been upset by thoughts that you aren't muscular or big enough?"
"Have your concerns about your weight or shape caused problems for you socially or with work, school, or other activities?"

You should also ask the patient about excessive, compulsive behaviors such as the following:

- Exercising more than 1 hour a day more than six times per week, continuing to exercise even when injured, or missing important activities in order to exercise.
- Repetitive and excessive weight lifting.
- Dieting or using diet pills or stimulants to lose weight.
- Using anabolic steroids or other substances to gain muscle mass.

- Eating a special diet (e.g., a high-protein, low-fat diet) or using nutritional supplements (e.g., creatine, amino acids, protein powders) to boost muscularity.
- Attempting to hide his body from others (e.g., by avoiding locker rooms, avoiding wearing a swimsuit, wearing baggy or oversized clothes), or to make his body look larger with layers of clothes.

If your patient is actually overweight, you will need to use your judgment about whether this module is appropriate. It may be helpful if the patient is only slightly overweight but overestimates how overweight he is. We recommend not using this module if a patient is significantly overweight, as the recommended exposures could provoke unpleasant scrutiny or ridicule. If patients who are actually obese want to lose weight, we suggest referring them to a weight loss program.

Session Structure

The standard agenda outlined in earlier chapters for all CBT-BDD sessions should be followed.

SESSION SUMMARY

☐ Check mood and BDD symptoms.
☐ Briefly review the previous session.
☐ Set the agenda jointly with the patient.
☐ Review homework.
☐ Work on the agenda.
  ☐ Gather information about preoccupation with weight, shape, or muscularity.
  ☐ Provide psychoeducation.
  ☐ Engage the patient in cognitive restructuring focused on weight/shape/muscularity.
  ☐ Help the patient begin exposure and response prevention focused on weight/shape/muscularity.
☐ Assign homework.
☐ Ask for summary of/feedback on the session.

SESSION FORMS AND HANDOUTS

BDI-II (or other depression inventory)
Personal Session Form (Form 2.1)
Therapist Session Form (Form 6.1)
Information about Body Shape and Weight Concerns (Handout 16.1)
Information about Muscle Dysmorphia (Handout 16.2)
Information about Anabolic Steroid Use (Handout 16.3)
Information about Other Body-Shaping Substances (Handout 16.4)
Examples of Cognitive Errors Associated with Weight, Shape, and Muscularity Concerns (Handout 16.5)
Completed *Your Personal BDD Model* (Form 7.1)

Thought Record (plus several extra copies for homework) (Form 9.1)
Ritual-Monitoring Form (Form 11.1)
Ritual Hierarchy List (Form 11.2)
Exposure and Response Prevention Worksheet (plus several extra copies for homework) (Form 11.3)

INTRODUCTION TO THIS SESSION

This module has the following goals:

- To help the patient feel comfortable with a healthy and realistic body weight and/or shape, rather than trying to achieve an excessively thin or muscular body.
- To increase the patient's awareness of the factors that influence the desire to change body shape and weight, and to recognize that body shape and weight are not completely under personal control.
- To help the patient identify cognitive distortions, beliefs, and assumptions that trigger and maintain avoidance, as well as compulsive behaviors designed to alter body shape and weight.
- To help the patient decrease avoidance and compulsive behaviors related to body shape and weight, and develop healthier shape/weight-related behaviors.

One to two sessions usually suffice, but more sessions may be needed for severe symptoms. (Most of the treatment described in this chapter focuses on muscle dysmorphia and is designed for patients for whom this is the main concern.) Material from this module can also be woven into other sessions. For example, exposure to wearing more appropriately sized clothing or fewer layers of clothes, and response prevention aimed at rituals like excessive exercise or weight lifting, will probably need to be continued over a number of sessions. Future assignments may include using copies of the *Thought Record* (Form 9.1) to assess and modify beliefs about body weight/shape and related rituals—for example, "If I miss one workout, my thighs will turn to Jell-O."

The general therapy approach for this module is shown in Figure 16.1.

- Establish that weight and shape concerns are actually due to BDD and not to an eating disorder. When an eating disorder is the patient's main problem, use a treatment developed for that disorder.
- Acknowledge that not all exercise is bad. In fact, moderate exercise (approximately 30 minutes daily) can improve mood, energy, and physical health. Encourage healthy physical activity.
- Identify avoidance behaviors, such as hiding body parts because of weight and shape concerns.
- Identify compulsive urges and behaviors, such as excessive exercise and other means to lose weight or increase muscle mass.
- Educate patients about the potential risks of using body-enhancing substances. Avoid scare tactics, and instead educate patients about the real dangers.
- Be patient. Many patients believe that they can alter their appearance if only they work hard enough through diet and exercise, but in fact what needs to change is on the inside, not the outside.

FIGURE 16.1. General approach for weight, shape, and muscularity concerns.

Check Mood and BDD Symptoms

Check the BDI-II (or other depression inventory) the patient has completed in the waiting room, and check the score on the suicidality item as usual, responding as appropriate. Briefly explore the patient's general mood, and discuss BDD symptoms since the last session. Hand out the *Personal Session Form* (Form 2.1), so that the patient can record information he finds significant during the session.

Briefly Review the Previous Session

Briefly check in with the patient regarding his perception and understanding of the previous session.

Set the Agenda Jointly with the Patient

Convey the topics you'd like to cover during the session, and ask the patient whether there are any items he would like to include in the agenda.

Review Homework

Discuss your patient's homework from the previous session.

Work on the Agenda

Gather Information about Preoccupation with Weight, Shape, or Muscularity

Distinguish BDD from an Eating Disorder

Ask your patient to further describe his concerns with being too fat or weighing too much. It's a challenge at times to distinguish weight and shape concerns attributable to BDD from those of an eating disorder, such as bulimia nervosa or anorexia nervosa (Grant & Phillips, 2004; Phillips, 1996). According to DSM-IV-TR (American Psychiatric Association, 2000), BDD should not be diagnosed if the symptoms are better accounted for by another disorder, such as an eating disorder. For example, if a patient's only body image concern is about being too fat, and the patient meets full criteria for anorexia nervosa, BDD would not be diagnosed. However, if a patient is obsessed with body weight/shape (e.g., a protruding stomach) but does not meet criteria for an eating disorder, BDD would be the more appropriate diagnosis. Furthermore, many patients meet criteria for both disorders. In fact, approximately 15% of patients with BDD also have lifetime anorexia nervosa or bulimia nervosa. One study found that among women hospitalized for anorexia nervosa, 39% also had BDD (Grant, Kim, & Eckert, 2002).

Identify Muscle Dysmorphia

If you suspect that a patient may have muscle dysmorphia, listen for comments about feeling "small" or "not muscular enough." Behaviors include mirror checking, reassurance seeking about body size, and attempts to camouflage a "small" body the patient feels embarrassed about. Ask also about the length of workouts and weight-lifting sessions, and whether the patient follows a regimented diet aimed at gaining muscle and losing fat. Find out as well whether personal and professional relationships suffer because your patient is consumed with working out.

For example, Steve was a muscular 30-year-old male who was convinced that he looked "tiny" and weak. He obsessed about his "puniness" for hours a day. To try to bulk up, he ate 10 meals a day, including 10 protein bars and several high-protein shakes. He avoided eating fat. He worked out for 3–4 hours a day. Although his trainer said he was working out too much and was at risk of injuring himself, Steve felt that he couldn't stop. To become more muscular, he had tried anabolic steroids, which he'd obtained illegally. However, he was no longer using them because they made him irritable and aggressive, and his girlfriend had threatened to leave him if he didn't stop. Nonetheless, he still took various supplements (e.g., creatine, DHEA) in the hope of becoming bigger. As a result of his muscularity concerns, Steve often avoided social events and sometimes missed work because he was too embarrassed to have others see him. He also frequently checked mirrors and wore several layers of clothes, even on hot summer days, in an attempt to look bigger.

Gather Information about Abuse of Steroids and Use of Other Substances

You should ask patients who feel they are too small or not muscular enough whether they have ever used—or are currently using or are thinking about using—substances to get bigger or more muscular. About 20% of men with muscle dysmorphia have abused or become dependent on dangerous anabolic steroids in an attempt to increase their muscularity. Such patients may be reluctant to disclose this, because they don't want to stop using the drugs and because they are usually obtained illegally. If a patient does not disclose steroid use, you might suspect this if the person is overly muscular, especially in the upper torso. It's virtually impossible to obtain a supermuscular look with ordinary weight lifting and dietary supplements alone. Additional clues to steroid use, including illustrative photographs, are included in *The Adonis Complex* (Pope, Phillips, & Olivardia, 2000).

Provide Psychoeducation

Psychoeducation is an important tool for combating distorted beliefs about body shape and weight. Below we recommend handouts and suggest educational information you can discuss with your patient.

Provide Informational Materials

Provide your patient with one or more of the following informational handouts pertinent to his symptoms:

- *Information about Body Shape and Weight Concerns* (Handout 16.1)
- *Information about Muscle Dysmorphia* (Handout 16.2)
- *Information about Anabolic Steroid Use* (Handout 16.3)
- *Information about Other Body-Shaping Drugs* (Handout 16.4)

Ask the patient for his thoughts about the information, and discuss any issues or questions the handouts raise. If the patient has used compulsive exercise, dieting, or substances to change weight, shape, or muscularity, discuss this experience and how similar or different it was from how most people he knows relate to food and physical activity.

Discuss How the Media Distort Body Images

Images of Women

If your patient is a woman, discuss the media's distorted view of the ideal female body shape. Print ads, television, billboards, the Internet, and movies constantly barrage women with the message that if they can become thin enough, they will finally be happy. As we have noted in Chapter 7, the ideal female form epitomized by cultural icons such as fashion models, celebrities, and beauty pageant contestants has become increasingly slim over the last several decades. The thin female ideal promoted by Hollywood, magazines, and children's toys (e.g., the Barbie doll) is virtually impossible to achieve.

You can point out that it isn't surprising that comparing one's own figure to these images feeds BDD symptoms and usually makes women feel worse about how they look. Moreover, our culture often depicts thinness as going hand in hand with beauty, and this union is equated with happiness and success. Unfortunately, many women have gotten the media's take-home message: "To be successful and loved, you must be thin." Tell your patient that research studies have found that most men actually prefer a more ordinary-looking female body to a super-thin one.

Discuss with your patient that many people (both women and men) internalize unrealistic media messages, find a discrepancy between the way they look and the way they think they "should" look, and judge themselves negatively as a result. Ask your patient if they think they might do this. Also discuss that it is easy to ignore other positive traits. Moreover, the ideal is unattainable for most people. Models in magazines are airbrushed and made slimmer than they really are. It isn't realistic for women to try to look like them.

Images of Men

If you are working with a male patient, discuss the unrealistic media messages that men receive, just as women do. These messages tell them that the bigger and more muscular they are, the better. Print ads, television, billboards, the Internet, and movies increasingly barrage men with the message that if they can get muscular enough, they'll finally be happy. Men who internalize these unrealistic media messages focus on the difference between their appearance and how they think they "should" look, and judge themselves negatively as a result. Unfortunately, in so doing, they can easily ignore their positive traits. Discuss with your patient whether he thinks this might be true for him.

One problem with this message is that most women actually prefer a more ordinary male body, rather than a supermuscular one. Surprisingly, the body that men *think* women like is typically about 15–20 pounds more muscular than what women *actually* like (Pope et al., 2000). In addition, remind your patient that many of the supermuscular men in magazines and advertisements for supplements actually owe their muscularity to anabolic steroids. Most men cannot put on that much muscle mass simply by working out; it isn't physiologically possible. Also, each man is genetically programmed to attain a certain body size. The regular use of anabolic steroids carries many risks, both physical and legal (since these drugs are often illegally obtained), and excessive working out can cause damage to joints, tendons, and muscles.

Discuss Diet and Exercise

Help the patient understand the problems caused by restrictive dietary regimens and exercise plans. Rigid patterns of exercise and diets are extremely difficult to maintain in the long run. This behavior often begins with thinking about food or exercise in extremes—for example, viewing some foods as "forbidden" (e.g., carbs, cookies, ice cream) and others as "safe" (e.g., salads, carrots, proteins). This way of thinking sets people up for failure because a highly restricted diet cannot be maintained forever. So the weight initially lost on a restrictive diet inevitably returns after a person stops the diet. Also, for some people, considering certain foods as "forbidden" just increases craving. It's important to help the patient acknowledge that some biological and hereditary factors that play a role in weight and shape are not under individual control.

Acknowledge the benefits of moderate physical activity, but also inform the patient of problems caused by excessive physical activity. Moderate physical activity (about 30 minutes daily, four to five times a week) has many physical and psychological benefits, including lower blood pressure and cholesterol; reduced risk of stroke, heart disease, diabetes, and osteoporosis; and reduced stress, depression, and anxiety. Too much exercise, however, can be problematic. Overexercise puts strain on the body and leaves people at risk for infections and other ailments. Excessive weight lifting, in particular, can damage muscles and joints. Compulsive exercise can also interfere with other aspects of life, taking time away from healthy engagement with family, friends, work, and other leisure activities. Discuss strategies that will promote long-term health, and emphasize *moderate* amounts of activity, since the perfectionism of many patients with BDD may make it difficult for them to accept moderation as a goal.

Engage the Patient in Cognitive Restructuring Focused on Weight/Shape/Muscularity

Cognitive restructuring for this module is similar to that described in Chapters 9 and 13, except that you will explicitly focus on beliefs about body shape, fat, and muscularity. The goals of cognitive restructuring are to help a patient (1) develop more accurate and helpful beliefs about body size and shape; and (2) identify the negative automatic thoughts, beliefs, and assumptions underlying the behaviors related to altering body shape and weight.

Have the patient complete a *Thought Record* (Form 9.1) that focuses on thoughts and beliefs about weight or body shape. Giving the patient *Examples of Cognitive Errors Associated with Weight, Shape, and Muscularity Concerns* (Handout 16.5) may be helpful, especially if the patient has trouble identifying cognitive errors. Ask the patient to rate his degree of conviction (0–100) and to examine the evidence for and against his thinking. Be sure to question the quality of evidence that supports the beliefs.

For example, one patient's negative automatic thought was "If I eat a donut, my stomach will stick out and I'll look terrible." The therapist's questioning laid the groundwork for the patient to begin cognitive restructuring:

THERAPIST: How much do you believe that your stomach will stick out and you'll look terrible if you eat that donut?

PATIENT: Completely.

THERAPIST: Completely? Is that 100% certainty, or is it less than that?

PATIENT: Maybe 90%. I'm not 100% certain.

Figure 16.2 provides an example of a completed *Thought Record* for this particular thought.

You can also use more advanced cognitive strategies to work on related underlying assumptions/rules or core beliefs. For example, some men with muscle dysmorphia are very concerned about not being "manly" or "masculine" enough. It's important to ask about this; the downward arrow technique is often useful in identifying underlying beliefs, which can then be addressed through cognitive restructuring or some of the advanced techniques described in Chapter 13. For example, the patient might try taking another perspective by considering what he would say to a son (or imagined son) of his who said he didn't want to go to school because he was "too puny" and "not masculine enough." The patient might also draw a self-esteem pie, with "manliness" and appearance concerns put in last. You could also engage in a discussion about the definition of masculinity. Is it really based just on muscles, or is it based on other traits, like being a loyal friend, making clear decisions, tolerating discomfort, or persevering at an activity? Even so-called "feminine" traits can be considered masculine—for example, being considerate, thoughtful, and helpful to others.

Date/time: Tuesday, 9:00 A.M.
Situation: I'm at the office and Jan has brought in a box of donuts.
Thoughts: If I eat a donut, my stomach will stick out and I'll look terrible.
Believability of thoughts (0–100):
Cognitive errors: All-or-nothing thinking, fortune telling, labeling, emotional reasoning
Feelings and intensity (0–100): Anxious (55), angry (40)
Questions: What's the evidence for my thought? What's the evidence against it? Which is more convincing? Am I really 100% certain that . . . or is this just one out of many possibilities? What's the worst that could happen if my fears came true? Could I live through it? What would I tell a friend in this situation?
Rational Response: One donut won't make my stomach stick out. Rationally, this wouldn't be possible. A donut isn't that big. I'm using emotional reasoning; just because I may *feel* it sticks out and looks terrible doesn't mean that this is really true. I'd tell a friend not to freak out over one donut. One donut isn't an entire box.
Believability of rational response (0–100): 80
Feelings: Anxious (35), angry (20)

FIGURE 16.2. Sample completed *Thought Record* for a weight/shape-related thought.

Help the Patient Begin Exposure and Response Prevention Focused on Weight/Shape/Muscularity

The goal of response prevention as used in this module is gradually to reduce and eventually to eliminate repetitive behaviors related to weight, fat, or muscularity concerns. Consistent with the strategies described in Chapters 10 and 11, use exposure to decrease avoidance (of healthy behaviors, social situations, work or school, etc.), and use response prevention to stop compulsive behaviors. You will want to target all avoidance and all typical BDD behaviors (such as mirror checking, comparing, and clothes changing) that are related to weight, shape, or muscularity concerns. Additional behaviors that require response prevention may include frequent weighing and body measuring, wearing clothes that are too small or too large, wearing many layers of clothes to look bigger, eating a restricted diet, adhering to a rigid or excessive exercise regimen, and using substances to lose fat and/or gain muscle. The dialogue that follows illustrates the introduction of these methods:

THERAPIST: We're now going to turn to exposure and response prevention and apply some of the skills you've already learned to address your worries about your body size. Let's look back at *Your Personal BDD Model* [completed Form 7.1] and review which types of avoidance and rituals are related to your weight and shape concerns.

PATIENT: (*Looks at Form 7.1.*) Well, I exercise a few hours a day, and I never eat certain foods like chocolate. I also wear big, baggy clothes to cover myself up so I don't look so fat. And sometimes I don't eat out with friends, because I'm afraid I'll eat fattening restaurant food and gain lots of weight.

THERAPIST: So let's take a few minutes to think about the consequences of these behaviors. Do they cause any problems for you?

If your patient has trouble identifying disadvantages associated with the avoidance or the compulsive behaviors, you could ask him to write down both the pros and cons on a piece of paper. Make one column for the pros, and another column for the cons, as in the *Pros and Cons Worksheets* in Chapter 15 (Forms 15.1–15.2). This may be necessary with potentially ego-syntonic behaviors such as excessive exercise. Without appearing too biased, help your patient think through some of the problematic aspects of his avoidance and rituals, such as not seeing friends, spending too much time on rituals, physical injury, or bingeing on forbidden foods as a result of excessive restraint. As illustrated by the completed copy of *Your Personal BDD Model*, these behaviors feed the BDD symptoms. You can say to the patient:

"So what's your sense of how frequently you do these behaviors and how distressed they make you? It helps to know this as we plan an exposure and response prevention exercise that focuses on these behaviors."

If it seems helpful, ask your patient to fill out the *Ritual-Monitoring Form* (Form 11.1) and the *Ritual Hierarchy List* (Form 11.2), to get a better sense of the frequency and triggers of these behaviors. Thereafter, use of the *Exposure and Response Prevention Worksheet* (Form 11.3) can help incorporate cognitive restructuring, exposure, and ritual prevention. Figures 16.3 and 16.4 present Sarah's and Mike's completed worksheets.

FILL OUT THIS PART *BEFORE* THE EXPOSURE/RESPONSE PREVENTION

My Exposure and/or Response Prevention situation (Be specific):
Going out to dinner this week with Susan and John and eating in a restaurant.

What aspect of the situation causes me the most distress?
Seeing fattening foods on the menu.
Being with people—they might think my face and thighs look fat.

What subtle ways of avoiding do I need to watch out for?
Wearing my really baggy pants.
Turning my face away from people.

Preparing My Thoughts

Negative thoughts/predictions
Everyone will be thinking that my thighs and my face are really fat.
If I don't work out for 2 hours before dinner, it will be a disaster.

Alternative thoughts
I can't read people's minds. They'll probably be focusing on enjoying their meal and the company.
A healthy amount of exercise will be enough.

Goals for the Exposure/Response Prevention (How will I know I did well?)
1. *Order a normal meal, including a healthy dessert.*
2. *Work out just a normal amount before dinner (under 1 hour).*
3. *Be sure I go to dinner—don't cancel at the last minute or make an excuse and leave early.*
4. *Wear my jeans, not my really baggy pants.*
5. *Face people and look at them directly when I talk with them.*

FILL OUT THIS PART *AFTER* THE EXPOSURE/RESPONSE PREVENTION

Distress Rating: Beginning *80* **Half-time** *60* **Ending** *40*

Evaluating My Efforts

Did I reach my goal?
Yes!

Did my negative thoughts/predictions come true?
No—the evening went fine and I ate a healthy dinner. No one seemed to focus on how I looked. They seemed to enjoy my company.

What did I learn?
That a normal amount of exercise and eating a healthy meal with my friends is OK. My face and thighs didn't get fatter from one meal.

How will I reward myself?
Buy a new book.

Adapted with permission of the publisher from Wilhelm, S. (2006). *Feeling Good about the Way You Look: A Program for Overcoming Body Image Problems*. New York: Guilford Press.

FIGURE 16.3. Sarah's sample completed *Exposure and Response Prevention Worksheet.*

FILL OUT THIS PART *BEFORE* THE EXPOSURE/RESPONSE PREVENTION

My Exposure and/or Response Prevention Situation (Be Specific):
Seeing people at work in our weekly meeting.

What aspect of the situation causes me the most distress?
Everyone's going to think I look puny and tiny. They'll think I'm shrinking and letting myself go.

What subtle ways of avoiding do I need to watch out for?
Wearing three T-shirts plus a sweater and my big plaid shirt.
Being quiet at the meeting (not speaking up) and sitting in the back of the room so no one will see me.

Preparing My Thoughts
Negative thoughts/predictions
Everyone will think I look tiny.
They'll laugh at me.

Alternative thoughts
I can't read people's minds.
They will probably be focusing on the meeting.
The meeting isn't about my muscles; it's about the project.
They might want my input on the project. I have some good ideas.

Goals for the Exposure/Response Prevention (How will I know I did well?)
1. *Sit at the conference table with everyone else.*
2. *Go to the meeting without wearing my big plaid shirt.*
3. *Speak up at least once—tell them my ideas about the marketing plan.*

FILL OUT THIS PART *AFTER* THE EXPOSURE/RESPONSE PREVENTION

Distress Rating: Beginning *70* **Half-time** *60* **Ending** *50*

Evaluating My Efforts

Did I reach my goal?
Yes!

Did my negative thoughts/predictions come true?
No—they liked my marketing plan ideas. I didn't see anyone laugh at me.

What did I learn?
That I can participate at meetings without wearing so many layers, and that people want to hear my ideas.

How will I reward myself?
Call my friend Lisa.

FIGURE 16.4. Mike's sample completed *Exposure and Response Prevention Worksheet.*

The sections below discuss some examples of ritualistic behaviors that can be the targets of response prevention exercises.

Frequent Weighing and Body Measuring

Ask how often the patient checks his weight. More than once a week (unless advised by a doctor) is excessive. Educate the patient about normal fluctuations in weight over the course of a day or week. Body weight is affected by many factors, including time of day, salt intake, menstrual cycle (for women), fluid intake, and clothing. Instruct the patient how to use weight and body measurements in a healthy way—by weighing himself not more than once a week and at the same time of day, with the same clothes, and on the same scale. Help a patient who is weighing himself several times a day to identify strategies to gradually reduce this frequency (e.g., removing the scale from sight, scheduling a specific time per week when body measurements can be taken). A good goal is gradual reduction to weighing and measuring only once a month. If the patient is using special tape measures or other measuring devices, encourage the use of stimulus control to minimize access to these things.

Wearing Clothes That Are Too Small

Women with weight and shape concerns may insist on wearing clothes that are a size or two smaller than they need. This behavior maintains the belief that they are overweight, even if they aren't (e.g., "See, I told you my stomach was too fat; it's hanging over the side of my pants"). These patients may also believe that someday they'll fit into a smaller size, even if this belief is unrealistic for their body types. Help such patients see that the size of their clothes does not determine who they are. Encourage them to find clothes that are fun or vibrant, or make them feel comfortable. Wearing clothes that showcase positive aspects of their appearance (e.g., hair and skin color, height) will help them feel more positive about their shape and will be more comfortable to wear.

Wearing Clothes That Are Too Large or Baggy

Alternatively, some patients who believe they are too fat—or too small, in the case of those with muscle dysmorphia—wear oversize clothing to camouflage body parts or give the illusion of being more muscular. Some men wear multiple layers of clothes (e.g., six T-shirts plus a sweater and a big lumberjack shirt) to try to look bigger. Again, help the patient wear clothes that fit instead of hiding perceived flaws. You can start by having him wear clothes that are the next size smaller, or by removing one layer of clothes, gradually working toward the patient's actual clothing size. If he has trouble doing this, identify the patient's beliefs about wearing appropriately sized clothes, look for flaws in this logic, and use other cognitive strategies to develop more accurate beliefs.

Dietary Restrictions

Adhering rigidly to a dietary plan only maintains erroneous beliefs about food. Encourage your patient to eat a well-balanced diet that includes all food groups. Gradually have the patient introduce "forbidden" foods in reasonable quantities into the dietary plan.

Rigid and Excessive Exercise Regimen

Try to find ways to increase flexibility in your patient's exercise regimen. Encourage alternative forms of less strenuous activity (such as yoga, stretching, or tai chi) if the patient is engaging in too much strenuous activity. Instead of going to the gym, add variation to the exercise routine, have the patient put on a favorite CD or iPod selection and dance in the kitchen, or play basketball with the kids. Try to help the patient recall a time when physical movement was simply fun, not a means of improving his appearance in some way. Have the patient try to bring joy back into physical activity.

If your patient appears to be damaging his body through excessive exercise, plan a new workout schedule to reduce overtraining and gradually reduce the amount of time spent in excessive exercise. As with other excessive behaviors, this may have to be done in a gradual, systematic way, as the patient may find it too anxiety-provoking to skip an entire day of exercise. For example, if a patient is working out several hours each day, help him first reduce the amount of time per day that he works out. During the newly freed time when the patient used to work out, have him plan some special self-care activity (e.g., massage, hot bath, or nonstrenuous activity such as yoga). As always, it is important to replace rituals with healthy and productive or enjoyable behaviors.

Comparison Rituals

As discussed in Chapter 11, patients with BDD compare their appearance to that of just about everyone—celebrities, strangers, friends, and family members. Help patients reduce time spent reading fashion and beauty magazines or muscle and fitness magazines, as the bodies presented in these publications are not typical of ordinary people, including very attractive ones. Comparisons a patient makes with these figures inevitably maintain negative thoughts about the patient's own shape and weight.

In addition, help patients see what is attractive in body types that are similar to their own, instead of focusing on people whose body type is different. Help a patient identify realistic goals for his own body by discussing what he has looked like over the course of his life and the appearance of family members. Reviewing the body shapes and weight of family members is often a useful exercise that enables the patient to see the lineage of family figures and clarify realistic expectations. To help the patient gradually cut down on comparing himself to others he considers more attractive, suggest the following:

- Spending less time watching TV shows or reading magazines that focus on unrealistic body images.
- Spend less time at the newsstand or in the library looking at magazines, and less time looking at unrealistic images online.
- Canceling subscriptions to such magazines.
- Spending more time watching TV shows or reading magazines that do not exalt beauty/muscularity or display unrealistic standards.

In addition, as described in Chapter 11, encourage patients to try to see the "big picture." Ask them to focus on other things in their environment, rather than the body parts of other people.

Use of Steroids, Diet Pills, and Others Substances

Help your patients eliminate the use of anabolic steroids, diet pills, or other substances intended for fat reduction/muscle enhancement. Ask whether your patient has been using high doses of anabolic steroids for long periods. If so, the patient may need to be carefully monitored, as withdrawal symptoms can occur (see Handouts 16.3 and 16.4).

ASSIGN HOMEWORK

- Assign appropriate readings from the handouts included in this module.
- Have the patient complete several copies of the *Thought Record* (Form 9.1).
- Assign exposure and response prevention exercises focusing on weight, shape, or muscularity preoccupations and associated rituals and avoidance behaviors.

ASK FOR SUMMARY OF/FEEDBACK ON THE SESSION

Ask the patient to briefly summarize the major points covered during the session. Also ask whether he had any concerns about the session or your behavior, and respond appropriately.

HANDOUT 16.1

Information about Body Shape and Weight Concerns

BDD and Excessive Worry about Weight and/or Shape

About 20–25% of people with BDD are excessively concerned with their weight or body shape. Women usually worry that they're too fat. Often they focus on the size of their hips, thighs, or buttocks. Usually they're also concerned about other body areas as well (e.g., their skin or hair).

How do you distinguish BDD from an eating disorder? BDD should not be diagnosed if the body image concerns are better accounted for by another disorder, such as bulimia nervosa or anorexia nervosa. For example, if a person's only body image concern is being "too fat," and the person has all of the features of anorexia nervosa, anorexia nervosa rather than BDD would be diagnosed. However, body image concerns in the absence of an eating disorder often signal the presence of BDD. Furthermore, many patients have both BDD *and* an eating disorder.

The Incredible Shrinking Woman

The ideal female form that's epitomized by cultural icons—fashion models, celebrities, and beauty pageant contestants—has become increasingly slimmer and less curvaceous over the last several decades. The thin female ideal we see in movies, magazines, and children's toys is virtually impossible to achieve. If the Barbie doll were as tall as a real woman, she'd have only a 14-inch waist!

Not surprisingly, many people with BDD compare their own figures to these unrealistic images. This compulsive comparing makes BDD symptoms worse and usually makes people feel worse about how they look. Moreover, our culture often portrays thinness and beauty as going hand in hand, and this union is equated with happiness, acceptance, and success. Unfortunately, many women have gotten this take-home message: "To be successful and loved, you must be thin."

(cont.)

Excessive Exercise, Dieting, and Use of Diet Pills

To become slimmer or bulk up, many people with BDD engage in the following behaviors:

- 19–24% have excessively exercised.
- 5–18% have excessively lifted weights.
- 30–37% have dieted.

There are many physical and psychological benefits to moderate physical activity. Exercising for approximately 30 minutes 5 days a week can lower blood pressure and cholesterol and can reduce the risk of stroke, heart disease, diabetes, and osteoporosis. In addition, moderate activity can reduce stress, mild to moderate depression, and anxiety. Too much exercise, however, can be problematic—and even worse than none at all. Overexercise can put more strain on the body and create a risk of infections and other ailments. Excessive weight lifting, in particular, can damage muscles and joints. Having a need to exercise compulsively can also interfere with the rest of life—for example, it can take time away from family, friends, work, and other activities. As with most behavior, the key is moderation!

What *Really* Is Attractive?

Both men and women err in estimating what the opposite sex would find attractive. Women underestimate the female body size that men tend to prefer. Men actually prefer a female body that's heavier than the body women think men like. Alternatively, men think women like a heavier and more muscular body than the body women actually like!

HANDOUT 16.2

Information about Muscle Dysmorphia

What Is Muscle Dysmorphia?

Muscle dysmorphia is a form of BDD that afflicts mostly men. About 10% of men with BDD have muscle dysmorphia, which consists of a distressing or impairing preoccupation with the idea that one's body isn't sufficiently lean and muscular. As detailed in the book *The Adonis Complex: The Secret Crisis of Male Body Obsession*, by H. G. Pope and colleagues, this increase in muscle dysmorphia parallels the media's increasing focus on the male body, and the increasing discontent with appearance among men in the general population.

In addition to obsessing about their perceived "smallness," men with muscle dysmorphia engage in many BDD behaviors, such as mirror checking, camouflaging their bodies because they're embarrassed to be seen, and seeking reassurance from other people that they look OK. In addition, most men with this form of BDD work out excessively and lift weights, and many have very regimented diets. Typically, they're so consumed with working out that their personal and professional relationships suffer.

What *Really* Is Attractive?

According to *The Adonis Complex*, the body that men *think* women like is typically about 15–20 pounds more muscular than what women *actually* like! Women actually prefer a more ordinary male body to a supermuscular body.

Excessive Exercise, Dieting, and Use of Diet Pills

To become slimmer or bulk up, many men with muscle dysmorphia engage in the following behaviors:

- About two-thirds have exercised excessively.
- Nearly three-quarters have excessively lifted weights.
- Nearly three-quarters have dieted.

(cont.)

There are many physical and psychological benefits to moderate physical activity. Exercising for approximately 30 minutes 5 days a week can lower blood pressure and cholesterol and can reduce the risk of stroke, heart disease, diabetes, and osteoporosis. In addition, moderate activity can reduce stress, mild to moderate depression, and anxiety. Too much exercise, however, can be problematic—and even worse than none at all. Overexercise can put more strain on the body and create a risk of infections and other ailments. Excessive weight lifting, in particular, can damage muscles and joints. A need to exercise compulsively can also interfere with the rest of life—for example, it can take time away from family, friends, work, and other activities. As with most behavior, the key is moderation!

The Dangers of Anabolic Steroid Abuse

Some men with muscle dysmorphia use anabolic steroids to build muscle. Unfortunately, many are unaware of the physical and psychological damage that steroids can cause. (See separate informational handout on steroids.)

Some men use other drugs and substances in an attempt to build muscle or lose fat. The dangers of these substances are less well established; nonetheless, they have some potential risks. (See separate informational handout on these other substances.)

HANDOUT 16.3

Information about Anabolic Steroid Use

Possible Increased Risk for Medical Problems

- Heart disease
- Increase in LDL, or "bad" cholesterol
- Decrease in HDL, or "good" cholesterol
- Stroke
- Prostate cancer
- Liver disease or cancer
- Increase in breast tissue under nipples (gynecomastia)
- Acne
- Shrinking testicles
- HIV/AIDS, hepatitis B and C, abscesses, infections (as results of needle use)

Note: The long-term use of high-dose steroids could potentially take *10 or 20 years* off your life expectancy.

Greater Danger of Psychiatric Hazards

- Irritability
- Aggression
- Depression
- Dependence; possible gateway to other injectable drugs
- Impaired judgment
- Mania and delusions (e.g., paranoia)

Withdrawal Syndrome on Stopping Use

- Depression
- Lethargy
- Decreased appetite
- Suicide

Note. We are referring to the type of steroids that are used for building muscle, not the type of steroids that are used to treat a variety of medical illnesses, such as allergies and certain auto immune diseases.

HANDOUT 16.4

Information about Other Body-Shaping Substances

Additional Potentially Dangerous Body-Shaping Drugs

- **Stimulants** (e.g., theophylline, over-the-counter cold preparations, ephedrine or ma huang; taken to burn fat)
  - Can increase blood pressure and cause palpitations and seizures.
  - Ephedrine or ma huang has caused death and can be habit-forming.
- **Clenbuterol** (used mostly by vets; burns fat and builds muscle)
  - Can cause potentially fatal heart problems.
- **Diuretics** (water pills; make body look sharper and more defined)
  - Occasionally cause sudden death due to heart problems.
- **Anticatabolics** (supposed to decrease muscle breakdown)
- **Narcotic agonist–antagonists** (e.g., buprenorphine, nalbuphene)
  - Can be habit-forming.
- **Testosterone stimulants** (e.g., human chorionic gonadotropin)
  - May elevate risk of prostate cancer.
- **Adrenal hormones** (DHEA, androstenedione, androstenedione derivatives; these hormones are chemically related to testosterone and are partially metabolized into testosterone to a limited degree)
  - May have little value for muscle gain.
  - May increase cholesterol and promote large breasts.
  - Dangers of long-term use at high doses are unknown.
- **Other hormones or neurochemicals** (e.g., insulin, thyroid hormone, human growth hormone, gamma hydroxybutyrate, levodopa)
  - Can be dangerous.

Most Common Supplements

- **Protein supplements** (powders and bars)
  - Little evidence exists that these are superior to ordinary food.
  - Long-term use of very high doses of protein may cause kidney damage.
- **Creatine** (a natural substance in foods like beef)
  - May increase lean body mass by a few pounds, but some of this gain may be water.
  - Dangers of long-term use at high doses are unknown.

Note. Some of these are prescription medications, which are usually safe when taken as prescribed.

HANDOUT 16.5

Examples of Cognitive Errors Associated with Weight, Shape, and Muscularity Concerns

1. **Discounting the positives:** Ignoring the positive aspects and only focusing on the negative aspects of weight, shape, and muscularity.

   Example: "I don't care how pretty my face is. I hate my flabby thighs; these fat thighs have to go!"

   Example: "My nice personality doesn't count. My calf muscles are so puny, it's amazing I can walk around!"

2. **All-or-nothing thinking:** Viewing situations as all or nothing, black or white, without seeing shades of gray.

   Example: "I can't ever eat more than 10% of my diet from carbs, because my face will get fat."

   Example: "I have to exercise 90 minutes morning and in the evening; otherwise I'll turn to mush."

3. **"Should" statements:** Having overly rigid rules about the way things "should be."

   Example: "I can't get rid of any of my clothes from high school. I should be able to wear a size 2."

   Example: "For someone my height, I should weigh 125 pounds."

4. **Mind reading:** Making assumptions about what others think.

   Example: "I know that girls laugh at me because I'm too small and puny-looking."

   Example: "Ted didn't call me back after our date because he thought my stomach was too big."

5. **Emotional reasoning:** Reasoning based purely on feelings.

   Example: "I feel like I have the fattest thighs in the school, so I must have."

   Example: "I feel like I'm a toothpick, so it must be true."

6. **Unfair comparisons:** Comparing oneself to unrealistic or extreme standards.

   Example: "The guy on the cover of *GQ* has six-pack abs; I totally look like a fat slob compared to him."

   Example: "I have to look like ____________ [model, actor, athlete] to be popular."

CHAPTER 17

COSMETIC TREATMENT

DOES YOUR PATIENT NEED THIS MODULE?

This optional module is intended for patients who are currently receiving cosmetic treatment for BDD or are considering getting such treatment. "Cosmetic treatment" as we define it includes surgical, dermatological, dental, paraprofessional (e.g., electrolysis), or any other type of treatment intended solely to improve appearance. You can use the following criteria to determine whether this module is needed:

- A patient has an elevated score on the BDD-SS (≥5 for the questions about cosmetic treatment).
- The patient thinks about getting such treatment at least occasionally (e.g., one or two times a month).
- The patient has gathered information about a desired procedure or treatment (e.g., on the Internet, from books).
- The patient has already consulted with a provider (e.g., a surgeon) to discuss treatment options, or has scheduled a consultation or actual treatment.
- The patient is saving money to obtain cosmetic treatment.
- You, as your patient's clinician, feel that the module is relevant.

If any of the criteria above are met, this should prompt discussion of whether this module should be used with the patient.

SESSION STRUCTURE

The standard agenda outlined in earlier chapters for all CBT-BDD sessions should be followed.

SESSION SUMMARY

☐ Check mood and BDD symptoms.
☐ Briefly review the previous session.

☐ Set the agenda jointly with the patient.
☐ Review homework.
☐ Work on the agenda.
  ☐ Provide psychoeducation.
  ☐ Evaluate the pros and cons of cosmetic treatment.
  ☐ Engage the patient in cognitive restructuring focused on cosmetic treatment.
  ☐ Help the patient begin response focused on cosmetic treatment.
  ☐ Deal with current treatments or planned cosmetic procedures on a case-by-case basis.
  ☐ Counsel a patient who wants to get cosmetic treatment instead of CBT-BDD.
☐ Assign homework.
☐ Ask for summary of/feedback on the session.

SESSION FORMS AND HANDOUTS

BDI-II (or other depression inventory)
Personal Session Form (Form 2.1)
Therapist Session Form (Form 6.1)
Information about Cosmetic Treatment for BDD (Handout 17.1)
Pros and Cons Worksheet for Cosmetic Treatment (Form 17.1)
Completed *Your Personal BDD Model* (Form 7.1)
Thought Record (plus several extra copies) (Form 9.1)
Examples of Cognitive Errors Involving Cosmetic Treatment (Handout 17.2)

INTRODUCTION TO THIS SESSION

Goals

The goals of this module are to help your patient do the following:

- More rationally assess the potential pros and cons of cosmetic treatment, and understand that such treatment is unlikely to diminish her BDD concerns.
- Recognize that cosmetic treatment won't change her life or fix all of her problems.
- Understand the need to change what is on the inside (how she feels about herself), not on the outside (her appearance). In other words, the patient's body image, not her appearance, needs to change.
- Understand that there are far more effective treatments for BDD, and that it is better to defer or avoid cosmetic treatment.

One session should usually suffice for this module, but patients who are very intent on receiving cosmetic treatment in the near future may benefit from an additional session. Material from this session can also be woven into future core sessions as needed. For example, core sessions on cognitive strategies may include negative automatic thoughts pertaining to cosmetic treatments (e.g., "If I don't get surgery right away, I'll never find a boyfriend.").

Information on Cosmetic Treatment for BDD

Some of the information in this section can be incorporated into your discussion with the patient when you are reviewing the handout *Information about Cosmetic Treatment for BDD* (Handout 17.1).

First, about 75% of people with BDD seek cosmetic treatment for their BDD concerns, and about two-thirds actually receive it. Many health care providers refuse to provide such treatment for patients with BDD, because the patients look normal and/or because the providers detect BDD. However, most of those with BDD who seek such treatment eventually succeed in obtaining it. Some patients have surgery after surgery. These treatments can be a real financial strain, even depleting life savings and leading to bankruptcy. Occasional patients with BDD even attempt their own surgery, sometimes in concerning ways, as described in Chapter 1. Many other patients buy unproven potions (e.g., hair growth potions) obtained over the Internet. Take a look at Table 17.1, which shows the percentages of patients with BDD who receive various types of cosmetic treatments, and discuss relevant details with your patient.

Because ordinary people who do not have BDD often get these treatments as well, it becomes important to distinguish BDD-related concerns from those of patients for whom such cosmetic treatments don't present a problem. The main difference is that people with BDD seek surgery to correct imagined defects that do not exist, or have concerns about minimal flaws that are clearly excessive. They desperately want surgery or other cosmetic treatments to fix their negative image of themselves. Their distress is out of proportion with their perceived flaws. In contrast, "normal" seekers of cosmetic treatments do not meet diagnostic criteria for BDD, and typically they aim to repair more obvious flaws in their features or to enhance their appearance for various purposes (e.g., pursuing careers as public performers).

Second, cosmetic treatment usually appears to be ineffective for BDD, and it can even make BDD symptoms worse. Body image dissatisfaction motivates individuals to seek cosmetic surgery and other appearance enhancing procedures. In a general study of patients receiving

TABLE 17.1. Nonpsychiatric Treatment Received by Patients with BDD

Treatment type	% of patients with BDD who receive the treatment	Most common treatments
Dermatological	40–50%	• Topical acne agents • Oral acne agents (antibiotics) • Accutane (also known an isotretinoin; a medication for severe acne)
Surgical	20–25%	• Rhinoplasty (nose job) • Breast augmentation/lift
Dental	5–10%	• Tooth whitening • Braces • Oral surgery
Paraprofessional	10–15%	• Electrolysis • Facials/heat wraps

Note. Data from Crerand et al. (2005) and Phillips et al. (2001).

cosmetic surgery, 87% were satisfied a year later and reported improvements in both their overall body image and the body feature altered (Sarwer et al., 2005). However, though individuals who do not suffer from BDD may benefit from cosmetic surgery, patients with BDD who obtain cosmetic treatments are rarely satisfied (Veale, 2000). Of 450 patients with BDD who received a total of 1,313 nonpsychiatric treatments, only about 5% of all treatments diminished the patients' concern about the treated body parts *and* improved BDD symptoms overall (Crerand et al. 2005; Phillips, Grant, et al., 2001). In some cases, preoccupation with the treated body parts diminishes, but BDD does not improve overall, because the patients' concern shifts to another body area. In another study of 50 patients, 81% were dissatisfied or very dissatisfied with past medical consultation or surgery (Veale et al., 1996).

In our clinical experience, the outcome tends to be worse for patients who are very perfectionistic (i.e., who expect a "perfect" outcome) or who want an unusual "look." In the latter case, the surgeon may create a look that is consistent with more traditional ideas of beauty, but that may not be consistent with the patient's desires. Sometimes the outcome is disastrous. We have known disappointed patients who became suicidal and needed urgent hospitalization. Sometimes patients end up blaming their doctors and even threaten to harm or sue them after receiving cosmetic treatments they considered disappointing. *Thus, at this time, we do not recommend these treatments for individuals with BDD.*

Finally, surgery and other cosmetic treatments can be risky. Cosmetic surgery is often portrayed as risk-free, even glamorous. However, "before" and "after" photos and TV reality shows usually omit the unpleasant recuperation phase and the occasional bad outcomes. As detailed in the book *The Smart Woman's Guide to Plastic Surgery* (Loftus, 2008), the risks are very real. For example, after rhinoplasty (a nose job), the implant can extrude through the skin or into the nasal cavity; in addition, severe bleeding and even death can occur, albeit rarely. Anesthesia can be very risky for occasional patients. Though most surgeries go well, patients need to be aware that there are potential risks.

General Approach

We suggest that your therapeutic approach in this module should include the following:

- Educate patients that they are likely to be disappointed with cosmetic treatment (according to the scientific evidence above) and that surgery has risks. However, be aware that simply educating patients probably won't stop them from pursuing cosmetic treatment.
- Recognize that patients may feel very driven to get the treatment; view their efforts as compulsive behaviors.
- Be nonjudgmental. Cosmetic treatments aren't inherently "bad." The problem is that they don't seem to work for BDD.
- Recognize that desire for such treatment is a manifestation of the poor insight that most patients with BDD have—the belief that their problem is a physical one.
- Acknowledge that whether patients obtain cosmetic treatment is their choice. At the same time, we don't recommend facilitating such treatment; for example, don't give the green light for surgery to a surgeon who is requesting your input. Instead, we suggest you use this module to emphasize that most people with BDD are disappointed with cosmetic treatment, and to convey that there are more helpful and effective ways to deal with appearance concerns—especially the skills that patients learn in CBT-BDD.

Check Mood and BDD Symptoms

Check the BDI-II (or other depression inventory) the patient has completed in the waiting room, and check the score on the suicidality item as usual, responding as appropriate. Briefly explore the patient's general mood, and discuss BDD symptoms since the last session. Hand out the *Personal Session Form* (Form 2.1), so that the patient can record information she finds significant during the session.

Briefly Review the Previous Session

Briefly check in with the patient regarding her perception and understanding of the previous session.

Set the Agenda Jointly with the Patient

Convey the topics you'd like to cover during the session, and ask the patient whether there are any items she would like to include in the agenda.

Review Homework

Discuss your patient's homework from the previous session.

Work on the Agenda

Provide Psychoeducation

Have the patient read the handout *Information about Cosmetic Treatment for BDD* (Handout 17.1). You can read through it with her and can amplify the information in the handout with some of the information provided above, but try to avoid lecturing the patient. Ask the patient what her thoughts are about the information. Discuss any issues or questions the handout raises.

When you are working with a patient who has had cosmetic treatment in the past, discuss her experience and how similar or different it was from how most people respond to cosmetic treatment. Ask what the patient learned from her experience.

Evaluate the Pros and Cons of Cosmetic Treatment

Have your patient think through and write down on the *Pros and Cons Worksheet for Cosmetic Treatment* (Form 17.1) as many pros (advantages) and cons (disadvantages) of cosmetic treatment as she can. She can do this for either treatment she is currently receiving or treatment she is considering receiving. In particular, ask the patient to consider pros and cons she may not have considered previously. Pros may include a change in her appearance, trying something "definitive" for her BDD, and the hope that she will feel better about her appearance. Cons may include financial cost, the risks of surgery, a painful rehabilitation period, the chance of an unsatisfactory outcome in which surgery doesn't produce the desired physical change, and the possibility of continued dissatisfaction with appearance. If the patient has had past cosmetic treatment that she feels was unsuccessful, this is an important "con."

In this conversation, remember to avoid pressuring the patient, and use a Socratic style instead. In other words, ask questions that express curiosity or wonder, rather than posing leading questions you know the answers to and are waiting for the patient to figure out. Attempt to subtly minimize or undermine the advantages, and to emphasize and reinforce the disadvantages, while being thoughtful and balanced in your approach.

Some patients will be reluctant to think through the pros and cons, or even to discuss the topic of cosmetic treatment with you, because they're so intent on getting such treatment. With such a patient, it may be helpful to convey that the point of focusing on cosmetic treatment in this session isn't to try to talk the patient out of getting the treatment, but rather to help her think through it more carefully and thoughtfully, including both the pros and cons. It may be helpful to use an addiction metaphor, noting that it's hard to think clearly about this treatment option when the urge to get it is so strong.

Ask whether the handout the patient has just reviewed (*Information about Cosmetic Treatment for BDD*, Handout 17.1) includes any additional information about pros and cons that could be included on the patient's *Pros and Cons Worksheet for Cosmetic Treatment* (Form 17.1). For example, the patient may not have heard before that surgery doesn't work for most people with BDD. You can also refer back to the patient's completed copy of *Your Personal BDD Model* (Form 7.1) and ask her about how getting cosmetic treatment might affect her BDD thoughts and beliefs. Usually cosmetic surgery intensifies the BDD problem by keeping a patient focused on how she looks—for example, "Do I look better now or worse?" "Will the swelling go down?" "Let me check out my new nose in the mirror." By using Socratic questioning here, you can help the patient see that such treatment may well reinforce her BDD symptoms by keeping her "BDD-focused" and by preventing her from learning that she can feel better without such drastic measures.

If the patient includes an unlikely benefit in the pros list (e.g., that it will make her appearance problems disappear), you could say:

> "We don't know for certain how the surgery will affect you, but let's look at how most people do according to the handout you just read [Handout 17.1]. What are your thoughts about that?"

Engage the Patient in Cognitive Restructuring Focused on Cosmetic Treatments

Cognitive restructuring for this module is done in the same way as described earlier in this manual, except that the focus here is specifically on beliefs about cosmetic treatment. The goal of this cognitive restructuring is to help the patient develop more accurate and helpful beliefs about cosmetic treatments, such as the following:

> "Cosmetic treatment won't change my life or fix all of my problems."
> "What needs to change is the inside (how I feel about myself), not the outside."
> "There are far more effective treatments for BDD."

Have the patients complete a copy of the *Thought Record* (Form 9.1) that focuses on thoughts and beliefs about cosmetic treatments:

- To help the patient identify automatic thoughts, think back to your previous discussion with the patient about *Information about Cosmetic Treatment for BDD* (Handout 17.1). This may have yielded some automatic thoughts that you could use here. Or use thoughts about cosmetic treatments that the patient may have recently had or is planning.
- To help the patient identify cognitive errors, especially if she has trouble recognizing erroneous thinking, it may be helpful to use *Examples of Cognitive Errors Involving Cosmetic Treatments* (Handout 17.2).
- Figure 17.1 is an example of a completed *Thought Record* (Form 9.1) for a patient who was afraid that she would always be alone if she didn't get a nose job.

Date/time: Wednesday, 8:30 P.M.
Situation: Seeing myself in the mirror.
Thoughts: If I don't get a nose job, I'll always be alone. Looking good is the only thing that matters.
Believability of thoughts (0–100): 80 for first one, 85 for second
Feelings and intensity (0–100): Anxiety, panic, depression (80)
Cognitive errors: Fortune telling, catastrophizing, all-or-nothing thinking
Questions: What would my friends say about whether I need a nose job? Are there other things besides my appearance that someone might love/like about me?
Rational response: I may not be perfect, but how do I know I'll always be alone? I can't predict the future. There are plenty of women with less than perfect noses who have boyfriends or husbands. Plus, people tell me they like lots of things about me, like I'm nice, I'm fun to be with, and I do a good job at work.
Believability of rational response (0–100%): 60
Feelings and intensity (0–100): Anxiety, depression (40)

FIGURE 17.1. Sample completed *Thought Record* for a patient who wanted a nose job. Based on J. S. Beck (2011).

Help the Patient Begin Response Prevention Focused on Cosmetic Treatment

The goal of response prevention in this module is for the patient to gradually cut down and stop repetitive behaviors related to seeking or obtaining cosmetic treatments. The approach is the same as that discussed in Chapter 11 on ritual prevention. Using response prevention that targets cosmetic treatment may be helpful for patients who are doing any of the following:

- Seeking information about cosmetic treatments on the Internet, in books, or elsewhere.
- Involved in Internet chat rooms with other treatment seekers/users.
- Scheduling a consultation to receive the cosmetic treatment.
- Saving money for cosmetic treatment.

As described in Chapter 11, you can develop a hierarchy involving these behaviors, and then plan response prevention strategies that target the behaviors. For example, the patient could gradually decrease the amount of time she spends on the Internet researching such treatments, buy fewer books on cosmetic treatments, delay a surgical consultation, or stop saving money for the treatment and save it for retirement instead. The patient could also cut back on conversations with family members in which she pleads with them to pay for surgery, and could cut back on mirror checking focusing on what she might look like after a cosmetic procedure.

Deal with Current Treatments or Planned Cosmetic Procedures on a Case-by-Case Basis

A tricky issue is how to handle a patient's current treatment or already planned treatment from a care provider. Examples include a scheduled surgery or ongoing antibiotic treatment for minimal or nonexistent acne. In many cases, it may be in the patient's best interest for you to "take a stand," whereas in some cases, it may be best to let the patient come to her own conclusion about whether to continue the treatment. We suggest that you address this situation on a case-by-case basis.

If a patient concludes, after completing this module, that she wants to stop ongoing or planned cosmetic treatment, reinforce this decision and encourage her to speak directly to her care provider about her decision to stop treatment. You can also offer to speak with the care provider if the patient would like. However, in our experience most patients will not want you to do this, and remember that you will need their written consent to do this.

If a patient decides to continue with ongoing or planned treatment that is "drastic" or potentially risky (such as surgery or dermabrasion), we suggest that you continue using this module to help her think more rationally about her options. For example, repeating the pros and cons approach may be helpful. You can also try Socratic questioning such as the following:

> "You have talked about how all the surgery in the past never helped you. In fact, you thought you looked worse after you had it. I'm wondering what makes you think it will be any different this time?"

You can then use cognitive restructuring with a belief such as "It will definitely turn out better this time," or "This time it will change my life." Help the patient examine the evidence, identify cognitive errors (e.g., all-or-nothing thinking, fortune telling), and come up with a more rational alternative thought—for example, "I can't predict the future, but none of my past surgeries have helped. There's no reason to think it will turn out better this time. Maybe I should work harder in CBT-BDD instead."

You can also offer to talk with the patient's care provider about the treatment and express your concern about it. Again, however, you will need the patient's consent to do this.

One approach we have found helpful with some patients is to encourage them to delay getting the treatment. Some patients are desperate for surgery or dermatological treatment, and cannot tolerate the anxiety they would feel if they agreed never to have it. You could ask such a patient whether she could delay getting it for a certain amount of time and then reconsider when that time comes. When the time comes, you might need to seek a further delay.

> "I know how anxious it makes you to think about never having another surgery, even though none of your surgeries have ever helped you feel any better. What would you think about delaying the next surgery for 3 months and reconsidering at that time? In the meantime, we can do more therapy together and see if after 3 months you feel better about your body image."

If a patient wants to continue a cosmetic treatment that is relatively benign (such as a topical drying agent), or if the patient actually has a mild condition (e.g., acne) and is receiving a benign treatment, you may not want to intervene. Or if a patient has other severe symptoms to work on, it may not be worthwhile to expend all your efforts on cosmetic treatment at this time. On the other hand, if other symptoms are much improved, you might consider spending more time on this module.

Counsel a Patient Who Wants to Get Cosmetic Treatment instead of CBT-BDD

Have the patient carefully consider and write down all the pros and cons of the cosmetic treatment on Form 17.1, as described above. Again, you can refer to Handout 17.1 and have the patient consider and incorporate some of the cons of cosmetic treatment into her list. Then have the patient write down the pros and cons of continuing CBT-BDD. Using Socratic questioning, guide the patient toward seeing that CBT-BDD has more pros than cosmetic treatment. To help the patient think through some of the pros of CBT-BDD, you can review what brought her to see you in the first place. Focus on the suffering that brought her in, and then ask her to make a real effort with CBT-BDD. You can say something like this:

> "I can understand that you want to change how you look, but you wanted to participate in this treatment and work on your BDD. What do you think about postponing the surgery and giving this treatment a try first? You might as well give it a shot. Why don't you commit 100% to CBT-BDD to see if it really works? To see if it will work, you'll need to really try it."

If the patient is discouraged with her progress, you can remind her that it typically takes time and lots of practice to improve with CBT-BDD. Some patients start getting a lot better toward the end of the treatment.

You can also ask the patient to complete copies of the *Thought Record* (Form 9.1) for thoughts such as "This treatment [CBT-BDD] will never work." Have the patient identify cognitive errors (such as fortune telling and catastrophizing), and develop a more helpful and rational responses.

If techniques such as these are not effective in persuading the patient, we suggest that you use some of the MI techniques discussed in Chapter 5.

ASSIGN HOMEWORK

- Ask your patient to review her *Pros and Cons Worksheet for Cosmetic Treatment* (Form 17.1) and add any more pros and/or cons she can think of. You can review these at the next session.
- Have the patient complete additional copies of the *Thought Record* (Form 9.1) to observe and dispute irrational thinking involving cosmetic procedures.
- Ask your patient to use response prevention to stop behaviors associated with seeking or obtaining cosmetic treatments.

ASK FOR SUMMARY OF/FEEDBACK ON THE SESSION

Ask the patient to briefly summarize the major points covered during the session. Also ask whether the patient had any concerns about the session or your behavior, and respond appropriately.

FORM 17.1

Pros and Cons Worksheet for Cosmetic Treatment

Pros	Cons

HANDOUT 17.1

Information about Cosmetic Treatment for BDD

1. What is cosmetic treatment for BDD? By "cosmetic treatment," we mean any surgical, medical, or "medical-like" treatment. This includes surgery, dermatological treatment, dental treatment, other medical treatment (such as hormone treatment for body hair), or "medical-like" treatment such as electrolysis.

2. You aren't alone in wanting cosmetic treatment. In fact, the majority of people with BDD try to get, and actually get, cosmetic treatment. Surgery and dermatological treatment are most commonly received. With all of the infomercials and plastic surgery TV shows, this desire may become even more common.

3. Cosmetic treatments don't seem to work for BDD.

- Cosmetic treatment isn't inherently "good" or "bad." Some people do well with it, whereas others don't.
- The problem is that, as far as we can tell, cosmetic treatment doesn't help people with BDD feel better about how they look. It doesn't seem to matter how good the surgeon or the dermatologist is. In fact, studies have found that only a very small percentage (about 5%) of people with BDD find that their BDD symptoms overall get better after cosmetic treatment. So even though many people who don't have BDD are happy with cosmetic treatment, this doesn't seem to be the case for people with BDD.
- Some people with BDD feel devastated after they get cosmetic treatment. They feel they look much worse and wish they'd never had it.
- Some people with BDD feel the cosmetic treatment helped—but only for a little while. After some time passes, they no longer like the result.
- Other people think that their treated body parts look better, but overall their BDD doesn't improve. What often happens is their concern shifts to another body area. This makes sense, because the problem in BDD isn't with how a person's body actually looks. The problem is with body image and the tendency to obsess and worry about minor imperfections. This is a "mind problem" that surgery won't fix.

4. Cosmetic treatments can be very costly. Although the expense will vary, depending on the procedure, these treatments are usually expensive—often costing many thousands of dollars.

(cont.)

5. Cosmetic treatment can be risky. Most procedures go fine, but not always. There is always a risk, such as scarring or excessive bleeding. For example, after a nose job, the implant can extrude through your skin or into your nasal cavity; severe bleeding can also occur. Occasionally people die from anesthesia. Also, the glamorous makeover shows tend to skip the recuperation period, which can be lengthy and painful.

6. Cosmetic treatment won't fix your problems or change your life for the better.

- Some people, especially those with BDD, hope or assume that cosmetic treatment will fix everything that isn't right in their lives. They think that if their nose (or other body part of concern) looks better, they'll get a boyfriend/girlfriend or find a better job. But cosmetic treatment only changes one small aspect of how you look—not your personality, intelligence, drive, or all the other things that affect how your life goes.
- Research has found that people who expect cosmetic treatment to fix their problems or change their lives are more likely to be disappointed with the results, because it doesn't actually accomplish these things.

7. What needs to change is the inside, not the outside. The problem in BDD isn't how you look—it's your body image. In other words, the problem is with how you think you look and how you feel about your appearance. Surgery and other cosmetic treatments won't change this, whereas CBT-BDD will.

8. CBT-BDD appears much more effective for BDD—and much less risky—than cosmetic treatment.

- There's much more evidence that CBT-BDD (and certain medications) helps BDD. Most people improve with this treatment. In contrast, it appears that almost no one with BDD gets better with cosmetic treatment.
- CBT-BDD is very unlikely to make your BDD worse, whereas this is not uncommon with cosmetic treatment.
- CBT-BDD isn't irreversible, the way cosmetic treatment often is. Certain cosmetic treatments are drastic and very hard to reverse if you aren't happy with them. Some patients end up living with permanent changes to their appearance that they detest.
- CBT-BDD is "cosmetic surgery for the mind." It gives you the skills to change from the inside. This is what's needed to manage BDD successfully.

HANDOUT 17.2

Examples of Cognitive Errors Involving Cosmetic Treatment

- **All-or-nothing thinking:** "If I don't have this surgery, I'll still have the bump on my nose and will look totally ugly."
- **Should statement:** "I should have laser treatment so I'll have perfectly clear skin."
- **Mind reading:** "I know that guy is thinking I should get a hair transplant. Otherwise, why would he be looking at me like that?"
- **Fortune telling:** "If I don't get a facelift, everyone at the holiday party will be thinking how awful I look."
- **Catastrophizing**: "If I don't get electrolysis to get rid of all this ugly hair, no guy will *ever* want to go out with me!"
- **Personalization**: "Every time I turn on the TV, there's a show on makeovers. That's a sign that I have to get my lips plumped!"
- **Emotional reasoning:** "I feel this chin implant will change my life, so it must be true."
- **Labeling:** "If I don't get electrolysis, I'll always look like a gorilla and a freak."
- **Discounting the positives:** "It doesn't matter that I'm a nice person and a good teacher. The only thing that matters is having nice breasts, so I have to get breast augmentation."

CHAPTER 18

DEPRESSION

DOES YOUR PATIENT NEED THIS MODULE?

This optional module is intended for patients with severe depressive symptoms and suicidality. Most patients with BDD have some degree of depression, which often appears to be a direct result of their BDD symptoms. It is easy to understand why they feel depressed; their thoughts about their physical appearance would make most people feel sad and down. It's common for patients with BDD to say such things as "If you looked as hideous as I do, you'd be depressed, too," or "Of course I'm depressed because of how I look. Everyone avoids me because I look so ugly." In addition, many of the core beliefs typical of BDD have depressive themes: "I'm worthless," "I'm unlovable," and "I'm inadequate."

Not surprisingly, BDD symptoms and depressive symptoms tend to run hand in hand. If one set of symptoms worsens, the other often does as well; conversely, if one set improves, the other often does as well (Phillips & Stout, 2006). Mild to moderate levels of depressed mood may not interfere with progress in treatment and often respond well to standard CBT-BDD. In such cases, it is probably not necessary to use this module; simply continuing with the usual CBT-BDD methods is likely to reduce the depressed mood.

However, some patients with BDD experience depression that is more serious or that may be independent of their BDD symptoms. For these patients, depression can exacerbate BDD symptoms even when the source of the negative mood is not directly related to the BDD. It can also impair their ability to make progress in treatment. For example, seriously depressed patients may find it hard to come to treatment sessions or to do CBT-BDD homework because their energy and motivation are low. They may not be able to make themselves complete the work assigned, and/or they don't see the point of doing so because "nothing will help anyway" or "I don't deserve to get better."

Patients with more serious depression may also experience serious suicidal ideation and even report plans or attempts at suicide. In fact, rates of suicidal ideation and suicide attempts appear to be very high among patients with BDD (Phillips & Menard, 2006). Clinicians must be alert to this risk. This is especially true for patients who are seriously impaired by their BDD symptoms and who have comorbid posttraumatic stress disorder and/or a substance use disorder. When patients present with these features, it is essential to monitor their depressed mood and their suicidal thinking and behaviors throughout their treatment.

Suicidality can wax and wane or could develop during the treatment. This module is specifically designed for patients with more severe depressed mood and possible suicidal thinking that is likely to interfere with progress in treatment or to pose a safety risk. In these cases, the focus of treatment will be on the depression and suicidal ideation. When the patients' depressed mood is less severe and the risk of suicide is low, you can return to using CBT-BDD.

As described in Chapter 4, you can judge the degree of depression from the BDI-II or a similar depression measure. Consider using this module if a patient's score is 20 or above on the BDI-II, or in the range for clinical depression on any other depression measure. Also elicit your patient's input regarding depression symptoms, and use your own judgment as to whether the module is relevant.

Keep in mind that BDD is an unusually distressing disorder that often causes intense depressive thoughts, as patients feel reviled by others, isolated, humiliated, and ashamed. To address these powerful negative feelings, you will need to strike a delicate balance—encouraging patients to challenge themselves in treatment, while also recognizing that serious depression may make it difficult (if not impossible) for them to muster the energy and courage to do this. Several components of this module rely on cognitive techniques like those presented in Chapters 9 and 13. If you are using this module early in the treatment because depressive symptoms are severe enough to warrant this focus, be sure to read through those chapters before moving forward.

If a patient has severe depressive symptoms and suicidal thinking that do not improve with the treatment strategies described here, consider referring the patient to a higher level of care and/or for medication treatment.

Session Structure

The standard agenda outlined earlier for all CBT-BDD sessions should be followed.

SESSION SUMMARY

- ☐ Check mood and BDD symptoms.
- ☐ Briefly review the previous session.
- ☐ Set the agenda jointly with the patient.
- ☐ Review homework.
- ☐ Work on the agenda.
  - ☐ Monitor the patient's mood.
  - ☐ Engage the patient in cognitive restructuring for depressive symptoms.
  - ☐ Introduce activity scheduling.
  - ☐ Encourage the patient to increase pleasant and achievement-oriented activities.
  - ☐ Use motivational enhancement strategies as needed.
- ☐ Assign homework.
- ☐ Ask for summary of/feedback on the session.

SESSION FORMS AND HANDOUTS

BDI-II (or other depression inventory)

Personal Session Form (Form 2.1)

Therapist Session Form (Form 6.1)
Keeping Track of Your Thoughts (Form 8.1)
Thought Record (Form 9.1)
Examples of Cognitive Errors in Depressive Thoughts (Handout 18.1)
Activity-Scheduling Form (Form 18.1)
List of Pleasant Activities and Achievement-Oriented Activities (Form 18.2)
Completed *Your Personal BDD Model* (Form 7.1)

INTRODUCTION TO THIS SESSION

Goals

The goals of this module are to do the following in order reduce depressive symptoms that are interfering with CBT-BDD:

- Monitor ongoing depressive symptoms and their effects.
- Increase goal-directed, enjoyable, and achievement-oriented activities via activity scheduling.
- Engage in cognitive restructuring focused on depressive thoughts and beliefs.

If your patient is already reasonably physically and socially active each week, you can probably skip activity scheduling for simple activities (such as making breakfast) and just work on increasing the frequency of pleasant and achievement-oriented activities and on cognitive restructuring. However, if your patient is inactive because of depressive symptoms (e.g., spending lots of time in bed, staring at the television for much of the day), begin with activity scheduling based on smaller tasks, work on increasing pleasant and achievement-oriented activities, and then include cognitive restructuring. Generally, one or two sessions should suffice to introduce the techniques for this module, and thereafter you can weave the interventions described below into subsequent sessions as needed.

Assessing and Monitoring Suicidality

Pay special attention to high scores on the suicidality item of the BDI-II (or other depression measure), and be aware that some patients with BDD can be at real risk for suicide. Do not underestimate this risk! *This module, by itself, will not be adequate to manage highly suicidal patients.* Accordingly, we advise you to take these precautions:

- Evaluate the suicide risk in seriously depressed patients with BDD, to determine whether to retain them in CBT-BDD or consider referring them to a higher level of care and/or to treatment with medication.
- Regularly monitor these patients during treatment for suicidal ideation, intent, and plans, and for other serious symptoms of depression (e.g., hopelessness, self-denigration). This should be done weekly until you are confident that the risk is indeed reduced.

Inquire about current and past suicidal ideas, plans, and behaviors in a matter-of-fact manner that indicates you expect patients to respond honestly. Probe further if they indicate any recent suicidal intention, to determine whether this is a current concern and how far their thoughts, plans, and recent actions extend. If patients cannot state unequivocally that they will not engage in any suicidal planning or behaviors during the treatment process, you need to consider a higher level of care (e.g., hospitalization, day treatment setting) that would provide closer monitoring (see below).

If a depressed patient with BDD reports suicidal thinking, but no plans or behaviors that suggest serious suicidal risk at the time of evaluation, you will nonetheless want to continue monitoring the patient's suicidality. As noted throughout this book, patients should complete the BDI-II (or a similar depression measure) before each therapy session. Most likely, if you have considered starting CBT-BDD with any patient and administered the BDI-II, his original score on item ("Suicidal thoughts and wishes") was 0 or 1 ("I have thoughts of killing myself, but I would not carry them out"). If his score on this item rises to a 2 ("I would like to kill myself") or a 3 ("I would kill myself if I had the chance"), discuss this in detail with the patient during the mood and symptom check-in at the beginning of the session to determine the risk. Also ask your patient in detail about suicidal ideation whenever the topic arises during the session (e.g., when you are eliciting BDD-related thoughts).

Check Mood and BDD Symptoms

In addition to checking the BDI-II (or other depression inventory) and the score on the suicidality item as described above, briefly explore your patient's general mood, and discuss BDD symptoms since the last session. Hand out the *Personal Session Form* (Form 2.1), so that the patient can record information he finds significant during the session.

Briefly Review the Previous Session

Briefly check in with the patient regarding his perception and understanding of the previous session.

Set the Agenda Jointly with the Patient

Convey the topics you'd like to cover during the session, and ask the patient whether there are any items he would like to include in the agenda.

Review Homework

Discuss your patient's homework from the previous session.

Work on the Agenda

Monitor the Patient's Mood

Start by introducing the idea that together you will focus more on the patient's depressive symptoms, and introduce the concept of mood monitoring:

> "We've been talking about how your depression is a real problem for you and is getting in the way of work and getting errands done. It's also making it hard for you to do the homework for this treatment. It may help to become more aware of when your depression and feelings of hopelessness are occurring. During our check-in at the beginning of today's session, you talked about how you've been feeling very sad and hopeless during the past week, especially on Tuesday morning, when you had to go to work and felt too depressed to get out of bed. Were there any other situations in the past week when you felt especially depressed?"

The patient may describe another situation or two. For one of these situations or the one mentioned already, ask, "What was going through your mind at that time?" This question will remind the patient to identify the thoughts that triggered the depressive feelings. Next you can introduce *Keeping Track of Your Thoughts* (Form 8.1) as this applies to depression. This is a form of mood monitoring:

> "We're first going to use the skill of tracking your mood and thoughts that you've already learned, but instead of focusing on your appearance concerns, we'll apply it to your depression. This form will help us better identify how you're feeling and also what kinds of situations and thoughts make you feel more depressed. How does this sound to you?"

It is often helpful to refer back to the copy of *Your Personal BDD Model* (Form 7.1) your patient completed earlier in therapy. Apply it now to the patient's depression, and discuss how certain negative thoughts that may or may not be appearance-related can trigger feelings of depression.

Now work with the patient to complete a copy of *Keeping Track of Your Thoughts* (Form 8.1) for a recent situation that provoked depressive thoughts. If needed, you can also discuss the range of depressive emotions and determine what feelings fall into the category of depression for this particular patient.

Engage the Patient in Cognitive Restructuring for Depressive Symptoms

Cognitive restructuring in this module is carried out as described in Chapters 9 and 13, except that the focus here is on depressive thoughts and core beliefs, especially those concerned with hopelessness. The aim is to help the patient develop more accurate and helpful thoughts and core beliefs.

Ask your patient to complete a copy of the *Thought Record* (Form 9.1) that builds on one of the thoughts in the copy of *Keeping Track of Your Thoughts* (Form 8.1) he has just completed. Alternatively, the *Thought Record* (Form 9.1) can build on another depressive thoughts that the patient has recently mentioned. Ask the patient to do the following:

- Identify the automatic thought(s).
- Notice any cognitive errors from the list contained in *Examples of Cognitive Errors in Depressive Thoughts* (Handout 18.1). Give the patient this handout as a guide to identifying such cognitive errors, and open the discussion in this way:

THERAPIST: So it seems that you have several different depressive feelings, such as sadness, irritability, and gloominess. By filling out a few *Keeping Track of Your Thoughts* forms [Form 8.1], you've identified some situations in the past week and some negative thoughts that triggered these depressive feelings for you. Let's look at how you might apply some of the cognitive restructuring skills you've already learned to these thoughts.

PATIENT: OK. So it's kind of like what I did before for my thoughts about somebody thinking how awful I look when I don't trim my sideburns exactly right?

THERAPIST: Yes, it's very similar. This time we're focusing on thoughts that make you feel depressed. We can also use the idea of "maladaptive thinking" or "cognitive errors" here. The same errors may be relevant to your depressive thoughts. In fact, these errors apply to all kinds of thoughts we have, not just BDD-related ones. We all make these thinking errors in various situations in our lives. Why don't we look at this handout, which gives some examples of cognitive errors that are related to depressive thoughts, and see whether you think any of them may apply to you?

Now engage the patient in a discussion of the cognitive errors in Handout 18.1 that apply to him, soliciting additional examples that may be especially applicable. After this, help the patient complete a copy of the *Thought Record* (Form 9.1) that focuses on depressive cognitions/feelings and alternative thoughts. See Figure 18.1 for an example.

Introduce Activity Scheduling

Activity scheduling is appropriate for patients who are engaging in very few daily activities because of their depression. For severely depressed patients, it may be beneficial to do activity scheduling first, before working on their self-defeating thoughts (as described above). Patients who are already reasonably active (e.g., going to work, doing errands, leaving the house) can skip scheduling these basic activities and go directly to the next section of this module, on increasing pleasant and achievement-oriented activities.

THERAPIST: Now I'd like to discuss a new skill. This skill involves becoming more active. One of the best ways to feel better and improve your mood is by staying active and doing things. Even if you can't think of enjoyable things to do right now, it can help to simply be busy. Lying in bed or sitting around doing nothing gives depressive thoughts more opportunity to fill your mind so you just feel worse and worse. Does this ever happen to you?

PATIENT: Yes. When I just lie in bed and don't go to work, I just get more depressed. I just lie there thinking of everything that makes me upset, plus then I don't get anything done. My bills just pile up, and that stresses me out even more. And I get more and more behind at work, which makes me feel even worse.

THERAPIST: OK, so it just makes matters worse to lie in bed or sit around and do nothing. Do you find that when you actually do something, you feel a little better?

Here you can again refer to the copy of *Your Personal BDD Model* (Form 7.1) your patient completed earlier in therapy, and discuss how it is relevant to depression. For example, thinking negative, depressing thoughts that involve cognitive errors just feeds depressive symptoms. Avoiding activities and isolating himself just keeps the patient focused on his depressive thoughts and his misery. It keeps the vicious cycle going. In other words, doing nothing just feeds the depression, whereas changing behavior to stay active can combat depressive thoughts and feelings.

Date/time: *Tuesday, 7:30 A.M.*
Situation: *Lying in bed after the alarm goes off.*
Thoughts: *I'm too depressed to go to work today. If I go, I'll just do a totally lousy job anyway, and everyone will think I'm useless and wonder why they hired me.*
Believability of thoughts (0–100): *85*
Feelings and intensity (0–100): *Anxiety (50), sadness (80)*
Cognitive errors: *Fortune telling, catastrophizing, all-or-nothing thinking, labeling, mind reading*
Questions: *What is the evidence that I will do a lousy job? Can I really read their minds?*
Rational response: *It's probably better to go and just do my best, even if my work isn't perfect. Actually, my last performance evaluation was pretty good. I can't read people's minds anyway, so how will I really know what they're thinking? And once I get to work and get going, I usually feel a little better.*
Believability of rational response (0–100%): *50*
Feelings and intensity (0–100): *Anxiety (40), depression (60)*

FIGURE 18.1. Sample completed *Thought Record* for a very depressed patient with BDD. Based on J. S. Beck (2011).

PATIENT: Most of the time it does help to do something. It's really hard to get going, but once I do, I usually feel a little better. At least I might get something done, or be a little distracted to take my mind off my depression. But it's really hard to get myself to do things. And sometimes, even when I do, I just drag myself through it.

THERAPIST: That's understandable, because you feel so bad. But as you said, you usually feel better after doing something. One thing that can help is to actually make a schedule for yourself, so when the time comes you don't have to think about whether to do something or make a decision about it. When you schedule it ahead and make it part of your day, then it becomes something you simply do. This is a simple but powerful way to feel better. Are you willing to give this a try?

Now show the patient how to use the *Activity-Scheduling Form* (Form 18.1) to schedule homework involving doing activities for the next week.

- Emphasize the need to plan activities ahead of time. Making the decision now, ahead of time, often makes it easier to do them.
- Help the patient to select realistic activities and fill in specific times at which they'll be done. If the patient is spending most of the day in bed, you can begin by scheduling meals, showers, laundry, and other basic activities.
- Look for a few potentially pleasant activities (e.g., grocery shopping at an especially good market, baking cookies, going sailing) and achievement-oriented activities (e.g., completing a helpful task), as noted in the section below.
- Include a 1–10 rating scale that allows the patient to record how much pleasure or satisfaction he got out of completing each task. This may help you identify pleasant activities that can be increased (see below).
- Use cognitive restructuring (as described in Chapter 9) to address negative thinking that may interfere with task completion.

It's important for the patient to try to fill in as much of the *Activity-Scheduling Form* (Form 18.1) as possible, in order to minimize activities like sleeping all day, lying in bed all day, or staring at the TV. It's also important for the patient to schedule self-care activities like showering, buying food, and cooking if he isn't currently doing these things.

Encourage the Patient to Increase Pleasant and Achievement-Oriented Activities

Some patients are already reasonably active, but have difficulty coming up with tasks that would be pleasurable or provide them with a sense of mastery. In such a case, it's important to help the patient identify and increase activities he might possibly enjoy or feel good about accomplishing. A typical exchange might go as follows:

PATIENT: But how will I enjoy things if I'm so depressed?

THERAPIST: Well, you might not enjoy everything you do. Most of us don't enjoy everything we do. But you never know; you might enjoy some of them more than you expect. I wonder if this has been true for you in the past. Can you remember something you've done that you thought would be boring or awful, but when you did it, it wasn't so bad and you even enjoyed it a little?

If the patient can't come up with an example, offer one that seems relevant, based on what you know about the person (e.g., playing with a pet or completing a crossword puzzle). If the patient can't come up with anything, comment that this may be because he hasn't really tried to do things recently. Suggest that scheduling pleasant activities is worth a try, since the patient's current plan of not doing anything isn't helping him feel better.

Help the Patient Develop a List of Pleasant and Achievement-Oriented Activities

Work on helping the patient plan pleasant and achievement-oriented activities by having him fill out the *List of Pleasant Activities and Achievement-Oriented Activities* (Form 18.2). This list can include hobbies, everyday activities (e.g., taking a hot bath), doing things outside the home (e.g., going to the movies), calling a friend, playing a game, making an appointment, going to the bank, and so on. Try to come up with activities that are (1) potentially enjoyable and/or (2) give the patient a sense of accomplishment or pride. Discuss with the patient that it's most helpful to choose activities that are:

- Specific, realistic, and doable (e.g., gardening rather than going on vacation, unless going on vacation is realistic).
- Active rather than passive (e.g., playing sports rather than watching sports on TV).
- Easy to do frequently and easily (e.g., walking or playing with a pet).
- Not expensive (e.g., going to a movie rather than buying a new car).
- Not harmful (e.g., going for a walk rather than drinking a bottle of wine).
- Not dependent on other people's schedules or availability (activities with others are good choices, but the patient should try not to limit these to activities requiring the presence of people who may not be available).

Assist the Patient in Actually Doing Activities

Next, have your patient pick some activities to increase in the next week, and add some of these activities to his *Activity-Scheduling Form* (Form 18.1). Explain that these are things the patient is choosing to schedule, so that when the time arrives, he will not have to decide whether to do the activity or not; he will simply do it because it's in his schedule. If an activity is not possible for some reason (e.g., the weather won't permit an outdoor activity), have the patient substitute another activity from his list to do at that time instead. It may be most helpful to include both some pleasant activities and some achievement-oriented activities.

Before your patient begins scheduling the activities, ask him to think about which activities and how many of them he did in the past few days, and to write these on Form 18.1. Explain that this is the baseline number of activities, and that the goal is to increase this during the next week.

If your patient finds it hard to select activities, have him pick just a few to start with, especially ones that are easy, possible, and/or potentially most enjoyable. You may also want to have the patient build in rewards for completing the activity.

Encourage the patient to try the activities even if he doesn't think he will enjoy them. He may not, but this may also reflect maladaptive thinking (e.g., fortune telling, catastrophizing). You can adopt the same "scientist" or "detective" approach you've taken throughout treatment. For example, you can note that it's hard for the patient to know how he will feel until he actually gives the activity a try. If it seems appropriate, you can ask the patient to rate how much pleasure he expects to get from the activity (0 = none, 10 = very much), and then see how much pleasure he actually experiences after completing the activity. This helps provide objective evidence that the patient's expectations may not always match reality, and that doing an activity even when he doesn't feel like it can be helpful. You can also engage the patient in cognitive restructuring of interfering beliefs (e.g., "I'll never enjoy anything I do").

Use Motivational Enhancement Strategies as Needed

If depression is interfering with homework completion or attendance at therapy sessions, consider using some of the motivational enhancement strategies described in Chapter 5. If you've used these strategies before with some success, begin with the techniques that worked best at that time. If these are not helpful enough, try different motivational strategies from Chapter 5. The key is to find strategies that will increase your patient's participation in the treatment. If he misses sessions or doesn't do homework, the therapy is unlikely to be helpful.

ASSIGN HOMEWORK

- Ask the patient to complete several copies of the *Thought Record* (Form 9.1) focusing on depressive thoughts, interpretations, and feelings.
- Have the patient complete the *Activity-Scheduling Form* (Form 18.1).
- Have the patient complete the *List of Pleasant Activities and Achievement-Oriented Activities* (Form 18.2).

ASK FOR SUMMARY OF/FEEDBACK ON THE SESSION

Ask the patient to briefly summarize the major points covered during the session. Also ask whether the patient had any concerns about the session or your behavior, and respond appropriately.

FORM 18.1

Activity-Scheduling Form

Fill in the dates until the next therapy session across the top of the grid. Write each activity you schedule for a particular day in the column for that day. After you are done with an activity, rate on a scale from 0 (least) to 10 (most) in terms of *pleasure* (P) and in terms of *accomplishment* (A). For example, if your activity for 8–9 A.M. on the first day is making pancakes, and you rate this activity a 1 in terms of pleasure and a 7 in terms of accomplishment, write "Make pancakes: P = 1, A = 7" in the 8–9 A.M. space in the first column.

Hour	Date						
8–9 A.M.							
9–10 A.M.							
10–11 A.M.							
11 A.M.–Noon							
Noon–1 P.M.							
1–2 P.M.							
2–3 P.M.							
3–4 P.M.							
4–5 P.M.							
5–6 P.M.							
6–7 P.M.							
7–8 P.M.							
8–9 P.M.							
9–10 P.M.							
10–11 P.M.							

Adapted with permission of the publisher from Beck, J. S. (2011). *Cognitive Behavior Therapy: Basics and Beyond*. New York: Guilford Press.

FORM 18.2

List of Pleasant Activities and Achievement-Oriented Activities

Work on developing a list of pleasant and achievement-oriented activities. This list can include hobbies, everyday activities (such as sorting the mail), doing things outside the home (e.g., going to the grocery store), calling a friend, and so forth. Try to come up with activities that are (1) potentially enjoyable and/or (2) give you a sense of accomplishment or pride.

1. ______________________________

2. ______________________________

3. ______________________________

4. ______________________________

5. ______________________________

6. ______________________________

7. ______________________________

8. ______________________________

9. ______________________________

10. ______________________________

11. ______________________________

12. ______________________________

13. ______________________________

14. ______________________________

15. ______________________________

16. ______________________________

HANDOUT 18.1

Examples of Cognitive Errors in Depressive Thoughts

The following thinking errors are demonstrated in these examples of depressive thoughts:

- **All-or-nothing thinking:** "Everyone else is so happy. It isn't fair. I'm the only one who's miserable."
- **"Should" statements:** "I should be enjoying this holiday like everyone else."
- **Mind reading:** "I know everyone's thinking I'm a jerk."
- **Fortune telling:** "I'll always be depressed. I'll never get better."
- **Catastrophizing:** "My life is always going to be a total disaster."
- **Labeling:** "I'm a total loser."
- **Discounting the positive:** "Everything in my life is terrible."

References

Allen, A., Hadley, S. J., Kaplan, A., Simeon, D., Friedberg, J., Priday, L., et al. (2008). An open-label trial of venlafaxine in body dysmorphic disorder. *CNS Spectrums, 13*(2), 138–144.

Allen, A., & Hollander, E. (2004). Similarities and differences between body dysmorphic disorder and other disorders. *Psychiatric Annals, 34*(12), 927–933.

American Psychiatric Association. (2000). *Diagnostic and statistical manual of mental disorders* (4th ed., text rev.). Washington, DC: Author.

American Psychiatric Association. (2003). Practice guideline for the assessment and treatment of patients with suicidal behaviors. *American Journal of Psychiatry, 160*(11, Suppl.), 1–60.

Azrin, N., & Nunn, R. (1973). Habit-reversal: A method of eliminating nervous habits and tics. *Behaviour Research and Therapy, 11*(4), 619–628.

Beck, A. T., Steer, R. A., & Brown, G. K. (1996). *Beck Depression Inventory—II: Manual.* San Antonio, TX: Psychological Corporation.

Beck, J. S. (2011). *Cognitive behavior therapy: Basics and beyond* (2nd ed.). New York: Guilford Press.

Bögels, S. M., Sijbers, G. F. V. M., & Voncken, M. (2006). Mindfulness and task concentration training for social phobia: A pilot study. *Journal of Cognitive Psychotherapy, 20*(1), 33–44.

Bohne, A., Keuthen, N. J., Wilhelm, S., Deckersbach, T., & Jenike, M. A. (2002). Prevalence of symptoms of body dysmorphic disorder and its correlates: A cross-cultural comparison. *Psychosomatics, 43*(6), 486–490.

Bohne, A., Wilhelm, S., Keuthen, N. J., Florin, I., Baer, L., & Jenike, M. A. (2002). Prevalence of body dysmorphic disorder in a German college student sample. *Psychiatry Research, 109*(1), 101–104.

Buhlmann, U., Etcoff, N. L., & Wilhelm, S. (2006). Emotion recognition bias for contempt and anger in body dysmorphic disorder. *Journal of Psychiatric Research, 40*(2), 105–111.

Buhlmann, U., Etcoff, N. L., & Wilhelm, S. (2007). Facial attractiveness ratings and perfectionism in body dysmorphic disorder and obsessive-compulsive disorder. *Journal of Anxiety Disorders, 22*(3), 540–547.

Buhlmann, U., Glaesmer, H., Mewes, R., Fama, J. M., Wilhelm, S., Brähler, E., et al. (2010). Updates on the prevalence of body dysmorphic disorder: A population-based survey. *Psychiatry Research, 178*(1), 171–175.

Buhlmann, U., & Wilhelm, S. (2004). Cognitive factors in body dysmorphic disorder. *Psychiatric Annals, 34*(12), 922–926.

Buhlmann, U., Wilhelm, S., McNally, R. J., Tuschen-Caffier, B., Baer, L., & Jenike, M. A. (2002). Interpretive biases for ambiguous information in body dysmorphic disorder. *CNS Spectrums, 7*(6), 435–436, 441–443.

Burns, D. D. (1999). *Feeling good: The new mood therapy* (rev. ed.). New York: Avon.

Campisi, T. A. (1996). Exposure and response prevention in the treatment of body dysmorphic disorder. *Dissertation Abstracts International, 56*, 7036B.

Cash, T. F. (2008). *The body image workbook: An eight-step program for learning to like your looks* (2nd ed.). Oakland, CA: New Harbinger.

Chosak, A., Marques, L., Greenberg, J. L., Jenike, E., Dougherty, D. D., & Wilhelm, S. (2008). Body dysmorphic disorder and obsessive-compulsive disorder: Similarities, differences and the classification debate. *Expert Reviews in Neurotherapeutics, 8*(8), 1209–1218.

Conroy, M., Menard, W., Fleming-Ives, K., Modha, P., Cerullo, H., & Phillips, K. A. (2008). Prevalence and clinical characteristics of body dysmorphic disorder in an adult inpatient setting. *General Hospital Psychiatry, 30*(1), 67–72.

Cotterill, J. A. (1996). Body dysmorphic disorder. *Dermatologic Clinics, 14*(3), 457–463.

Cotterill, J. A., & Cunliffe, W. J. (1997). Suicide in dermatological patients. *British Journal of Dermatology, 137*(2), 246–250.

Crerand, C. E., Phillips, K. A., Menard, W., & Fay, C. (2005). Nonpsychiatric medical treatment of body dysmorphic disorder. *Psychosomatics, 46*(6), 549–555.

Deckersbach, T., Savage, C. R., Phillips, K. A., Wilhelm, S., Buhlmann, U., Rauch, S. L., et al. (2000). Characteristics of memory dysfunction in body dysmorphic disorder. *Journal of the International Neuropsychological Society, 6*(6), 673–681.

Feusner, J. D., Hembacher, E., & Phillips, K. A. (2009). The mouse who couldn't stop washing: Pathologic grooming in animals and humans. *CNS Spectrums, 14*(9), 503–513.

Feusner, J. D., Townsend, J., Bystritsky, A., & Bookheimer, S. (2007). Visual information processing of faces in body dysmorphic disorder. *Archives of General Psychiatry, 64*(12), 1417–1425.

First, M. B., Gibbon, M., Spitzer, R. L., Williams, J. B. W., & Benjamin, L. S. (1997). *Structured Clinical Interview for DSM-IV Axis II Personality Disorders (SCID-II).* Washington, DC: American Psychiatric Press.

First, M. B., Spitzer, R. L., Gibbon, M., & Williams, J. B. W. (1996). *Structured Clinical Interview for DSM-IV Axis I Disorders. Clinical Version (SCID-CV).* Washington, DC: American Psychiatric Press.

Foa, E. B. (1979). Failure in treating obsessive-compulsives. *Behaviour Research and Therapy, 17*(3), 169–176.

Fukuda, O. (1977). Statistical analysis of dysmorphophobia in outpatient clinic. *Japanese Journal of Plastic and Reconstructive Surgery, 20*, 569–577.

Geremia, G., & Neziroglu, F. (2001). Cognitive therapy in the treatment of body dysmorphic disorder. *Clinical Psychology and Psychotherapy, 8*, 241–251.

Grant, J. E., Kim, S. W., & Crow, S. J. (2001). Prevalence and clinical features of body dysmorphic disorder in adolescent and adult psychiatric inpatients. *Journal of Clinical Psychiatry, 62*(7), 517–522.

Grant, J. E., Kim, S. W., & Eckert, E. D. (2002). Body dysmorphic disorder in patients with anorexia nervosa: Prevalence, clinical features and delusionality of body image. *International Journal of Eating Disorders, 32*(3), 291–300.

Grant, J. E., & Phillips, K. A. (2004). Is anorexia nervosa a subtype of body dysmorphic disorder?: Probably not, but read on. *Harvard Review of Psychiatry, 12*(2), 123–126.

Greenberg, J., Markowitz, S., Petronko, M., Taylor, C., Wilhelm, S., & Wilson, T. (2010). Cognitive behavioral therapy for adolescent body dysmorphic disorder. *Cognitive and Behavioral Practice, 17*(3), 248–258.

Gunstad, J., & Phillips, K. A. (2003). Axis I comorbidity in body dysmorphic disorder. *Comprehensive Psychiatry, 44*(4), 270–276.

Hayes, S., Strosahl, K., & Wilson, K. (1999). *Acceptance and commitment therapy: An experiential approach to behavior change.* New York: Guilford Press.

Hollander, E., & Allen, A. (2006). Beauty is in the eye of the beholder: New insights in imagined ugliness. *Primary Psychiatry, 13*(7), 37–38.

Hollander, E., Allen, A., Kwon, J., Aronowitz, B., Schmeidler, J., Wong, C., et al. (1999). Clomipramine vs. desipramine crossover trial in body dysmorphic disorder: Selective efficacy of a serotonin reuptake inhibitor in imagined ugliness. *Archives of General Psychiatry, 56*(11), 1033–1039.

Hollander, E., & Aronowitz, B. R. (1999). Comorbid social anxiety and body dysmorphic disorder: Managing the complicated patient. *Journal of Clinical Psychiatry, 60*(Suppl. 9), 27–31.

Ishigooka, J., Iwao, M., Suzuki, M., Fukuyama, Y., Murasaki, M., & Miura, S. (1998). Demographic features of patients seeking cosmetic surgery. *Psychiatry and Clinical Neurosciences, 52*(3), 283–287.

Keuthen, N. J., Stein, D. J., & Christensen, G. A. (2001). *Help for hair pullers: Understanding and coping with trichotillomania.* Oakland, CA: New Harbinger.

Koblenzer, C. S. (1994, March–April). The broken mirror: Dysmorphic syndrome in the dermatologist's practice. *Fitzgerald's Journal of Clinical Dermatology*, pp. 14–19.

Koran, L. M., Abujaoude, E., Large, M. D., & Serpe, R. T. (2008). The prevalence of body dysmorphic disorder in the United States adult population. *CNS Spectrums, 13*(4), 316–322.

Ladee, G. A. (1966). *Hypochondriacal syndromes.* Amsterdam: Elsevier.

Linehan, M. M. (1993). *Skills training manual for treating borderline personality disorder.* New York: Guilford Press.

Loftus, J. (2008). *The smart woman's guide to plastic surgery* (updated 2nd ed.). New York: McGraw-Hill.

Mancuso, S., Knoesen, N., & Castle, D. J. (2010). Delusional vs. nondelusional body dysmorphic disorder. *Comprehensive Psychiatry, 51*(2), 177–182.

Marques, L., Weingarden, H., LeBlanc, N., & Wilhelm, S. (2011). Treatment utilization and barriers to treatment engagement among people with body dysmorphic symptoms. *Journal of Psychosomatic Research, 70*(3), 286–293.

McKay, D., Todaro, J., Neziroglu, F., & Campisi, T. (1997). Body dysmorphic disorder: A preliminary evaluation of treatment and maintenance using exposure with response prevention. *Behaviour Research and Therapy, 35*(1), 67–70.

Miller, W. R., & Rollnick, S. (1991). *Motivational interviewing: Preparing people to change addictive behavior.* New York: Guilford Press.

Miller, W. R., & Rollnick, S. (2002). *Motivational interviewing: Preparing people for change* (2nd ed.). New York: Guilford Press.

Miller, W. R., & Rollnick, S. (2013). *Motivational interviewing: Helping people change addictive behavior* (3rd ed.). New York: Guilford Press.

Morselli, E. (1891). *Sulla dismorfofobia e sulla tafefobia* (Vol. 6). Genoa, Italy: Bolletinno della R Accademia di Genova.

Mulkens, S., Bögels, S. M., & deJong, P. J. (1999). Attentional focus and fear of blushing: A case study. *Behavioural and Cognitive Psychotherapy, 27*(2), 153–164.

National Collaborating Centre for Mental Health. (2006). Core interventions in the treatment of obsessive-compulsive disorder and body dysmorphic disorder (a guideline from the National Institute for Health and Clinical Excellence, National Health Service). Retrieved from *http://www.nice.org.uk/page.aspx?o=289817*

Neziroglu, F., Anderson, M. C., & Yaryura-Tobias, J. A. (1999). An in-depth review of obsessive-compulsive disorder, body dysmorphic disorder, hypochondriasis, and trichotillomania: Therapeutic issues and current research. *Crisis Intervention and Time Limited Treatment, 5*(1–2), 59–94.

Neziroglu, F., McKay, D., Todaro, J., & Yaryura-Tobias, J. A. (1996). Effect of cognitive behavior therapy on persons with body dysmorphic disorder and comorbid Axis II diagnosis. *Behavior Therapy, 27*(1), 67–77.

Neziroglu, F., & Yaryura-Tobias, J. A. (1997). A review of cognitive behavioral and pharmacological treatment of body dysmorphic disorder. *Behavior Modification, 21*(3), 324–340.

O'Sullivan, R. L., Phillips, K. A., Keuthen, N. J., & Wilhelm, S. (1999). Near-fatal skin picking from delusional

body dysmorphic disorder responsive to fluvoxamine. *Psychosomatics, 40*(1), 79–81.
Perugi, G., Akiskal, H., Giannotti, D., Frare, F., Di Vaio, S., & Cassano, G. (1997). Gender-related differences in body dysmorphic disorder (dysmorphophobia). *Journal of Nervous and Mental Disease, 185*(9), 578–582.
Perugi, G., Giannotti, D., Di Vaio, S., Frare, F., Saettoni, M., & Cassano, G. (1996). Fluvoxamine in the treatment of body dysmorphic disorder (dysmorphophobia). *International Clinical Psychopharmacology, 11*(4), 247–254.
Phillips, K. A. (1991). Body dysmorphic disorder: The distress of imagined ugliness. *American Journal of Psychiatry, 148*(9), 1138–1149.
Phillips, K. A. (1996). *The broken mirror: Understanding and treating body dysmorphic disorder.* New York: Oxford University Press.
Phillips, K. A. (2000). Quality of life for patients with body dysmorphic disorder. *Journal of Nervous and Mental Disease, 188*(3), 170–175.
Phillips, K. A. (2002). Body image and body dysmorphic disorder. In C. G. Fairburn & K. D. Brownell (Eds.), *Eating disorders and obesity: A comprehensive handbook* (2nd ed., pp. 113–117). New York: Guilford Press.
Phillips, K. A. (2004). Psychosis in body dysmorphic disorder. *Journal of Psychiatric Research, 38*(1), 63–72.
Phillips, K. A. (2005). *The broken mirror: Understanding and treating body dysmorphic disorder* (rev. and expanded ed.). New York: Oxford University Press.
Phillips, K. A. (2006a). An open-label study of escitalopram in body dysmorphic disorder. *International Clinical Psychopharmacology, 21*(3), 177–179.
Phillips, K. A. (2006b). The presentation of body dysmorphic disorder in medical settings. *Primary Psychiatry, 13*(7), 51–59.
Phillips, K. A. (2009). *Understanding body dysmorphic disorder: An essential guide.* New York: Oxford University Press.
Phillips, K. A., Albertini, R. S., & Rasmussen, S. A. (2002). A randomized placebo-controlled trial of fluoxetine in body dysmorphic disorder. *Archives of General Psychiatry, 59*(4), 381–388.
Phillips, K. A., Albertini, R. S., Siniscalchi, J. M., Khan, A., & Robinson, M. (2001). Effectiveness of pharmacotherapy for body dysmorphic disorder: A chart-review study. *Journal of Clinical Psychiatry, 62*(9), 721–727.
Phillips, K. A., Coles, M. E., Menard, W., Yen, S., Fay, C., & Weisberg, R. B. (2005). Suicidal ideation and suicide attempts in body dysmorphic disorder. *Journal of Clinical Psychiatry, 66*(6), 717–725.
Phillips, K. A., & Diaz, S. F. (1997). Gender differences in body dysmorphic disorder. *Journal of Nervous and Mental Disease, 185*(9), 570–577.
Phillips, K. A., Didie, E. R., & Menard, W. (2007). Clinical features and correlates of major depressive disorder in individuals with body dysmorphic disorder. *Journal of Affective Disorders, 97*(1–3), 129–135.
Phillips, K. A., Didie, E. R., Menard, W., Pagano, M. E., Fay, C., & Weisberg, R. B. (2006). Clinical features of body dysmorphic disorder in adolescents and adults. *Psychiatry Research, 141*(3), 305–314.
Phillips, K. A., Dwight, M. M., & McElroy, S. L. (1998). Efficacy and safety of fluvoxamine in body dysmorphic disorder. *Journal of Clinical Psychiatry, 59*(4), 165–171.
Phillips, K. A., Grant, J., Siniscalchi, J., & Albertini, R. S. (2001). Surgical and nonpsychiatric medical treatment of patients with body dysmorphic disorder. *Psychosomatics, 42*(6), 504–510.
Phillips, K. A., Gunderson, C. G., Mallya, G., McElroy, S. L., & Carter, W. (1998). A comparison study of body dysmorphic disorder and obsessive-compulsive disorder. *Journal of Clinical Psychiatry, 59*(11), 568–575.
Phillips, K. A., & Hollander, E. (2008). Treating body dysmorphic disorder with medication: Evidence, misconceptions, and a suggested approach. *Body Image, 5*(1), 13–27.
Phillips, K. A., Hollander, E., Rasmussen, S. A., & Aronowitz, B. R. (1997). A severity rating scale for body dysmorphic disorder: Development, reliability, and validity of a modified version of the Yale–Brown Obsessive Compulsive Scale. *Psychopharmacology Bulletin, 33*(1), 17–22.
Phillips, K. A., & Kaye, W. H. (2007). The relationship of body dysmorphic disorder and eating disorders to obsessive-compulsive disorder. *CNS Spectrums, 12*(5), 347–358.
Phillips, K. A., & Kelly, M. M. (2009). Suicidality in a placebo-controlled fluoxetine study of body dysmorphic disorder. *International Clinical Psychopharmacology, 24*(1), 26–28.
Phillips, K. A., & McElroy, S. L. (2000). Personality disorders and traits in patients with body dysmorphic disorder. *Comprehensive Psychiatry, 41*(4), 229–236.
Phillips, K. A., McElroy, S. L., Keck, P. E., & Pope, H. G. (1993). Body dysmorphic disorder: 30 cases of imagined ugliness. *American Journal of Psychiatry, 150*(2), 302–308.
Phillips, K. A., & Menard, W. (2006). Suicidality in body dysmorphic disorder: A prospective study. *American Journal of Psychiatry, 163*(7), 1280–1282.
Phillips, K. A., & Menard, W. (2009). A prospective pilot study of levetiracetam for body dysmorphic disorder. *CNS Spectrums, 14*(5), 252–260.
Phillips, K. A., Menard, W., & Fay, C. (2006). Gender similarities and differences in 200 individuals with body dysmorphic disorder. *Comprehensive Psychiatry, 47*(2), 77–87.
Phillips, K. A., Menard, W., Fay, C., & Pagano, M. E. (2005). Psychosocial functioning and quality of life in body dysmorphic disorder. *Comprehensive Psychiatry, 46*(4), 254–260.
Phillips, K. A., Menard, W., Fay, C., & Weisberg, R. (2005). Demographic characteristics, phenomenology, comorbidity, and family history in 200 individuals with body dysmorphic disorder. *Psychosomatics, 46*(4), 317–325.
Phillips, K. A., Menard, W., Pagano, M. E., Fay, C., & Stout, R. L. (2006). Delusional versus nondelusional body dysmorphic disorder: Clinical features and course of illness. *Journal of Psychiatric Research, 40*(2), 95–104.
Phillips, K. A., & Najar, F. (2003). An open-label study of citalopram in body dysmorphic disorder. *Journal of Clinical Psychiatry, 64*(6), 715–720.
Phillips, K. A., Nierenberg, A. A., Brendel, G., & Fava, M. (1996). Prevalence and clinical features of body dysmorphic disorder in atypical major depression. *Journal of Nervous and Mental Disease, 184*(2), 125–129.
Phillips, K. A., Pagano, M. E., Menard, W., & Stout, R. L. (2006). A 12 month follow-up study of the course of body dysmorphic disorder. *American Journal of Psychiatry, 16*(3), 907–912.

Phillips, K. A., & Rasmussen, S. A. (2004). Change in psychosocial functioning and quality of life of patients with body dysmorphic disorder treated with fluoxetine: A placebo-controlled study. *Psychosomatics, 45*(5), 438–444.

Phillips, K. A., Siniscalchi, J. M., & McElroy, S. L. (2004). Depression, anxiety, anger, and somatic symptoms in patients with body dysmorphic disorder. *Psychiatric Quarterly, 75*(4), 309–320.

Phillips, K. A., & Stout, R. L. (2006). Associations in the longitudinal course of body dysmorphic disorder with major depression, obsessive compulsive disorder, and social phobia. *Journal of Psychiatric Research, 40*(4), 360–369.

Phillips, K. A., & Taub, S. L. (1995). Skin picking as a symptom of body dysmorphic disorder. *Psychopharmacology Bulletin, 31*(2), 279–288.

Pope, H. G., Phillips, K. A., & Olivardia, R. (2000). *The Adonis complex: The secret crisis of male body obsession*. New York: Simon & Schuster.

Rief, W., Buhlmann, U., Wilhelm, S., Borkenhagen, A., & Brähler, E. (2006). The prevalence of body dysmorphic disorder: A population-based survey. *Psychological Medicine, 36*(6), 877–885.

Rosen, J. C. (1995). The nature of body dysmorphic disorder and treatment with cognitive behavior therapy. *Cognitive and Behavioral Practice, 2*(1), 143–166.

Rosen, J. C. (1998). Cognitive behavior therapy for body dysmorphic disorder. In V. E. Caballo (Ed.), *International handbook of cognitive and behavioural treatments for psychological disorders* (pp. 363–391). Oxford, UK: Pergamon/Elsevier Science.

Rosen, J. C., & Ramirez, E. (1998). A comparison of eating disorders and body dysmorphic disorder on body image and psychological adjustment. *Journal of Psychosomatic Research, 44*(3–4), 441–449.

Rosen, J. C., Reiter, J., & Orosan, P. (1995). Cognitive-behavioral body image therapy for body dysmorphic disorder. *Journal of Consulting and Clinical Psychology, 63*(2), 263–269.

Rush, A. J., Giles, D. E., Schlesser, M. A., Fulton, C. L., Weissenburger, J. E., & Burns, C. T. (1986). The Inventory of Depressive Symptomatology (IDS): Preliminary findings. *Psychiatry Research, 18*, 65–87.

Rush, A. J., Gullion, C. M., Basco, M. R., Jarrett, R. B., & Trivedi, M. H. (1996). The Inventory of Depressive Symptomatology (IDS): Psychometric properties. *Psychological Medicine, 26*, 477–486.

Rush, A. J., Trivedi, M., Ibrahim, H., Carmody, T., Arnow, B., Klein, D., et al. (2003). The 16-item Quick Inventory of Depressive Symptomatology (QIDS) Clinician Rating (QIDS-C) and Self-Report (QIDS-SR): A psychometric evaluation in patients with chronic major depression. *Biological Psychiatry, 54*, 573–583.

Sarwer, D. B., Gibbons, L. M., Magee, L., Baker, J. L., Casas, L. A., Glat, P. M., et al. (2005). A prospective, multi-site investigation of patient satisfaction and psychosocial status following cosmetic surgery. *Aesthetic Surgery Journal, 25*(3), 263–269.

Sarwer, D. B., Wadden, T. A., Pertschuk, M. J., & Whitaker, L. A. (1998). Body image dissatisfaction and body dysmorphic disorder in 100 cosmetic surgery patients. *Plastic and Reconstructive Surgery, 101*(6), 1644–1649.

Saxena, S., Winograd, A., Dunkin, J. J., Maidment, K., Rosen, R., Vapnik, T., et al. (2001). A retrospective review of clinical characteristics and treatment response in body dysmorphic disorder versus obsessive-compulsive disorder. *Journal of Clinical Psychiatry, 62*(1), 67–72.

Spitzer, R. L., Williams, J. B., Gibbon, M., & First, M. B. (1992). The Structured Clinical Interview for DSM-III-R (SCID): I. History, rationale, and description. *Archives of General Psychiatry, 49*(8), 624–629.

Veale, D. (2000). Outcome of cosmetic surgery and 'DIY' surgery in patients with body dysmorphic disorder. *Psychiatric Bulletin, 24*(6), 218–221.

Veale, D. (2009). *Body dysmorphic disorder*. New York: Oxford University Press.

Veale, D., Boocock, A., Gournay, K., & Dryden, W. (1996). Body dysmorphic disorder: A survey of fifty cases. *British Journal of Psychiatry, 169*(2), 196–201.

Veale, D., Gournay, K., Dryden, W., Boocock, A., Shah, F., Willson, R., et al. (1996). Body dysmorphic disorder: A cognitive behavioural model and pilot randomised controlled trial. *Behaviour Research and Therapy, 34*(9), 717–729.

Wegner, D. M. (1989). *White bears and other unwanted thoughts*. New York: Viking.

Wells, A. (1997). *Cognitive therapy of anxiety disorders: A practice manual and conceptual guide*. Chichester, UK: Wiley.

Wilhelm, S. (2006). *Feeling good about the way you look: A program for overcoming body image problems*. New York: Guilford Press.

Wilhelm, S., Keuthen, N. J., Deckersbach, T., Engelhard, I. M., Forker, A. E., Baer, L., et al. (1999). Self-injurious skin picking: Clinical characteristics and comorbidity. *Journal of Clinical Psychiatry, 60*(7), 454–459.

Wilhelm, S., & Neziroglu, F. (2002). Cognitive theory of body dysmorphic disorder. In R. Frost & G. Steketee (Eds.), *Cognitive approaches to obsessions and compulsions: Theory, assessment, and treatment* (pp. 203–214). Amsterdam: Pergamon/Elsevier Science.

Wilhelm, S., Otto, M. W., Lohr, B., & Deckersbach, T. (1999). Cognitive behavior group therapy for body dysmorphic disorder. *Behaviour Research and Therapy, 37*, 71–75.

Wilhelm, S., Otto, M. W., Zucker, B. G., & Pollack, M. H. (1997). Prevalence of body dysmorphic disorder in patients with anxiety disorders. *Journal of Anxiety Disorders, 11*(5), 499–502.

Wilhelm, S., Phillips, K. A., Fama, J. M., Greenberg, J. L., & Steketee, G. (2011). Modular cognitive behavioral therapy for body dysmorphic disorder. *Behavior Therapy, 42*, 624–633.

Wilhelm, S., Phillips, K. A., Steketee, G., Didie, E., Fama, J. M., & Buhlmann, U. (2009, November). *A randomized controlled trial of CBT for body dysmorphic disorder*. Paper presented at the 43rd annual conference of the Association for Behavioral and Cognitive Therapies, New York.

Wilhelm, S., & Steketee, G. (2006). *Cognitive therapy for obsessive-compulsive disorder*. Oakland, CA: New Harbinger.

Woods, D. W., & Twohig, M. P. (2008). *Trichotillomania: An ACT-enhanced behavior therapy approach: Workbook*. New York: Oxford University Press.

INDEX